Endorsements

Amanda and Stewart have produced a carefully researched and eminently practical handbook for using the plant-based diet in clinical practice.

—Helmuth Fritz, MD. Adjunct Professor of Medicine, Loma Linda University, CA

Finally, a book that covers the wide range of pathologies that can be prevented and treated with a plant-based diet. This book will be invaluable to me in my practice.

—Lynn Fioretti DO, Family Medicine, Veterans Administration, Silverdale, WA

Amanda and Stewart have responded to the many requests for a compendium of pathologies that can be prevented or treated with a plant-based diet, by compiling this invaluable book of their well-researched articles.

—Esther Park-Hwang, MD, Obstetrician and Gynecologist, Multicare Women's Center, Tacoma, WA, and Assistant Clinical Professor, University of Washington

The PREVENTION and TREATMENT of DISEASE with a PLANT-BASED DIET

Published, evidence-based, review articles to guide the physician in prescribing a plant-based diet

STEWART ROSE

and

AMANDA STROMBOM

The Prevention and Treatment of Disease with a Plant-Based Diet

First Edition
Plant-Based Diets in Medicine
12819 SE 38th St, #427
Bellevue, WA 98006
USA
pbdmedicine.org

Library of Congress Control Number: 2021900460

ISBN: 978-1-09834-327-9 (softcover)
ISBN: 978-1-09834-328-6 (eBook)

Table of Contents

Introduction

Long gone are the days when the prevention and treatment of disease with a plant-based diet (vegan diet) was based on anecdote or educated guess. Today, the prevention and treatment of disease with a plant-based diet is based on the bedrock of extensive research and now is considered evidence-based medicine.

Yet, it may be the least utilized tool in the physician's toolbox. There are two main reasons for this. First is that although diet remains the number one risk factor for disease and disability in the United States, (1) exceedingly little attention is given to nutrition in medical school and almost none is given to the prevention and treatment of disease with a plant-based diet.

The most recent survey during the 2012-2013 academic year included 121 medical schools, with an average of 19 hours (SD =13.7) of nutrition education in their curriculum. The survey showed that 71% of medical schools failed to meet the minimum recommendation of 25 hours, 36% provided 12 or fewer hours, and 9% provided none. (2)

We hear many complaints from patients that their doctors don't know nearly enough about nutrition. This concern prompts many physicians to complain in return that they weren't taught enough about the science of nutrition or its applications as a therapeutic in their medical school education. This situation is hardly surprising for according to one study, over 90% of doctors feel that their training in nutrition was inadequate to meet their needs. (3)

This lack of education disempowers doctors from offering the best preventative and therapeutic measures to their patients, and deprives their patients from effective therapies resulting in unnecessary morbidity and mortality, while greatly increasing healthcare costs for both their patients and the entire nation.

Another reason for the lack of application of a plant-based diet by physicians is the lack of a comprehensive book that covers the wide range of a pathologies that can be prevented and treated with a plant-based diet. While the amount of research is considerable, to our knowledge, there is no resource which gathers this research together in one place and includes clinical considerations such as enhancing patient compliance, integrating with standard treatment and lab work. It is this deficiency that this book seeks to overcome.

Both as a treatment or prophylaxis the plant-based diet has no side effects, adverse reactions and no contraindications. It can be used as a monotherapy or as an adjunct to medication and surgery. It can also treat several comorbidities at once. While some physicians may be aware of treating coronary artery disease and type II diabetes with a plant-based diet, few are aware of its efficacy in treating other pathologies such as rheumatoid arthritis and Crohn's disease.

A growing number of patients are not waiting for their doctors to learn about the role of a plant-based diet in human health, and so they treat themselves using information from the internet and other potentially unreliable sources, without the knowledge and experience that one would expect their physician to have. (4) In our experience, they would much rather be able to include their physicians on their healthcare team, but they feel they can't because their doctors have so little knowledge in nutritional medicine.

Treating patients with a plant-based diet has the advantage of being an extremely low-cost method of treatment, thus saving patients and society as a whole an enormous amount of money which could be better used elsewhere. In fact, a Mutual of Omaha study determined that for every dollar spent on the Dean Ornish program, a very successful treatment for coronary artery disease utilizing vegetarian nutritional medicine, there was an immediate savings of $5.55 for every dollar spent. (5)

While a plant-based diet is particularly effective as a preventive measure, it is often when disease strikes that patients are most open to the idea of making lifestyle changes, placing the physician in the perfect position to encourage a change of diet. The idea of being a vegetarian or a vegan is no longer viewed as exotic or obscure. The rapid rise in sales of meat and dairy substitute products in mainstream grocery stores and restaurants shows that the public is open to the idea of trying new foods and diets. Evidence shows most patients will switch to a plant-based diet, once their doctor explains and prescribes it. (6)

This book is an accumulation of articles we have written over the past few years, many of which have been published in medical journals. As such, the references for each article are provided at the end of the article. We are continuing to write and publish articles covering additional pathologies not yet addressed in this edition. These can be found on our website Plant-Based Diets in Medicine, pbdmedicine.org, and will be published in future editions of this book.

It's time for medical schools to start teaching the effectiveness of a plant-based diet to treat and prevent disease, and for physicians to start prescribing it to their patients. We hope that this book will aid physicians in learning the efficacy of a plant-based diet, and how to effectively prescribe a plant-based diet for their patients.

Definitions

In medical research, the terms vegetarian, vegan, and plant-based, have no standard definitions, and therefore are used inconsistently throughout the literature.

A vegetarian diet is a diet free of meat, poultry, and fish. Total vegetarian or vegan diets are a subset of this group that exclude all animal products. Lacto-ovo vegetarian diets include dairy and eggs.

In our writing, we prefer to use the term "plant-based diet" to refer to a diet based only on plant foods, such as fruits, vegetables, whole grains, nuts and legumes, that includes no foods derived from animals. This may also be called a total vegetarian or vegan diet.

When referring to specific research, we have used the terminology chosen by the researchers, if their use of it appears to be consistent with these definitions. We used more accurate terms if their research reports were not consistent with the terminology they used.

References

1. Murray CJL, et al. (2013) The State of US Health, 1990-2010 Burden of Diseases, Injuries, and Risk Factors. *JAMA* 310(6):591-606.
2. Adams K, Butsch W, Kohlmeier M. (2015) The State of Nutrition Education at US Medical Schools. *J Biomed Educ* 2015:1-7.

3. Vetter M, Herring S, Sood M, et al. (2008) What Do Resident Physicians Know about Nutrition? An Evaluation of Attitudes, Self-Perceived Proficiency and Knowledge. *Journal of the American College of Nutrition* 27(2):2877-298.
4. Schwartz K, Roe T, Northrup J, et al. (2006) Family Medicine Patients' Use of the Internet for Health Information: A MetroNet Study. *Journal of American Board of Family Medicine* 19(1):39-45.
5. Ornish D. (2010) *Dr Dean Ornish's Program for Reversing Heart Disease.*: Random House.
6. Drozek D, Diehl H, Nakazawa M, Kostohryz T, Morton D, et al. (2014) Short-term effectiveness of a lifestyle intervention program for reducing selected chronic disease risk factors in individuals living in rural appalachia: a pilot cohort study. *Advances in Preventive Medicine* 2014:798184.

Journal of
Cardiology & Cardiovascular Therapy
ISSN: 2474-7580

Juniper Publishers
key to the Researchers

Review Article

Volume 12 Issue 5 - December 2018

DOI: 10.19080/JOCCT.2018.12.555847

J Cardiol & Cardiovasc Ther

A Comprehensive Review of the Prevention and Treatment of Heart Disease with a Plant-Based Diet

Stewart Rose* **and Amanda Strombom**

Plant-Based Diets in Medicine, USA

Submission: November 22, 2018; **Published:** December 14, 2018

***Corresponding author:** Stewart Rose, Plant-Based Diets in Medicine, 12819 SE 38th St, #427, Bellevue, WA 98006, USA

Abstract

Epidemiological studies show that vegetarians have a much lower risk of myocardial infarction. Reductions of risk factors and comorbidities such as angina, hypercholesterolemia, hypertension, diabetes, metabolic syndrome and obesity have also been shown.

A low-fat plant-based diet can reverse or prevent further progression of coronary atheroma, improve endothelial dysfunction and is effective even in cases of severe stenosis. Studies show that in addition to regression, there is a remolding of the geometry of the stenosis with consequent improvement in coronary flow reserve.

Those following a plant-based diet have much lower total cholesterol and LDL. They also have lower levels of cardio-reactive protein, apolipoprotein (a) and apolipoprotein (b), plus levels of MPO, MMP-9, MMP-2 and MMP-9/TIMP-1 ratios. In addition, studies have determined that vegans produce less TMAO than their omnivorous counterparts after dietary challenge.

Long term exposure to persistent organic pollutants can drastically affect the circulatory system. The consumption of animal products is the greatest source of exposure of these toxins, due to bioaccumulation of these lipophilic toxins in animal tissues.

Interventional studies confirm that a plant-based diet is as effective in lowering cholesterol as statin drugs. Interventional studies show that a plant-based diet can help treat heart failure and is very efficacious in treating angina pectoris. Vegetarians also show better improvements in cardiac rehab. Follow-up studies at one and four years confirm continued benefit to the patient, and patient compliance has been demonstrated over several years. Treatment with a plant-based diet is devoid of side effects and contraindications.

1. Introduction

It has long been known from epidemiological studies that vegetarians have lower incidences of several common chronic diseases including ischemic heart disease. Epidemiological studies have also shown that they have lower incidences of risk factors for ischemic heart disease such as hypercholestrolemia, type 2 diabetes and essential hypertension.

This prompted research on using a vegetarian diet as a treatment for coronary artery disease. For over 45 years, evidence from interventional studies have strongly indicated that a low-fat plant-based diet is both safe and efficacious in the treatment of coronary artery disease (CAD). It's particularly effective in the treatment angina pectoris. Interventional studies have shown that a low-fat plant-based diet is a safe and efficacious alternative to other treatments.

This treatment can be used alone or in combination with standard treatment regimens, including medication, stenting and CABG. Treatment with the plant-based diet has the distinct advantages of having no adverse reactions or contraindications, is affordable, effectively treats common comorbidities and has been shown to have a high patient compliance.

2. Reducing hypercholesterolemia

Hypercholesterolemia is a well-known risk factor for Coronary Artery Disease (CAD). Dietary saturated fat and cholesterol intake are shown to be strongly correlated with serum cholesterol levels. Less well-known is the fact that Apolipoproteins (a) and (b) are significant risk factors for CAD. While statin drugs are effective at lowering serum cholesterol levels, they are not effective at lowering Lp(a).

2.1 Epidemiology

Vegetarians, and most especially vegans, have a much lower risk of hypercholesterolemia (for both total cholesterol and LDL) and a less atherogenic profile. They have been found to have lower total and LDL cholesterol levels on average. The following chart shows the average cholesterol levels among three dietary groups. (1, 2) Vegans, or total vegetarians, have the lowest levels.

How to cite this article: Rose S, Strombom A. A comprehensive review of the prevention and treatment of heart disease with a plant-based diet. J Cardiol & Cardiovasc Ther. 2018; 12(5): 555847. DOI: 10.19080/JOCCT.2018.12.555847.

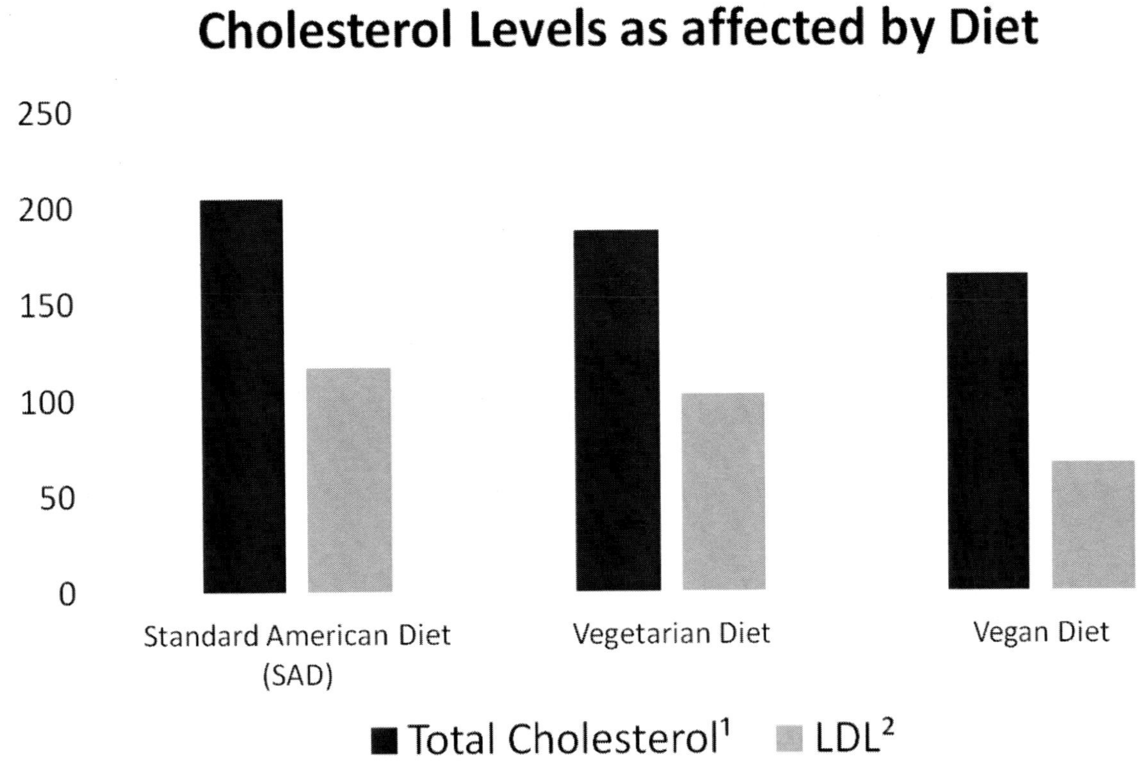

The main reason for this is that animal products are high in both saturated fats and cholesterol. While saturated and trans fat intake have the greatest effect on blood cholesterol concentrations, serum cholesterol concentrations also rise in response to dietary cholesterol intake. This relationship is linear within the range of cholesterol intakes in typical omnivorous diets, but at higher cholesterol intakes, the relationship is curvilinear; changes in dietary cholesterol have less impact on serum cholesterol. (3)

Another reason why low-fat vegetarian and vegan diets result in lower serum cholesterol levels is that they improve insulin sensitivity, which in turn can reduce cholesterol synthesis. This may account for a portion of the lower prevalence of hypercholesterolemia among vegetarians and vegans and for the results obtained in interventional studies. (4, 5)

The fact that vegetarians and especially vegans have lower cholesterol levels, and better cholesterol ratios, leads to much less atherosclerosis. One of the important mechanisms whereby LDL cholesterol results in atherosclerotic lesions involves the oxidation of LDL cholesterol. (6, 7) There is evidence that the LDL cholesterol in vegetarians is much less oxidizable. (8)

Vegans have also been found to have better regulation of the metabolism of triglyceride-rich lipoproteins than omnivores, because they are more efficient in removing remnants that are potentially atherogenic. In addition, the diminished cholesteryl ester transfer shown in the study, and the diminished LDL cholesterol levels that have been previously documented in other published studies, clearly suggest that a vegan diet offers some protection against atherogenesis. (9) A vegetarian diet also results in lower levels of C-reactive protein. (10, 11)

In a cross-sectional study of apparently healthy vegetarian and non- vegetarian men, all over 35 years old, the vegetarian men had lower body mass index, systolic and diastolic blood pressures, fasting serum total cholesterol, LDL and non-HDL-cholesterol, apolipoprotein B, glucose and glycated hemoglobin values in comparison with non- vegetarian men. The vegetarian men had better arterial function as measured by arterial stiffness determined by carotid-femoral pulse wave velocity, relative carotid distensibility and carotid intima-media thickness than non-vegetarian men. (12)

2.2 Apolipoproteins

Apolipoprotein (a)

Several large population studies have shown a strong independent relationship between high apolipoprotein (a) (Lp(a)) levels and heart disease. This has led to the consensus agreement that it is a very important risk factor for cardiovascular disease, even when cholesterol levels and other classical risk factors such as elevated cholesterol, hypertension and diabetes have been taken into account. It is thought to increase the risk of cardiovascular disease by two different mechanisms:

1. It promotes atherosclerosis. Research studies have shown that Lp(a) may accelerate atherosclerotic damage. It is thought to increase the size of plaque atheroma in artery walls, causing inflammation, instability and growth of smooth muscle cells. It is retained in the artery wall more than LDL cholesterol as it binds to the artery lining through its "sticky" apolipoprotein.
2. It can trigger blockage of arteries by formation of clots. Lp(a) is thought to increase risk of heart attacks by interfering with clotting mechanisms and therefore promoting clot development on the inner surface of blood vessels. Lp(a) appears similar to proteins involved in clotting, such as plasminogen. It is thought to form a link between lipids and the coagulation system by preventing fibrinolysis.

Existing data show that elevated apolipoprotein(a) (Lp[a]) levels are associated with increased risk of CHD, stroke, peripheral arterial disease, and calcific aortic valve stenosis. (13, 14, 15) In a recent individual-patient data meta-analysis of statin-treated patients, elevated baseline and on-statin Lp(a) showed an independent approximately linear relation with cardiovascular disease risk. This study provides a rationale for lowering Lp(a) even in statin-treated patients. (16)

Not only does a plant-based diet reduce serum cholesterol, but a recent study showed that Lp(a) could also be reduced. In a four-week study on patients following a plant-based diet, significant reductions were observed for serum Lp(a) with an average reduction of -32.0 nmol/L. Lp(a) is considered resistant to change by lifestyle modification making this result very notable. (17) In contrast, initiation of statin therapy reduced LDL cholesterol (mean change −39% [95% CI −43 to −35]) without a significant change in Lp(a). (16)

Apolilipoprotein (b)

It is also evident that an increased serum apolipoprotein (b) (Lp(b)) concentration is an

How to cite this article: Rose S, Strombom A. A comprehensive review of the prevention and treatment of heart disease with a plant-based diet. J Cardiol & Cardiovasc Ther. 2018; 12(5): 555847. DOI: 10.19080/JOCCT.2018.12.555847.

important coronary heart disease (CHD) risk factor. (18) Lp(b) is the primary apolipoprotein of chylomicrons, VLDL, intermediate-density lipoprotein, and LDL particles. Prospective studies suggest that concentrations of Lp(b) are indicators of vascular heart disease and CVD risk. (19, 20)

Studies have also shown that vegetarians and vegans have lower Lp(b) than meat eaters. (21) Several studies show that a low-fat vegetarian diet reduces Lp(b) concentrations. (22, 23) When a low-fat vegetarian diet is introduced, Lp(b) levels are reduced more than by other diets such the Atkins and South Beach diets. (24)

2.4 Hypercholesterolemia Intervention

Vegetarian and vegan diets can be very efficacious in reducing serum cholesterol. Patients in a 4-week plant-based diet program had significant reductions in total cholesterol (34mg/dl), LDL-C (25 mg/dl), triglycerides (20mg/dl), hs-CRP (2.5 mg/dl), systolic BP (16 mmHg), and diastolic BP (9 mmHg). (25)

One study showed that a low-fat vegetarian diet was as effective at lowering serum cholesterol as the Standard Heart Association diet plus Lovostatin. (26) This study is notable because it contains nuts in the treatment regimen. (See Clinical Considerations for more information about the benefit of including nuts in the diet.)

Another study examining children and their adult parents found that a plant-based, or vegan, diet reduced total cholesterol, LDL cholesterol and C-reactive protein more than the American Heart Association diet. This study is especially important given the recent increase in the incidence of hypercholesterolemia in children and the fact that atherosclerosis seems to start early in life. (27)

3. Persistent Organic Pollutants

3.1 Epidemiology

The increasing deterioration of the natural environment is having serious consequences on human health. The circulation system is the major organ exposed to xenobiotics and endobiotics during metabolic homeostasis, (28, 29, 30) and exposure to persistent organic pollutants can drastically alter this system, resulting in cardiovascular diseases such as hypertension, atherosclerosis, and ischemic heart disease. (30, 31, 32, 33, 34, 35, 36)

Exposure to persistent organic pollutants such as dioxins and dioxin-like polychlorinated biphenyls (PCBs) is associated with increased risk of multiple pro-inflammatory human diseases including diabetes, cancer, and cardiovascular disease (37, 38, 39, 40, 41, 42, 43, 44, 45)

High quality studies found consistent and significant dose-related increases in ischemic heart disease with dioxin. (46) Given the large worldwide burden of CAD, the potential role of dioxin exposure as a preventable risk factor could be of substantial public health and clinical interest. (46)

3.2 Mechanism A – The Aryl-Hydrocarbon Receptor

The aryl-hydrocarbon receptor (AhR) is a well-known environmental sensor. Because many environmental pollutants contain exogenous AhR ligands, increasing attention is being given to the relationship between AhR and cardiovascular diseases. Recent evidence from gene knock-out studies and clinical trials suggests that not only does AhR have a major impact on general physiological functions, including immune responses, reproduction, oxidative stress, tumor promotion, the cell cycle, and proliferation, but also influences cardiovascular physiological functions. (31, 32, 33, 34, 35, 36)

AhR is a ligand activated transcription factor that mediates the cellular response to environmental contaminants, including dioxin and polycyclic aromatic hydrocarbons (PAH) (from meat or cigarette smoke), and has recently been associated with CAD. (47, 48) Exposure to pollutants containing ligands of AhR, such as dioxins, Tetrachlorodibenzo-p-dioxin (TCDD), PAH, and benzo(α)pyrene, is thought to promote the development and progression of atherosclerosis, indicating that AhR may play a role in the regulation of atherosclerosis. (37) These environmental toxins, as well as endogenous activators such as ox-LDL, activate the AhR pathway, leading to increased inflammatory burden in the plaque. (47)

Studies have shown that dioxin-like PCBs may also increase oxidative stress and subsequent chronic inflammatory states which can lead to glucose intolerance, alterations of lipid and cholesterol homeostasis, and other risk factors for multiple metabolic diseases (37, 49)

3.3 Mechanism B – TMAO

Dioxin-like PCBs can lead to increased levels of the known pro-atherogenic nutrient biomarker Trimethylamine N-oxide (TMAO). (50) A strong link between plasma levels of nutrient-derived TMAO and coronary artery disease has been identified. Dietary precursors of TMAO include carnitine and phosphatidylcholine, which are abundant in animal-derived foods. (50)

TMAO levels are strongly linked to human diseases, and plasma concentrations are correlated to dietary choices. (51, 52) For example, diets high in red meat, and specifically L-carnitine, produce TMAO and accelerate atherosclerosis. (53, 54) However, human studies have determined that vegans and vegetarians produce less TMAO than their omnivorous counterparts after dietary challenge. (53)

3.4 The Diet Connection

Significant exposure of human populations to persistent organic pollutants (POPs) such as PCBs and dioxin occurs through consumption of fat-containing food such as fish, dairy products, and meat, (55, 56, 57) with the highest POP concentrations being commonly found in fatty fish. (55, 56, 58, 59, 60, 61, 62)

Humans bioaccumulate these lipophilic pollutants in their adipose tissues for many years because POPs are highly resistant to metabolic degradation. (57, 63) This is likely to be one of the factors reducing the risk of CAD for vegans.

4. Coronary Artery Disease

4.1 Epidemiology

Epidemiological studies show a 40% risk reduction of ischemic heart disease (64) and a 50% risk reduction of coronary heart disease mortality (65) for vegetarians.

4.2 Pathophysiology

Myeloperoxidase (MPO) is a leukocyte-derived pro-oxidant enzyme that is released from granules of neutrophils and monocytes. (66) MPO and its oxidant products, nitrotyrosine and chlorotyrosine, have been identified in atherosclerotic plaque and at the site of plaque rupture, and play important role in the genesis of atherosclerosis. (66) MPO promotes a number of pathological events involved in plaque formation and rupture, including uptake

How to cite this article: Rose S, Strombom A. A comprehensive review of the prevention and treatment of heart disease with a plant-based diet. J Cardiol & Cardiovasc Ther. 2018; 12(5): 555847. DOI: 10.19080/JOCCT.2018.12.555847.

of oxidized lipid by macrophages and impaired nitric oxide bioavailability. MPO levels independently predict outcomes in patients presenting with acute coronary syndromes or for evaluation of chest pain of suspected cardiac etiology and endothelial dysfunction. (66)

Matrix metalloproteinases (MMPs) are extracellular enzymes that are important in many physiologic and pathologic processes. Their activity is regulated mainly by tissue inhibitors of metalloproteinases (TIMPs). Their expression is associated with classical cardiovascular risk factors as well as with inflammation. They play a central role in atherosclerosis, plaque formation, platelet aggregation, acute coronary syndrome, restenosis, aortic aneurysms and peripheral vascular disease. Many studies have shown that commonly prescribed antihypertensive medications, glitazones and statins, may influence MMPs activity. (67)

It is known that the arterial wall consists of collagen types I and III, macrophages and smooth muscle cells. The evolution of the atherosclerotic plaque from the fatty streak to advanced plaque is associated with an increase in its content of collagen, (68) in the number of smooth muscle cells, (69) and in MMP-9 levels. (69) Increased levels of MMP-9 are found more often in patients with unstable angina compared with those with stable angina. (70) Human coronary plaques that are less likely to rupture demonstrate lower MMP-9 expression. (69) In patients with coronary artery disease, higher MMP-9 levels are an independent risk factor of cardiovascular mortality. (71) Increased TIMP-1 levels have been reported consistently in human atherosclerotic plaques, mainly in relation to areas of calcification. (72) Increased circulating TIMP-1 levels have also been related to stable coronary, (73) carotid, (74) and peripheral artery atherosclerosis. (74)

One study of circulating cardiovascular biomarker profiles compared the plasma concentrations of myeloperoxidase (MPO), matrix metalloproteinases MMP-9 and MMP-2, and tissue inhibitors of MMP TIMP-1 and TIMP-2, between healthy vegetarians and healthy omnivores. The study found significantly lower concentrations of MPO, MMP-9, MMP-2 and MMP-9/TIMP-1 ratio in vegetarians compared to omnivores. Moreover, MMP-9 concentrations were correlated positively with leukocyte and neutrophil counts in both groups. Therefore, a vegetarian diet is associated with a healthier profile of cardiovascular biomarkers compared to omnivores. (75)

E-selectin (cE-Selectin) is a cell adhesion molecule expressed only on endothelial cells activated by cytokines. Like other selectins, it plays an important role in inflammation. (76)

The intercellular adhesion molecule-1 (cICAM-1) is an Ig-like cell adhesion molecule expressed by several cell types, including leukocytes and endothelial cells. It can be induced in a cell-specific manner by several cytokines, for example, tumor necrosis factor alpha, interleukin 1, and interferon gamma, and inhibited by glucocorticoids. (77)

Upregulation of leukocyte adhesion molecules under atherogenic conditions is accompanied by the release of soluble forms of adhesion molecules into the bloodstream. (78) One study assessed the levels of circulating E-selectin (cE-selectin) and circulating intercellular adhesion molecule-1 (cICAM-1), in both vegetarians and subjects from the general population. (78)

In this study vegetarians were characterized by a significantly lower cE-selectin levels. Vegetarians also showed a tendency towards lower cICAM-1 levels in comparison with control subjects. (78) Low cE-selectin levels of vegetarians may reflect the favorable cardiovascular risk profile of this group.

The lower levels of myeloperoxidase, matrix metalloproteinases and cE-selectin combine to give vegetarians a less atherogenic profile and helps explain their lower levels of atherosclerotic plaque.

4.3 General Intervention

For over 45 years, evidence from interventional studies has strongly indicated that a low-fat plant-based diet is both safe and efficacious in the treatment of coronary artery disease (CAD). Researchers have investigated using a very low-fat vegan or nearly vegan diet to treat CAD of varying severity, and have achieved very positive results.

A moderately low-fat vegetarian diet was studied as an intervention for CAD as early as 1960. Morrison placed 50 patients with confirmed CAD on a moderately low-fat (25 g/day) vegetarian diet and followed them, and the 50 patients with CAD in the control group, for 12 years. While none of the patients in the control group survived for that length of time, 38% of the patients in the treatment group did. (79) It should be noted that since in 1960 neither stent, nor CABG surgery, nor cholesterol-reducing drugs, were available this was a very notable finding.

More recently in 1990, a prospective, randomized, controlled trial was done to determine whether comprehensive lifestyle changes affect coronary atherosclerosis after one year. Twenty-eight patients were assigned to an experimental group (very-low-fat vegetarian diet, healthy lifestyle and stress management) and 20 to a standard care control group. 195 coronary artery lesions were analyzed by quantitative coronary angiography. The average percentage diameter stenosis regressed from an average 40.0% to 37.8% in the experimental group, yet progressed from an average of 42.7% to 46.1% in the control group. When only lesions greater than 50% stenosed were analyzed, the average percentage diameter stenosis regressed from an average of 61.1% to 55.8% in the experimental group, and progressed from an average of 61.7% to 64.4% in the control group. Overall, 82% of experimental-group patients had an average change towards regression. (23) In evaluating the regression, it is very important to keep in mind that blood flow increases by the radius raised to the 4th power according to Poiseuille's Law, so small changes make a big difference.

This landmark study provided compelling evidence that a low-fat vegetarian diet can not only halt the progression of CAD, but even result in modest regressions in arterial stenosis. Given that CAD culminating in myocardial infarction is the leading cause of death in the developed world, and a tremendous burden on the health care system as well as on the patients themselves, the importance of this finding can hardly be overstated.

Following up on these results, researchers then looked to see if the treatment effects were sustained for longer periods of time, and if even further improvements could be obtained. The answer to both questions seems to be yes.

In a group of patients who participated in a 4-year follow up, the average percent diameter stenosis at baseline decreased 1.75 absolute percentage points after 1 year (a 4.5% relative improvement) and by 3.1 absolute percentage points after 4 years (a 7.9% relative improvement). In contrast, the

How to cite this article: Rose S, Strombom A. A comprehensive review of the prevention and treatment of heart disease with a plant-based diet. J Cardiol & Cardiovasc Ther. 2018; 12(5): 555847. DOI: 10.19080/JOCCT.2018.12.555847.

average percent diameter stenosis in the control group increased by 2.3 percentage points after 1 year (a 5.4% relative worsening) and by 11.8 percentage points after 4 years (a 27.7% relative worsening).

Patients in the experimental group lost 10.9 kg (23.9 lbs) at 1 year, and sustained a weight loss of 5.8 kg (12.8 lbs) at 4 years, whereas weight in the control group changed little from baseline. In the experimental group, LDL cholesterol levels decreased by 40% at 1 year and remained 20% below baseline at 4 years. Experimental group patients also had a 91% reduction in reported frequency of angina after 1 year, and a 72% reduction after 4 years. (80) It is important to note that for the results obtained above were dose dependent. The more closely patients adhered to the dietary regimen the better their results.

A smaller study also showed good results. 17 patients with CAD treated with a low-fat vegan diet, were followed for 5 years. Lesion analysis by percent stenosis showed that of 25 lesions, 11 regressed and 14 remained stable. Mean arterial stenosis decreased from an average of 53.4% to 46.2%. (81)

A larger study, though with only a 3.7 year follow up, also showed positive results. 198 patients were placed on a low fat vegan, or total vegetarian diet. 93% of patients experienced improvement or resolution of angina symptoms during the follow up period. Radiographic or stress testing results documented disease reversal in 22% of patients. 99.4% of adherent patients avoided major cardiac events. 89% patients were adherent to the treatment regimen. However, this was not a controlled study and the self-selected patients were very motivated. (82)

An Indian study examined 360 coronary lesions in 123 such patients. Results were dose dependent. In CAD patients with the greatest adherence to a low-fat vegetarian diet, percent diameter stenosis regressed by an average of 18.23 absolute percentage points. 91% of all patients showed a trend towards regression, and 51.4% lesions regressed by more than 10 absolute percentage points. (83)

A Dutch interventional study took patients who had at least one 50% obstruction and placed them on a vegetarian diet, although not as low in fat and cholesterol as other studies. After 2 years, 46% of patients showed no progression of the stenosis. Dietary changes were associated with a significant increase in linoleic acid content of cholesteryl esters, and a significant lowering of body weight, systolic blood pressure, serum total cholesterol, and the ratio of total to high-density lipoprotein (total/HDL) cholesterol. (84)

4.4 Coronary Perfusion Study

As might be expected, patients on a low-fat vegetarian diet experience improvements in coronary perfusion as well. In one study after 4 years, the size and severity of perfusion abnormalities on dipyridamole PET images decreased after risk factor modification in the experimental group, compared with an increase of size and severity in controls. The percentage of left ventricle perfusion abnormalities outside 2.5 SDs of those of normal persons, on the dipyridamole PET image of normalized counts, worsened in controls by an average of 10.3% and improved in the experimental group by an average of 5.1%. The percentage of left ventricle with activity less than 60% of the maximum activity worsened in controls by an average 13.5%, and improved in the experimental group 4.2%. The myocardial quadrant on the PET image with the lowest average activity, expressed as a percentage of maximum activity, worsened in controls by an average of 8.8% and improved in the experimental group by an average of 4.9%. The size and severity of perfusion abnormalities on resting PET images were also significantly improved in the experimental group as compared with controls. The relative magnitude of changes in size and severity of PET perfusion abnormalities was comparable to, or greater than, the magnitude of changes in percent diameter stenosis, absolute stenosis lumen area, or stenosis flow reserve documented by quantitative coronary arteriography. (85)

4.5 Stenotic Morphology Study

In 1992, an interesting study looked at the change of the geometric shape of the stenosis, in addition to the degree of stenosis, and their combined effect on flow reserve. Percent stenosis is an incomplete measure of stenosis because length, absolute lumen area and shape effects are not accounted for, and correlate poorly with the functional measure of coronary stenosis, coronary reserve flow. (86) Patients treated with a low-fat vegetarian diet show complex stenosis shape change, with profound effects on fluid dynamic severity, not accounted for by simple percent narrowing in a dose dependent manner. This effect is most pronounced with patients with severe pretreatment stenosis, with stenosis flow reserve less than 3. In this study, the minimal diameter increased by 18%. Patients with a pretreatment average of 67% stenosis showed a 14% improvement in diameter. (87) As mentioned earlier, coronary blood flow effects are a function of arterial radius raised to the 4th power, so small changes in the radius have proportionately much larger effects on flow capacity and functional severity of stenosis, thus contributing to the greater significance of stenosis flow reserve as a measure of change in severity.

5. Angina Pectoris

An all-too-common comorbidity, angina, can also be treated with a low-fat plant-based diet. One study examined over 100 patients with CAD at 22 different clinics throughout the U.S. After 12 weeks, 74% of these patients on a plant-based diet were angina free and an additional 9% moved from limiting to mild angina. (88) Another study of patients placed on a vegetarian diet found that 91% of patients had a reduction in the frequency of angina episodes. (80) Using a purely vegan diet, one small study found complete remission of symptoms in all patients by the 6th month. (89)

6. Heart Failure

Several epidemiological investigations have identified risk factors for heart failure (HF). The key risk factors are: increasing age, hypertension, coronary artery disease, diabetes, obesity, valvular heart disease, and the metabolic syndrome. (90)

Coronary artery disease, which can lead to heart failure, may be the underlying cause in most cases of heart failure patients with low ejection fraction. Coronary artery disease may also play a role in the progression of heart failure through mechanisms such as endothelial dysfunction, ischemia, and infarction, among others.

Since those following a plant-based diet are at lower risk of coronary artery disease, diabetes and obesity, they can be expected to be at lower of heart failure as well. Several population-based cohort studies that have demonstrated an inverse relationship between increased consumption of

How to cite this article: Rose S, Strombom A. A comprehensive review of the prevention and treatment of heart disease with a plant-based diet. J Cardiol & Cardiovasc Ther. 2018; 12(5): 555847. DOI: 10.19080/JOCCT.2018.12.555847.

plant-based foods and incidence of heart failure. (91, 92, 93, 94, 95)

Five prospective studies examined the association between meat consumption and HF incidence in separate medium to large, middle-aged cohorts. All of these studies found increased HF risk with meat consumption. (96, 97, 98, 99, 100)

In a prospective cohort study of 21,275 participants from the Physicians' Health Study I, consumption of one egg a day increased the risk of heart failure by 28% and consuming two eggs a day increased the risk of heart failure by 64%. (101) In another prospective study of over 15,000 participants, those who ate a plant-based diet most of the time had a 42% reduced risk of heart failure. (102)

The beneficial effects of a low-fat vegetarian diet are indicated for patients at risk of heart failure and who also have CAD. One study showed significant improvements in such patients with documented CHD, regardless of ejection fraction, in lifestyle behaviors, body weight, body fat, blood pressure, resting heart rate, total and LDL-cholesterol, exercise capacity, and quality of life by 3 months. Most improvements were maintained over 12 months. (103)

A recent case report demonstrated the effects of a plant-based diet in a 79-year-old male with documented triple vessel disease (80–95 % stenosis) and left ventricular systolic dysfunction (ejection fraction 35%) in the context of progressive dyspnea. Two months of the plant-based diet led to clinically significant reductions in body weight and lipids, with improved exercise tolerance and ejection fraction (+15 %) (95)

7. Post Op Cardiac Rehabilitation Studies

Researchers have also studied the effects of a low-fat vegetarian diet on patients who had already had standard treatments and were ready for post op cardiac rehabilitation.

One study compared patients in cardiac rehabilitation programs using either the standard treatment or a low-fat vegetarian diet (combined with stress reduction). Low-fat vegetarian program participants had significantly greater reductions in anginal frequency, body weight, body mass index, systolic blood pressure, total cholesterol, low-density lipoprotein cholesterol, glucose and dietary fat. (104)

Another study looked at psychosocial risk factors and quality of life variables for patients in cardiac rehabilitation programs, using either the standard treatment or a low-fat vegetarian program. At 3 and 6 months, vegetarian participants demonstrated significant improvements in all 12 outcome measures, while the standard rehabilitation group improved in only 7 of the 12. (105)

8. Clinical Considerations

Substantial evidence indicates that plant-based diets can play an important role in preventing and treating CVD and its risk factors. (106) This suggests that a plant-based diet should be recommended as a prophylaxis to all patients, given that CAD is such a frequent cause of disability and death.

Dietary intervention is an extremely cost effective treatment, and may be the only viable treatment for those patients struggling with the affordability of other options. Some patients are either unwilling, fearful of or not good candidates for surgery. This treatment also offers them a non-surgical option of proven efficacy.

One of the key advantages of the treatment of coronary heart disease with a low fat vegetarian diet is the very low restenosis rate. One study reports the following average restenosis rates: balloon angioplasty 30-60%, bare metal stents, 16-44%, drug eluting stents <10%. (107) Compare this with the low-fat vegan diet, which resulted in a zero-percentage restenosis rate in a study by Dean Ornish. (108)

A low-fat vegetarian treatment regimen has also been shown suitable for diabetics with CAD. In a one year study, diabetic patients with comorbid CAD showed good adherence to the treatment, and improvements in both cardiovascular and diabetic parameters, as demonstrated by significant improvements in weight, body fat, LDL cholesterol, and exercise capacity. About 20% of these patients were able to reduce or discontinue diabetic medications such as insulin or oral anti-hyperglycemics. (109)

The problem of depression is a common concomitant of heart disease. A study using a low-fat plant-based diet in cardiac rehab patients, found that 80% saw very significant reductions in depression by 12 weeks, and the improvement was maintained for at least one year. (110) Another study of patients at high risk also showed an improvement in depressive symptoms. (111)

While the interventional studies stressed a low-fat dietary regimen, there is good evidence that the inclusion of tree nuts, despite their fat content, reduces cardiac risk. (112, 113) The research has been accumulating on the value of nuts in the prevention and treatment of a variety of diseases, including cardiovascular, indicating that the low-fat regimen now more commonly employed may be enhanced by moderate amounts of tree nuts. In one study, nut consumption was associated with reduced prevalence of high cholesterol and high blood pressure; having a history of heart attack, diabetes and gallstones; and markers of diet quality. In this cross-sectional analysis, higher nut consumption was also associated with lower body mass index and waist circumference. (114)

8.1 Fish Oil Supplementation

There has been an unfortunate tendency amongst some physicians to recommend fish oils to their patients. However, this has not been borne out by the evidence. One metastudy conducted on the supposed benefits of fish oil reported, "*All of the studies included were the gold-standard kind of clinical trial — with people assigned at random to either take fish oil or a placebo. The studies ranged in length from one to nearly five years. The authors detected no reduction in any cardiovascular events, such as heart attacks, sudden death, angina, heart failures, strokes or death, no matter what dose of fish oil used.*" (115)

A recent meta-analysis of 10 randomized clinical trials also demonstrated that randomization to trial showed that fish oil had no significant effect on either of fatal CHD, nonfatal MI, stroke, revascularization events, or any major vascular events. Likewise, the study showed no significant association of omega-3 FA supplementation with all-cause mortality or cancer. (116)

In patients with established cardiovascular disease or an increased risk of cardiovascular disease, omega-3 fatty acid supplementation also had no effect on major adverse cardiac events, all-cause mortality, sudden cardiac death, coronary artery revascularization, or hypertension. (117) In addition, a large, long-term randomised trial showed

How to cite this article: Rose S, Strombom A. A comprehensive review of the prevention and treatment of heart disease with a plant-based diet. J Cardiol & Cardiovasc Ther. 2018; 12(5): 555847. DOI: 10.19080/JOCCT.2018.12.555847.

that fish oil supplements do not reduce the risk of cardiovascular events in patients with diabetes. (118)

There has also been a mistaken notion that the Eskimo had a lower incidence of coronary heart disease, by virtue of their high fish oil consumption. This also turns out to not be the case. One report states, "*Greenland Eskimos and the Canadian and Alaskan Inuit have CAD as often as the non-Eskimo populations.*" (119) Another study states, "*Eskimos have CHD despite high consumption of omega-3 fatty acids.*" (120)

9. Discussion

9.1 Treatment Advantages

Interventional studies have shown that a low-fat (<10% of calories) plant-based diet is a viable and highly advantageous alternative to other interventional strategies. The low-fat vegetarian diet also has no surgical risk of mortality, morbidity, no post op complications, and no adverse reactions or contra-indications. The cost to the patient is minimal, and also both treats and lowers the risk of common comorbidities such as hypertension, diabetes and certain forms of cancer. It can serve as a monotherapy or as an adjunct to standard treatment regimens, including medication, stenting and CABG.

9.2 Cost-Effective Treatment

The treatment of CAD with a plant-based diet has been shown to be very cost effective. Highmark's Blue Cross estimated cost savings per participant in the Ornish low-fat vegetarian cardiac program is $16,186 measured in 1999 dollars. (121) Estimated savings would likely be much higher today. A Mutual of Omaha Insurance study, also conducted in the 1990s, determined that for every dollar spent on the Ornish program there was a savings of $5.55 in health care costs that would have otherwise accrued. (122)

According to a Kaiser Family Foundation/New York Times survey, among people with health insurance, one in five (20%) working age Americans report having had problems paying medical bills in the past year, often causing serious financial challenges and changes in employment. The situation is even worse among people who are uninsured or underinsured: half (53%) face problems with medical bills, bringing the overall total to 26 percent. (123) Many people struggle with copayments and have high deductibles.

Coronary artery disease takes a tremendous toll in both lives and money. Heart disease remains the leading cause of death for both men and women. (124) CAD costs the United States $108.9 billion each year. (125, 126) Clearly, a more cost-effective treatment to Percutaneous Coronary Intervention and CABG is needed. As we have seen, treatment of CAD with a low-fat vegetarian diet would save a very considerable amount of money.

9.3 A Needed Treatment Option

As most physicians know, many patients these days attempt to gain health-related information and to treat themselves based upon what they read on the internet. Such information is often highly unreliable. (127) In our experience, most patients would rather get their health information and advice from their physicians, but turn to the internet when they can't. Therefore, to serve the best interests and needs of their patients, physicians should familiarize themselves with this treatment.

Research has documented the high rate of compliance with this treatment, especially when physicians explain the rationale behind the treatment and specifically prescribes it to their patients.

We live in an age of advanced medical technology. These advances have alleviated much suffering and saved countless lives. They have an unquestioned place in modern medicine. However, this can sometimes lead towards a kind of technological fundamentalism. Little notice is taken of treatments that, while lacking in technological sophistication, are nevertheless quite efficacious. This indeed seems to be the case with treating CAD with a low-fat vegetarian diet.

Fortunately, many doctors have already started to integrate therapeutic plant-based diets into their patients' prevention and treatment of CAD. The former president of the American College of Cardiology, Dr. Kim Williams, uses this modality of treatment for his patients. (128) In a recent article, he states:

"Unlike many of our cardiovascular prevention and treatment strategies, including antioxidants, vitamin E, folic acid and niacin to name a few, that have disintegrated over time, the "truth" (i.e., evidence) for the benefits of plant-based nutrition continues to mount. This now includes lower rates of stroke, hypertension, diabetes mellitus, obesity, myocardial infarction and mortality, as well as many non-cardiac issues that affect our patients in cardiology, ranging from cancer to a variety of inflammatory conditions. Challenges with the science are, however, less daunting to overcome than inertia, culture, habit and widespread marketing of unhealthy foods. Our goal must be to get data out to the medical community and the public where it can actually change lives—creating healthier and longer ones." (129)

References

1. Thorogood M, Carter R, Benfield L, et.al. Plasma and lipoprotein cholesterol concentrations in people with different diets in Britain. *British Medical Journal (Clin Res Ed)*. Aug 1987;295(6594):351–353.
2. Haddad E, Berk LKJ, et.al. Dietary intake and biochemical, hematologic, and immune status of vegans compared with nonvegetarians. *American Journal of Clinical Nutrition*. Sep 1999;70(3 Suppl):586S-593S.
3. Hopkins P. Effects of dietary cholesterol on serum cholesterol: a meta-analysis and review. *American Journal of Clinical Nutrition*. Jun 1992;55(6):1060-70.
4. Barnard N, Cohen J, Jenkins D, Turner-McGrievy G, Gloede L, et.al. A low-fat vegan diet improves glycemic control and cardiovascular risk factors in a randomized clinical trial in individuals with type 2 diabetes. *Diabetes Care*. Aug 2006;29(8):1777-83.
5. Tobin K, Ulven S, Schuster G, et.al. Liver X Receptors as Insulin-mediating Factors in Fatty Acid and Cholesterol Biosynthesis. *Journal of Biological Chemistry*. Mar 2002;277(12):10691-7.
6. Berliner J, Navab M, Fogelman A, et.al. Atherosclerosis: basic mechanisms. Oxidation, inflammation, and genetics. *Circulation*. May 1995;91(9):2488-96.
7. Li D, Mehta J. Oxidized LDL, a critical factor in atherogenesis. *Cardiovascular Research*. Dec 2005;68(3):353-4.
8. Lu S, Wu W, Lee C, et.al. LDL of Taiwanese vegetarians are less oxidizable than those of omnivores. *Journal of Nutrition*. Jun 2000;130(6):1591-6.
9. Vinagre J, Vinagre C, Pozzi F, et.al. Metabolism of triglyceride-rich lipoproteins and transfer of lipids to high-density lipoproteins (HDL) in vegan and omnivore subjects. *Nutrition, Metabolism and Cardiovascular Diseases*. Jan 2013;23(1):61-7.

How to cite this article: Rose S, Strombom A. A comprehensive review of the prevention and treatment of heart disease with a plant-based diet. J Cardiol & Cardiovasc Ther. 2018; 12(5): 555847. DOI: 10.19080/JOCCT.2018.12.555847.

10. Krajcovicova-Kudlackova M, Blazicek P. C-reactive protein and nutrition. *Bratisl Lek Listy*. 2005;106(11):345-7.

11. Chen C, Lin Y, Lin T, Lin C, Chen B, Lin C. Total cardiovascular risk profile of Taiwanese vegetarians. *Eur J Clin Nutr*. Jan 2008;62(1):138-44.

12. Acosta-Navarro J, Antoniazzi L, Oki A, et al. Reduced subclinical carotid vascular disease and arterial stiffness in vegetarian men: The CARVOS Study. *Int J Cardiol*. Mar 2017;230:562-566.

13. Tsimikas S. A test in context: lipoprotein(a): diagnosis, prognosis, controversies, and emerging therapies. *J Am Coll Cardiol*. Feb 2017;69(6):692-711.

14. Tsimikas S, Fazio S, Ferdinand K, et al. NHLBI Working Group recommendations to reduce lipoprotein(a)-mediated risk of cardiovascular disease and aortic stenosis. *J Am Coll Cardiol*. Jan 2018;71(2):177-192.

15. Yu B, Hafiane A, Thanassoulis G, et al. Lipoprotein(a) induces human aortic valve interstitial cell calcification. *JACC Basic Transi Sci*. Aug 2017;2(4):358-371.

16. Willeit P, Ridker P, Nestel P, et al. Baseline and on-statin treatment lipoprotein(a) levels for prediction of cardiovascular events: individual patient-data meta-analysis of statin outcome trials. *Lancet*. Oct 2018;392(10155):1311-1320.

17. Najjar R, Moore C, Montgomery B. Consumption of a defined, plant-based diet reduces lipoprotein(a), inflammation, and other atherogenic lipoproteins and particles within 4 weeks. *Clin Cardiol*. Aug 2018;41(8):1062-1068.

18. Contois J, McConnell J, Sethi A, et al. Apolipoprotein B and Cardiovascular Disease Risk: Position Statement from the AACC Lipoproteins and Vascular Diseases Division Working Group on Best Practices. *Clin Chem*. Mar 2009;55(3):407-19.

19. Sandhu P, Mus[illegible] Lipoprotein Biomarkers [illegible] Cardiovascular Disease: A Labora[illegible] Best Practices (LMBP) Systematic Review. [illegible] *Appl Lab Med*. Sep 2016;1(2):214-229.

20. Davidson M, Ballantyne C, Jacobson T, et al. Clinical utility of inflammatory markers and advanced lipoprotein testing: advice from an expert panel of lipid specialists. *J Clin Lipidol*. Sep-Oct 2011;5(5):338-67.

21. Bradbury K, Crowe F, Appleby P, et.al. Serum concentrations of cholesterol, apolipoprotein A-I, and apolipoprotein B in a total of 1694 meat-eaters, fish-eaters, vegetarians, and vegans. *European Journal of Clinical Nutrition*. Feb 2014;68(2):178-183.

22. Cooper R, Goldberg R, Trevisan M, et.al. The selective lipid-lowering effect of vegetarianism on low density lipoproteins in a cross-over experiment. *Atherosclerosis*. Sep 1982;44(3):293-305.

23. Ornish D, Brown S, Scherwitz L, et.al. Can lifestyle changes reverse coronary heart disease? The Lifestyle Heart Trial. *Lancet*. Jul 1990;336(8708):129-33.

24. Miller M, Beach V, Sorkin J, et.al. Comparative effects of three popular diets on lipids, endothelial function, and C-reactive protein during weight maintenance. *Journal of American Dietetic Assoc*. Apr 2009;109(4):713-7.

25. Najjar R, Moore C, Montgomery B. A defined, plant-based diet utilized in an outpatient cardiovascular clinic effectively treats hypercholesterolemia and hypertension and reduces medications. *Clin Cardiol*. Mar 2018;41(3):307-313.

26. Jenkins D, Kendall C, Marchie A, et.al. Direct comparison of a dietary portfolio of cholesterol-lowering foods with a statin in hypercholesterolemic participants. *American Journal of Clinical Nutrition*. Feb 2005;81(2):380-7.

27. Macknin M, Kong T, Weier A, et.al. Plant-Based, No-Added-Fat or American Heart Association Diets: Impact on Cardiovascular

...e of
...nune
...ure trends.
...14.

...man B, Flaws J. The ...ocarbon receptor in the ...tive system. *Niochem* ...eb 2009;77(4):547-59.

30. ...ng J, Zhu K, et al. Aryl Hydrocarbon ...eptor: A New Player of Pathogenesis and Therapy in Cardiovascular Diseases. *Biomed Res Int*. 2018;2018:11 pages.

31. Xiao L, Zhang Z, Luo X. Roles of xenobiotic receptors in vascular pathophysiology. *Circ J*. 2014;78(7):1520-30.

32. Chuang K, Yan Y, Chiu S, Cheng T. Long-term air pollution exposure and risk factors for cardio-vascular diseases among the elderly in Taiwan. *Occup Environ Med*. Jan 2011;68(1):64-8.

33. Oesterling E, Toborek M, Hennig B. Benzo[a] pyrene induces intercellular adhesion mole-cule-1 through a caveolae and aryl hydrocar-bon receptor mediated pathway. *Toxicol Appl Pharmacol*. Oct 2008;232(2):309-16.

34. Kopf P, Huwe J, Walker M. Hypertension, cardiac hypertrophy, and impaired vascular relaxation induced by 2,3,7,8-Tetrachlorodibenzo-p-Dioxin are associated with increased superoxide. *Cardiovasc Toxicol*. Dec 2008;8(4):181-93.

35. Savouret J, Berdeaux A, Casper R. The aryl hydrocarbon receptor and its xenobiotic ligands: A fundamental trigger for cardiovascu-lar diseases. *Nutr Metab Cardiovasc Dis*. Apr 2003;13(2):104-13.

36. Dalton T, Kerzee J, Wang B, et al. Dioxin exposure is an environmental risk factor for ischemic heart disease. *Cardiovasc Toxicol*. 2001;1(4):285-98.

37. Perkins J, Petriello M, Newsome B, Hennig B. Polychlorinated biphenyls and links to cardiovascular disease. *Environ Sci Pollut Res Int*. Feb 2016;23(3):2160-72.

38. Kim S, Kim K, Lee Y, Jacobs D, Lee D. Associations of organochlorine pesticides and polychlorinated biphenyls with total, cardio-vascular, and cancer mortality in elders with differing fat mass. *Environ Res*. Apr 2015;138:1-7.

39. Pavuk M, Olson J, Wattigney W, et al. Predictors of serum polychlorinated biphenyl concentrations in Anniston residents. *Sci Total Environ*. Oct 2014;496:624-634.

40. Pavuk M, Olson J, Sjödin A, et al. Serum concentrations of polychlorinated biphenyls (PCBs) in participants of the Anniston Community Health Survey. *Sci Total Environ*. Mar 2014;473-474:286-97.

41. Aminov Z, Haase R, Pavuk M, Carpenter D, Consortium AEHR. Analysis of the effects of exposure to polychlorinated biphenyls and chlorinated pesticides on serum lipid levels in residents of Anniston, Alabama. *Environ Health*. Dec 2013;12:108.

42. Silverstone A, Rosenbaum P, Weinstock R, et al. Polychlorinated biphenyl (PCB) exposure and diabetes: results from the Anniston Community Health Survey. *Environ Health Perspect*. May 2012;120(5):727-32.

43. Goncharov A, Bloom M, Pavuk M, Birman I, Carpenter D. Blood pressure and hypertension in relation to levels of serum polychlorinated biphenyls in residents of Anniston, Alabama. *J Hypertens*. Oct 2010;28(10):2053-60.

44. Langer P, Kocan A, Tajtáková M, et al. Multiple adverse thyroid and metabolic health signs in the population from the area heavily polluted by organochlorine cocktail (PCB, DDE, HCB, dioxin). *Thyroid Res*. Mar 2009;2(1):3.

45. Lind P, Orberg J, Edlund U, Sjöblom L, Lind L. The dioxin-like pollutant PCB 126 (3,3′,4,4′,5-pentachlorobiphenyl) affects risk factors for cardiovascular disease in female rats. *Toxicol Lett*. May 2004;150(3):293-9.

How to cite this article: Rose S, Strombom A. A comprehensive review of the prevention and treatment of heart disease with a plant-based diet. J Cardiol & Cardiovasc Ther. 2018; 12(5): 555847. DOI: 10.19080/JOCCT.2018.12.555847.

46. Humblet O, Birnbaum L, Rimm E, Mittleman M, Hauser R. Dioxins and Cardiovascular Disease Mortality. *Environ Health Perspect*. Nov 2008;116(11):1443-8.
47. Kim J, Pjanic M, Nguyen T, et al. TCF21 and the environmental sensor aryl-hydrocarbon receptor cooperate to activate a pro-inflammatory gene expression program in coronary artery smooth muscle cells. *PLoS Genet*. May 2017;13(5):e1006750.
48. Kim J, Pjanic M, Sazanova O, Wang T, Miller C, Quertermous T. TCF21 Regulates Coronary Artery Disease Causing Aryl-hydrocarbon Receptor Gene Expression and its Downstream Pathway Activation by Environmental Ligands. *Circulation*. Mar 2018;132(Suppl 3).
49. Murphy M, Petriello M, Han S, et al. Exercise protects against PCB-induced inflammation and associated cardiovascular risk factors. *Environ Sci Pollut Res Int*. Feb 2016;23(3):2201-11.
50. Petriello M, Hoffman J, Sunkara M, et al. Dioxin-like pollutants increase hepatic flavin containing monooxygenase (FMO3) expression to promote synthesis of the pro-atherogenic nutrient biomarker Trimethylamine N-oxide from dietary precursors. *J Nutr Biochem*. Jul 2016;33:145-53.
51. Wang Z, Klipfell E, Bennett B, et al. Gut flora metabolism of phosphatidylcholine promotes cardiovascular disease. *Nature*. Apr 2011;472:57-63.
52. Fogelman A. TMAO is both a biomarker and a renal toxin. *Circ Res*. Jan 2015;116(3):396-7.
53. Koeth R, Wang Z, Levison B, et al. Intestinal microbiota metabolism of L-carnitine, a nutrient in red meat, promotes atherosclerosis. *Nat Med*. May 2013;19(5):576-585.
54. Ufnal M, Jazwiec R, Dadlez M, Drapala A, Sikora M, Skrzypecki J. Trimethylamine-N-oxide: a carnitine-derived metabolite that prolongs the hypertensive effect of angiotensin II in rats. *Can J Cardiol*. Dec 2014;30(12):1700-5.
55. Walker P, Rhu[illegible] K, Lawrence R. Public [illegible] meat production and consumpti[illegible] *Health Nutrit*. Jun 2005;8(4):348-356.
56. Sasamoto T, Ushio F, Kikutani N, et al. Estimation of 1999-2004 dietary daily intake of PCDDs, PCDFs and dioxin-like PCBs by a total diet study in metropolitan Tokyo, Japan. *Chemosphere*. Jul 2006;64(4):634-41.
57. Fisher B. Most Unwanted. *Environmental Health Perspectives*. Jan 1999;107(1):A18-23.
58. Bocio A, Domingo J. Daily intake of polychlorinated dibenzo-p-dioxins/polychlorinated dibenzofurans (PCDD/PCDFs) in foodstuffs consumed in Tarragona, Spain: a review of recent studies (2001-2003) on human PCDD/PCDF exposure through the diet. *Environ Res*. Jan 2005;97(1):1-9.
59. Schecter A, Colacino J, Haffner D, et al. Perfluorinated compounds, polychlorinated biphenyls, and organochlorine pesticide contamination in composite food samples from Dallas, Texas, USA. *Environ Health Perspect*. Jun 2010;118(6):796-802.
60. Darnerud P, Atuma S, Aune M, Bierselius RGA, et.al. Dietary intake estimations of organohalogen contaminants (dioxins, PCB, PBDE and chlorinated pesticides, e.g. DDT) based on Swedish market basket data. *Food Chem Toxicol*. Sep 2006;44(9):1597-606.
61. Bergkvist C, Oberg M, Appelgren M, et al. Exposure to dioxin-like pollutants via different food commodities in Swedish children and young adults. *Food Chem Toxicol*. Nov 2008;46(11):3360-7.
62. Dougherty C, Henricks Holtz S, Reinert J, Panyacosit L, Axelrad D, et.al. Dietary exposures to food contaminants across the United States. *Environ Res*. Oct 2000;84(2):170-85.
63. Kiviranta H, Tuomisto J, Tuomisto J, et.al. Polychlorinated dibenzo-p-dioxins, dibenzofurans, and biphenyls in the general population in Finland. *Chemosphere*. Aug 2005;60(7):854-69.

):680-6.

zma J. ality among with differing dietary report. *Am J Clin Nutr.* uppl):S191-S198.

Emerging Risk Biomarkers in scular Diseases and Disorders. *Journal ids.* 2015;2015:Article ID 971453, 50 pages.

67. Papazafiropoulou A, Tentolouris N. Matrix metalloproteinases and cardiovascular diseases. *Hippokratia*. Apr-Jun 2009;13(2):76-82.
68. Stary H, Chandler A, Dinsmore R, et.al. A definition of advanced types of atherosclerotic lesions and a histological classification of atherosclerosis. A report from the Committee on Vascular Lesions of the Council on Arteriosclerosis, American Heart Association. *Circulation*. Sep 1995;92(5):1355-74.
69. Brown D, Hibbs M, Kearney M, Isner J. Differential expression of 92-kDa gelatinase in primary atherosclerotic versus restenotic coronary lesions. *American Journal of Cardiology*. Apr 1997;79(7):878-82.
70. Brown D, Hibbs M, Kearney M, et.al. Identification of 92-kD gelatinase in human coronary atherosclerotic lesions: association of active enzyme synthesis with unstable angina. *Circulation*. Apr 1995;91(8):2125-31.
71. Blankenberg S, Rupprecht H, Poirier O, et.al. Plasma concentrations and genetic variation of matrix metalloproteinase 9 and prognosis of patients with cardiovascular disease. *Circulation*. Apr 2003;107(12):1579-85.
72. Orbe J, Fernandez L, Rodríguez J, et.al. Different expression of MMPs/TIMP-1 in human atherosclerotic lesions. Relation to plaque features and vascular bed. *Atherosclerosis*. Oct 2003;170(2):269-76.
73. Noji Y, Kajinami K, Kawashiri M, et.al. Circulating matrix metalloproteinases and their inhibitors in premature coronary atherosclerosis. *Clinical Chemistry and Laboratory Medicine*. May 2001;39(5):380-4.
74. Beaudeux J, Giral P, Bruckert E, et.al. Serum matrix metalloproteinase-3 and tissue inhibitor of metalloproteinases-1 as potential markers of carotid atherosclerosis in infraclinical hyperlipidemia. *Atherosclerosis*. Jul 2003;169(1):139-46.
75. Navarro J, de Gouveia L, Rocha-Penha L, et.al. Reduced levels of potential circulating biomarkers of cardiovascular diseases in apparently healthy vegetarian men. *Clinica Chimica Acta*. Aug 2016;461:110-113.
76. Leeuwenberg J, Smeets E, Neefjes J, et.al. E-selectin and intercellular adhesion molecule-1 are released by activated human endothelial cells in vitro. *Immunology*. Dec 1992;77(4):543-9.
77. van de Stolpe A, van der Saag P. Intercellular adhesion molecule-1. *Journal of Molecular Medicine (Berlin)*. Jan 1996;74(1):13-33.
78. Purschwitz K, Rassoul F, Reuter W, et.al. [Soluble leukocyte adhesion molecules in vegetarians of various ages]. *Zeitschrift fur Gerontologie und Geriatrie*. Dec 2001;34(6):476-9.
79. Morrison LM. Diet in Coronary Atherosclerosis. *JAMA*. Jun 1960;173(8):884-888.
80. Ornish D, Scherwitz L, Billings J, et.al. Intensive Lifestyle Changes for Reversal of Coronary Heart Disease. *JAMA*. 1998;280(23):2001-7.
81. Esselstyn CJ, Ellis S, Medendorp S, Crowe T. A strategy to arrest and reverse coronary artery disease: a 5-year longitudinal study of a single physician's practice. *Journal of Family Practice*. Dec 1995;41(6):560-8.
82. Esselstyn CJ, Gendy G, Doyle J, et.al. A way to reverse CAD? *Journal of Family Practice*. Jul 2014;63(7):356-364b.
83. Gupta S, Sawhney R, Rai L, et.al. Regression of coronary atherosclerosis through healthy

lifestyle in coronary artery disease patients–Mount Abu Open Heart Trial.. *Indian Heart Journal*. Sept-Oct 2011;63(5):461-9.

84. Arntzenius A, Kromhout D, Barth J, et.al. Diet, Lipoproteins, and the Progression of Coronary Atherosclerosis — The Leiden Intervention Trial. *New England Journal of Medicine*. Mar 1985;312(13):805-11.
85. Gould K, Ornish D, Scherwitz L, et.al. Changes in myocardial perfusion abnormalities by positron emission tomography after long-term, intense risk factor modification. *JAMA*. Sep 1995;274(11):894-901.
86. Gould K. *Coronary arterial stenosis: a textbook of Coronary Pathophysiology, Quantitative Arteriography, Cardiac PET and reversal of Coronary Artery Disease*: Elsevier; 1990.
87. Gould K, Ornish D, Kirkeeide R, et.al. Improved stenosis geometry by quantitative coronary arteriography after vigorous risk factor modification. *American Journal of Cardiology*. Apr 1992;69(9):845-53.
88. Frattaroli J, Weidner G, Merritt-Worden T, et.al. Angina pectoris and atherosclerotic risk factors in the multisite cardiac lifestyle intervention program. *American Journal of Cardiology*. Apr 2008;101(7):911-8.
89. Ellis F, Sanders T. Angina and the Vegan Diet. *American Heart Journal*. Jun 1977;93(6):803–805.
90. Velagaleti R, Vasan R. Heart Failure in the 21st Century: Is it a Coronary Artery Disease Problem or Hypertension Problem? *Cardiol Clin*. Nov 2007;25(4):487-95.
91. Djoussé L, Driver J, Gaziano J. Relation between modifiable lifestyle factors and lifetime risk of heart failure. *JAMA*. Jul 2009;302(4):394-400.
92. Wang Y, Tuomilehto J, Jousilahti P, et al. Lifestyle factors in relation to heart failure among Finnish men and women. *Circ Heart Fail*. Sep 2011;4(5):607-12.
93. Pfister R, Sharp S, Luben R, Wareham N, Khaw K. Plasma vitamin C predicts incident heart failure in men and women in European Prospective Investigation into Cancer and Nutrition-Norfolk prospective study. *Am Heart J*. Aug 2011;162(2):246-53.
94. Rautiainen S, Levitan E, Mittleman M, Wolk A. Fruit and vegetable intake and rate of heart failure: a population-based prospective cohort of women. *Eur J Heart Fail*. Jan 2015;17(1):20-6.
95. Choi E, Allen K, McDonnough M, Massera D, Ostfeld R. A plant-based diet and heart failure: case report and literature review. *J Geriatr Cardiol*. May 2017;14(5):375-378.
96. Wirth J, di Giuseppe R, Boeing H, Weikert C. A Mediterranean style diet, its components and the risk of heart failure: a prospective population-based study in a non-Mediterranean country. *Eur J Clin Nutr*. Sep 2016;70(9):1015-21.
97. Nettleton J, Steffen L, Loehr L, Rosamond W, Folsom A. Incident heart failure is associated with lower whole-grain intake and greater high-fat dairy and egg intake in the Atherosclerosis Risk in Communities (ARIC) study. *J Am Diet Assoc*. Nov 2008;108(11):1881-7.
98. Ashaye A, Gaziano J, Djoussé L. Red meat consumption and risk of heart failure in male physicians. *Nutr Metab Cardiovasc Dis*. Dec 2011;21(12):941-6.
99. Kaluza J, Åkesson A, Wolk A. Long-term processed and unprocessed red meat consumption and risk of heart failure: a prospective cohort study of women. *Int J Cardiol*. Aug 2015;193:42-6.
100. Kerley C. A Review of Plant-based Diets to Prevent and Treat Heart Failure. *Card Fail Rev*. May 2018;4(1):54-61.
101. Djoussé L, Gaziano J. Egg consumption and risk of heart failure in the Physicians' Health Study. *Circulation*. Jan 2008;117(4):512-6.
102. Lara K, Levitan E, Guitterrez O, Shikany J, Safford MJS, Rosenson R. Dietary patterns and incident heart failure in adults with no known

coronary disease or heart failure: The REGARDS Cohort. *Circulation*. Nov 2017;136(Suppl 1).

103. Pischke C, Weidner G, Elliott-Eller M, Ornish D. Lifestyle changes and clinical profile in coronary heart disease patients with an ejection fraction of 40% in the Multicenter Lifestyle Demonstration Project.. *European Journal of Heart Failure*. Sep 2007;9(9):928-34.

104. Aldana S, Whitmer W, Greenlaw R, et.al. Cardiovascular risk reductions associated with aggressive lifestyle modification and cardiac rehabilitation. *Heart and Lung*. Nov-Dec 2003;32(6):374-82.

105. Aldana S, Whitmer W, Greenlaw R, et.al. Effect of intense lifestyle modification and cardiac rehabilitation on psychosocial cardiovascular disease risk factors and quality of life.. *Behavior Modification*. Jul 2006;30(4):507-25.

106. Patel H, Chandra S, Alexander S, Soble J, Williams KS. Plant-Based Nutrition: An Essential Component of Cardiovascular Disease Prevention and Management. *Curr Cardiol Rep*. Sep 2017;19(10):104.

107. Buccheri D, Piraino D, Andolina G, Cortese B. Understanding and managing in-stent restenosis: a review of clinical data, from pathogenesis to treatment. *J Thorac Dis*. Oct 2016;8(10):E1150-E1162.

108. Ornish D. Avoiding revascularization with lifestyle changes: The Multicenter Lifestyle Demonstration Project. *American Journal of Cardiology*. Nov 1998;82(10B):72T-76T.

109. Pischke C, Weidner G, Elliott-Eller M, et.al. Comparison of coronary risk factors and quality of life in coronary artery disease patients with versus without diabetes mellitus. *American Journal of Cardiology*. May 2006;97(9):1267-73.

110. Silberman A, Banthia R, Estay I, et.al. The effectiveness and efficacy of an intensive cardiac rehabilitation program in 24 sites. *American Journal of Health Promotion*. Mar-Apr 2010;24(4):260-2.

111. Pischke C, Frenda S, Ornish D, et.al.. Lifestyle changes are related to reductions in depression in persons with elevated coronary risk factors. *Psychology and Health*. Nov 2010;25(9):1077-100.

112. Gopinath B, Flood V, Burlutksya G, Mitchell P. Consumption of nuts and risk of total and cause-specific mortality over 15 years.. *Nutrition, Metabolism, and Cardiovascular Diseases*. Dec 2015;25(12):1125–1131.

113. Kris-Etherton P. Walnuts decrease risk of cardiovascular disease: a summary of efficacy and biologic mechanisms. *Journal of Nutrition*. Apr 2014;144(4 Suppl):547S-554S.

114. Brown R, Gray A, Tey S, et al. Associations between Nut Consumption and Health Vary between Omnivores, Vegetarians, and Vegans. *Nutrients*. Nov 2017;9(11):E1219.

115. Kwak S, Myung S, Lee Y, et.al. Efficacy of Omega-3 Fatty Acid Supplements in the Secondary Prevention of Cardiovascular Disease. *Archives of Internal Medicine*. May 2012;172(9):686-94.

116. Aung T, Halsey J, Kromhout D, et al. Associations of Omega-3 Fatty Acid Supplement Use With Cardiovascular Disease Risks: Meta-analysis of 10 Trials Involving 77 917 Individuals. *JAMA Cardiol*. Mar 2018;3(3):225-234.

117. Rogers T, Seehusen D. Omega-3 Fatty Acids and Cardiovascular Disease. *Am Fam Physician*. May 2018;97(9):562-564.

118. The ASCEND Study Collaborative Group. Effects of n−3 Fatty Acid Supplements in Diabetes Mellitus. *New Eng J Med*. Oct 2018;379:1540-1550.

119. Fodor J, Helis E, Yazdekhasti N, et.al. “Fishing” for the origins of the “Eskimos and heart disease” story: facts or wishful thinking?. *Canadian Journal of Cardiology*. Aug 2014;30(8):864-8.

120. Ebbesson S, Risica P, Ebbesson L, Kennish J. Eskimos have CHD despite high consumption of omega-3 fatty acids: the Alaska Siberia

How to cite this article: Rose S, Strombom A. A comprehensive review of the prevention and treatment of heart disease with a plant-based diet. J Cardiol & Cardiovasc Ther. 2018; 12(5): 555847. DOI: 10.19080/JOCCT.2018.12.555847.

project. *Internat Journal of Circumpolar Health*. Sep 2005;64(4):387-95.

121. Highmark Blue Cross Blue Shield. *Two-Year Results of Highmark Blue Cross Blue Shield's Dr. Dean Ornish Program For Reversing Heart Disease Demonstrates Outstanding Lifestyle Improvements By The Men and Women Who Took Bold Step in Quest For Longer, Better, Happier Lives*. Pittsburgh: PR Newswire; 1999.
122. Ornish D. *Dr Dean Ornish's Program for Reversing Heart Disease.*: Random House; 2010.
123. Kaiser Family Foundation. *New Kaiser/New York Times Survey Finds One in Five Working-Age Americans With Health Insurance Report Problems Paying Medical Bills*: kff.org; 2016.
124. Hasty R, Garbalosa R, Barbato V, et.al. Wikipedia vs peer-reviewed medical literature for information about the 10 most costly medical conditions. *Journal of American Osteopath Assoc*. May 2014;114(5):368-73.
125. Centers for Disease Control and Prevention, National Center for Health Statistics. *Underlying Cause of Death 1999-2013*: Wonder.CDC.gov/ucd-icd10.html; Accessed Feb 3, 2015.
126. Heidenreich P, Trogdon J, Khavjou O, et.al. Forecasting the future of cardiovascular disease in the United States: a policy statement from the American Heart Association.. *Circulation*. Mar 2011;123(8):933-44.
127. Schwartz K, Roe T, Northrup J, et.al. Family Medicine Patients' Use of the Internet for Health Information: A MetroNet Study. *Journal of American Board of Family Medicine*. Jan-Feb 2006;19(1):39-45.
128. Tuso P. Nutritional Update for Physicians: Plant-Based Diets. *The Permanente Journal*. Spring 2013;17(2):61-66.
129. Williams K. Introduction to the "A plant-based diet and cardiovascular disease" special issue. *J Geriatr Cardiol*. May 2017;14(5):316.

Open access Journal of
Neurology & Neurosurgery
ISSN: 2476-0501

Juniper Publishers
key to the Researchers

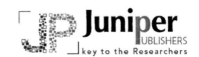

Review Article
Volume 14 Issue 2 – September 2020
DOI: 10.19080/OAJNN.2020.14.555882

Open Access J Neurol Neurosurg

Preventing Stroke with a Plant-Based Diet

Stewart Rose and Amanda Strombom*

Plant-Based Diets in Medicine, USA

Submission: August 05, 2020; **Published:** September 29, 2020

***Corresponding author:** Amanda Strombom, Plant-Based Diets in Medicine, 12819 SE 38th St, #427, Bellevue, WA 98006, USA

Abstract

Current known modifiable risk factors for stroke together account for more than 90% of population attributable risk. A plant-based diet has been shown to reduce the risk of stroke by 28-48%, and to significantly reduce the biggest risk factors – hypertension, coronary heart disease, and type 2 diabetes. Vegetarians have been found to have a 34-44% lower risk of developing hypertension, and a 40% reduced risk of ischemic heart disease. Vegans have a 78% lower risk of type 2 diabetes and a 75% reduced risk of hypertension compared to meat eaters with an otherwise healthy lifestyle. In addition, plant-based diets may reduce the likelihood of other risk factors that are associated with stroke, such as atrial fibrillation and heart failure.

One of the main goals in stroke risk reduction is to control vascular risk factors such as hypertension, diabetes, dyslipidemia, and smoking cessation. Changes in lifestyle such as a healthy diet and aerobic exercise are recommended strategies for all of these. Patient compliance on plant-based diets has been good in almost all studies, with the degree of compliance often very high. The patient should be informed that while a plant-based diet reduces the risk of stroke, it will also reduce the risk of a number of other diseases.

Keywords

Atrial fibrillation, hemorrhagic stroke, hypertension, ischemic stroke, plant-based diet, stroke, vegetarian, vegan

Abbreviations

AF: Atrial Fibrillation; ApoB/ApoA1: Apolipoprotein ratio; BP: Blood pressure; CAD: Coronary artery disease; CHD: Coronary heart disease; CRP: C-Reactive Protein; HDL: High density lipoprotein; HF: Heart failure; hsCRP: High sensitivity C-reactive protein; LDL: Low density lipoprotein; tPA; tissue plasminogen activator

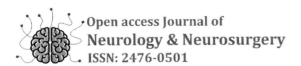

1. Introduction

Nearly 800,000 people suffer from a stroke each year in the United States. Stroke is the fifth leading cause of adult death and disability. With up to 40% of survivors not expected to recover independence from severe disabilities, it results in over $72 billion in annual cost in the US alone. (1)

Stroke results in immense human suffering, and an excessive financial burden on health systems worldwide. Treatment is difficult hence prevention strategies are all the more important. Therefore, physician education on stroke prophylaxis with a plant-based diet would be especially valuable in preventing the incidence of stroke.

Stroke is a heterogeneous, multifactorial disease regulated by modifiable and nonmodifiable risk factors. Modifiable factors include a history of hypertension, diabetes mellitus, C-reactive protein (CRP), high sensitivity CRP (hsCRP), and coronary heart disease amongst others. Nonmodifiable factors include age, sex and race. Other less-well documented risk factors include geographic location, socioeconomic status and alcoholism. Approximately 80% of stroke events could be reduced by making simple lifestyle modifications. (2)

The majority, 82–92%, of strokes are ischemic although the relative burden of hemorrhagic versus ischemic stroke varies among different populations. (3) Hemorrhagic strokes can be either primarily intraparenchymal or subarachnoid. Ischemic stroke can be further divided into what have been referred to as etiologic subtypes, or categories thought to represent the causes of the stroke: cardioembolic, atherosclerotic, lacunar, other specific causes (dissections, vasculitis, specific genetic disorders, others), and strokes of unknown cause. (4)

As far as treatment goes, the intravenous administration of tissue plasminogen activator (tPA) within 3 hours of stroke onset, or within 4.5 hours of stroke onset in select patients, is currently the only U.S. Food and Drug Administration (FDA)-approved therapy for ischemic stroke. (5) Because of the time-dependent nature of tPA therapy and a fear of hemorrhagic complications, only 1%–8% of potentially eligible patients have been treated with tPA. (6)

Mechanical thrombectomy may also be performed. Restoring blood flow can mitigate the effects of ischemia only if performed quickly. Mechanical clot disruption is an alternative for patients in whom fibrinolysis is ineffective or contraindicated. (7)

In the case of cardioembolism due to atrial fibrillation, mechanical valves, or cardiac thrombus, anticoagulation is the mainstay of therapy. (8)

In contrast to treatment for ischemic stroke, the recommendation for managing hemorrhagic stroke is supportive treatment, because no specific medication has been developed. (9, 10)

Therefore, treatments for acute ischemic and hemorrhagic stroke continue to be a major unmet clinical need, making prevention even more important.

2. Risk Factors

Some risk factors of stroke are nonmodifiable, such as older age and male sex. Current known modifiable risk factors — hypertension, current cigarette smoking, high waist-to-hip ratio, poor diet, lack of regular physical activity, diabetes mellitus, alcohol consumption, psychological factors,

How to cite this article: Rose S, Strombom A. Preventing stroke with a plant-based diet. Open Access J Neurol Neurosurg 2020; 14(2): 555882.
DOI: 10.19080/OAJNN.2020.14.555882

cardiac causes, and apolipoprotein (ApoB/ApoA1) ratio — together account for more than 90% of population attributable risk for stroke. (11, 12)

Risk factors for hemorrhagic and ischemic stroke are similar, but there are some notable differences. There are also differences in risk factors among the etiologic categories of ischemic stroke. Hypertension is a particularly important risk factor for hemorrhagic stroke, though it contributes to atherosclerotic disease that can lead to ischemic stroke as well. Hyperlipidemia, on the other hand, is a particularly important risk factor for ischemic strokes due to atherosclerosis of extracranial and intracranial blood vessels, just as it is a risk factor for coronary atherosclerosis. Recent evidence has firmly established heart failure as a risk factor for stroke, most commonly for ischemic stroke. (13)

Metabolic syndrome and high low-density lipoprotein (LDL) cholesterol have also been identified as risk factors for intracranial atherosclerosis, an important mechanistic step in the pathogenesis of ischemic stroke. (14)

Atrial fibrillation (AF) is also a risk factor for cardioembolic stroke. (11)

3. Impact of Diet

According to the American Heart Association statistical report of 2015, only 0.1% of Americans consume a healthy diet and only 8.3% consume a moderately healthy diet. (1)

Within the last decades, plant-based nutrition has experienced increased interest in the medical community, because it can reduce the risk factors of diseases such as hypertension (15), type 2 diabetes (16), and coronary heart disease (17).

Generally, a Mediterranean diet is a much more plant-rich diet than the standard American diet. In one Dutch cohort followed for 10–15 years, those with the highest adherence to the diet had an adjusted relative risk of incident stroke of 30% less than compared to those with the lowest adherence. (18)

In one study comparing vegetarians to nonvegetarians who otherwise practice a healthy diet, a 29% reduction in the risk of stroke was noted. (19) In another study, researchers found vegetarians had a 48% lower risk of overall stroke than non vegetarians, a 60% lower risk of ischemic stroke, and a 65% lower risk of hemorrhagic stroke. (20)

However, one study did show an increased risk of hemorrhagic stroke. (21) Nearly 80% of vegetarians in this study drank varying degrees of alcohol. Alcohol consumption (as measured by γ-glutamyl transferase) has been suggested in a previous cohort study to modify the effect of low serum cholesterol typical of vegetarians on hemorrhagic stroke risk. (22)

Dietary intake of fruits and vegetables may reduce the risk of stroke. These foods may protect against stroke through antioxidant mechanisms or by raising potassium levels (23, 24, 25).

4. Dyslipidemia

Vegetarians have a 40% reduced risk of ischemic heart disease. (19, 26)

Epidemiological research also points to the lower total cholesterol and LDL cholesterol levels in those already following plant-based diet. One study showed that vegans had on average a total cholesterol of only 142 mg/dl and an LDL cholesterol of only 69 mg/dl. (27) Other studies have also shown a much lower than average level of total cholesterol and LDL. (28, 29) One study showed am LDL/HDL ratio 1.63 for vegans compared to 2.27

for meat eaters. (28) Vegans have also been shown to have lower ratios of ApoB/Apo1 ratios. (17, 30, 31)

A newer area of research has focused on the role of the gut microbiota in the pathogenesis of atherosclerosis. It has been found that vegetarians and vegans have bacterial flora that produce less trimethylamine-N-oxide (TMAO), thought to be atherogenic, than the flora of meat eaters. (32)

Several studies found an association between high serum CRP level and development of stroke (33, 34, 35, 36, 37). Rooco et al. found an independent association between high serum CRP level with mortality and intercerebral hemorrhage after thrombolysed stroke (38).

Lower levels of hs-CRP were found in those following a vegetarian diet for more than 2 years. (39, 40) An interventional study found that after 8 weeks on a vegan diet hs-CRP was reduced 32% even more than the American Heart Association diet. (41)

5. Hypertension and Type 2 Diabetes

DASH (dietary approaches to stop hypertension) was developed by the National Heart, Lung, and Blood Institute to help people prevent high blood pressure. The plan focuses on eating plenty of fruits, vegetables, and whole grains while lowering salt. Adherence to the DASH-style diet is associated with a lower risk of stroke among middle-aged women during 24 years of follow-up. (42)

Studies have found that vegans and vegetarians have lower blood pressure than their meat-eating counterparts. Observational studies have found that vegetarian diets are associated with a 6.9 mmHg lower mean systolic blood pressure and 4.7 mmHg lower mean diastolic blood pressure compared to omnivorous diets. Clinical trials of vegetarian or vegan diets of at least 6 weeks duration resulted in mean decreases of 4.8 mmHg systolic BP and 2.2 mmHg diastolic BP. (43) This finding may, in part, be related to increased potassium intake from plant foods (particularly if accompanied by a low sodium intake). A high sodium to potassium ratio has been associated with increased risk of stroke. (15)

In a prospective cohort study of 1546 non-hypertensive subjects followed for three years, those consuming more phytochemical rich foods (plant-based foods) had lower risk of developing hypertension. (44) In a matched cohort study of 4109 non-hypertensive subjects followed for a median of 1.6 years, vegetarians had a 34% lower risk of developing hypertension than non-vegetarians. (45) In a study comparing black vegetarians with non-vegetarians who had a healthy lifestyle, the risk of hypertension was reduced 44%. (46)

Diabetes causes various microvascular and macrovascular changes often culminating in major clinical complications, one of which, is stroke. (47) Vegans have a 78% lower risk of type 2 diabetes and a 75% reduced risk of hypertension compared to meat eaters with an otherwise healthy lifestyle. (48)

6. Atrial Fibrillation

Atrial fibrillation can lead to thrombus development within the atria, (49) particularly the left atrial appendage (50, 51), which can cause thromboembolic events. Multiple risk factors and clinical conditions that are associated with the development and progression of AF have been identified in the last decades. (52, 53)

Although there are several nonmodifiable risk factors, such as gender or advancing age, a gradual

How to cite this article: Rose S, Strombom A. Preventing stroke with a plant-based diet. Open Access J Neurol Neurosurg 2020; 14(2): 555882.
DOI: 10.19080/OAJNN.2020.14.555882

shift in awareness toward modifiable predisposing conditions has been observed. (54) Conventional cardiovascular risk factors that are associated with atrial fibrillation include hypertension, coronary heart disease, heart failure, and valvular heart disease. (52, 55) Other well-established concomitant risk factors include diabetes, overweight, obesity, and hyperthyroidism. Additionally, there are a number of emerging and less well-researched risk factors, such as subclinical atherosclerosis, inflammation, obstructive sleep apnea, and chronic kidney disease. (56)

Plant-based diets may reduce the likelihood of many traditional risk factors that are associated with AF (56), including hypertension (43, 57, 58), hyperthyroidism (59), obesity (48), and diabetes. (16) One study showed that a vegan diet reduced the risk of hyperthyroidism by 51% while a vegetarian diet reduced the risk by 28% showing a dose response relationship. (60) Several lines of epidemiological research have also shown a lower risk of chronic kidney disease among vegetarians. It also shows a substantially increased risk among omnivores, especially those who eat red and processed meats. (61)

Contrary to recent interest, both fish and fish oil do not seem to have an antiarrhythmic effect or protect against atrial fibrillation. (62, 63)

7. Heart Failure

Traditionally, the following are the known causes of ischemic stroke: (a) embolism to the brain of cardiac or aortic origin (i.e., myocardial infarction, AF, valvular heart disease, complicated aortic plaque, or patent foramen ovale); (b) cerebral ischemia due to perfusion failure and artery-to-artery embolism (i.e., large artery atherosclerotic plaque, small vessel disease or occlusion, or vasculitis); and (c) thrombosis (prothrombotic state). Not surprisingly, heart failure (HF) comprises all of these. (13)

Several epidemiological investigations have identified the following key risk factors for heart failure: increasing age, hypertension, coronary artery disease, diabetes, obesity, valvular heart disease, and the metabolic syndrome. (64)

Since those following a plant-based diet are at lower risk of coronary artery disease, diabetes and obesity, they can be expected to be at lower of heart failure as well. Several population-based cohort studies that have demonstrated an inverse relationship between increased consumption of plant-based foods and incidence of heart failure. (65, 66, 67, 68, 69)

Five prospective studies examined the association between meat consumption and HF incidence in separate medium to large, middle-aged cohorts. All of these studies found increased HF risk with meat consumption. (70, 71, 72, 73, 74)

In a prospective cohort study of 21,275 participants from the Physicians' Health Study I, consumption of one egg a day increased the risk of heart failure by 28% and consuming two eggs a day increased the risk of heart failure by 64%. (75) In another prospective study of over 15,000 participants, those who ate a plant-based diet most of the time had a 42% reduced risk of heart failure. (76)

The beneficial effects of a low-fat vegetarian diet are indicated for patients at risk of heart failure and who also have CAD. One study showed significant improvements in such patients with documented CHD, regardless of ejection fraction, in lifestyle behaviors, body weight, body fat, blood pressure, resting heart rate, total and LDL-cholesterol, exercise capacity, and quality of life by 3 months. Most

How to cite this article: Rose S, Strombom A. Preventing stroke with a plant-based diet. Open Access J Neurol Neurosurg 2020; 14(2): 555882.
DOI: 10.19080/OAJNN.2020.14.555882

improvements were maintained over 12 months. (77)

A recent case report demonstrated the effects of a plant-based diet in a 79-year-old male with documented triple vessel disease (80–95% stenosis) and left ventricular systolic dysfunction (ejection fraction 35%) in the context of progressive dyspnea. Two months on a plant-based diet led to clinically significant reductions in body weight and lipids, with improved exercise tolerance and ejection fraction (+15%) (69)

In another case study, a 54-year-old female with grade 3 obesity (body mass index (BMI) 45.2 kg/m2) and type II diabetes (hemoglobin A1c 8.1%), coronary artery disease with a 30% proximal left anterior descending artery stenosis, a 25% proximal and a 60% distal left circumflex artery stenosis, and a 65% first obtuse marginal artery lesion. Echocardiography revealed a left ventricular ejection fraction of 25% without significant valvular pathology; heart failure was diagnosed.

After 5 months on a plant-based diet, her baseline dyspnea on exertion improved considerably. Repeat echocardiography revealed a normal left ventricular ejection fraction of 55% (78) Comorbid diabetes showed a reduction of HbA1c from her diabetes resolved, with her hemoglobin A1c falling from 8.1% to 5.7% without the use of diabetes medications.

8. Clinical Considerations

One out of four strokes is recurrent. Secondary stroke prevention starts with deciphering the most likely stroke mechanism. One of the main goals in stroke risk reduction is to control vascular risk factors such as hypertension, diabetes, dyslipidemia, and smoking cessation. Changes in lifestyle such as a healthy diet and aerobic exercise are recommended strategies for all of these. In general, a plant-based diet, low salt intake, and a limited intake of saturated fats and simple sugars are likely to have significant cardiovascular benefits in the secondary prevention of stroke. (8)

Patient compliance on plant-based diets has been good in almost all studies. The degree of compliance has often been very high. For instance, one study obtained a 99% compliance. (79) In a 22-week study 94% of subjects on a vegan diet were compliant. (80) In a somewhat longer study, 84% of the participants in each group completed all 24 weeks. (81) In studies of patients placed on plant-based diets for coronary artery disease, high compliance has been noted even over several years. For instance, one study of patients placed on a plant-based diet showed 89% compliance for 3.7 years. (82)

Compliance may be enhanced when the rationale for the treatment, and that the treatment is backed by research, is explained to the patient. (83) The doctor should prescribe the treatment by writing it down on a prescription form or other stationery with the physician's name on it. This written prescription is not only valuable to the patient, but can also be valuable in enlisting the support of family, friends and social contacts.

Vegetarian and vegan diets and food are not as uncommon as they used to be. The sales and availability of meat and dairy substitutes are have grown enormously in recent years. These products make dietary changes much easier in most cases, and when combined with a diet composed of vegetables, whole grains, fruits, legumes and nuts they can be very healthy. When starting the patient on a plant-based diet, foods with high levels of dietary

How to cite this article: Rose S, Strombom A. Preventing stroke with a plant-based diet. Open Access J Neurol Neurosurg 2020; 14(2): 555882.
DOI: 10.19080/OAJNN.2020.14.555882

fiber should be introduced slowly to avoid flatulence.

When prescribing a plant-based diet for the prevention of stroke, many patients may already be being treated with other medications for other pathologies. Patients concurrently being treated for type II diabetes, hypercholesterolemia, coronary artery disease, hypertension and other pathologies such as rheumatoid arthritis, ulcerative colitis and Crohn's disease, can be treated with a plant-based diet. Medications being prescribed for any of these pathologies may need to be titrated as the effects of the plant-based diet become evident.

For instance, a plant-based diet is more effective for treating type II diabetes than Metformin. The dosage may have to be titrated down as blood glucose is lowered. Similarly, a plant-based diet is as efficacious in treating hypercholesterolemia as Lovostatin. (84). The plant-based diet is also very effective for treating angina pectoris, with patients experiencing a 91% decrease in frequency. (85)

It may take several weeks to two months for the full effect to take place. Lab work should be done with this time factor in mind. A bit of patience on the part on the part of the patient is necessary for compliance to take place.

The patient should be informed that while a plant-based diet reduces the risk of stroke, it will also reduce the risk of a number of other diseases. This risk reduction of several diseases by one prescription may help maintain patient compliance as the perceived benefit is increased.

9. Discussion

The plant-based diet has the advantage of having no side effects, adverse reactions and no contraindications. It can also help prevent and treat a number of pathologies including common comorbidities of stroke patients. It is also very affordable for the patient.

We live in an age of advanced medical technology. These advances have alleviated much suffering and saved countless lives. They have an unquestioned place in modern medicine. However, this can sometimes lead towards a kind of technological fundamentalism. Little notice is taken of treatments that, while lacking in technological sophistication, are nevertheless quite efficacious.

Fortunately, many doctors have already started to integrate therapeutic plant-based diets into their patients' prevention and treatment of CAD. The former president of the American College of Cardiology, Dr. Kim Williams, uses this modality of treatment for his patients. In a recent article, he states:

"Unlike many of our cardiovascular prevention and treatment strategies, including antioxidants, vitamin E, folic acid and niacin to name a few, that have disintegrated over time, the "truth" (i.e., evidence) for the benefits of plant-based nutrition continues to mount. This now includes lower rates of stroke, hypertension, diabetes mellitus, obesity, myocardial infarction and mortality, as well as many non-cardiac issues that affect our patients in cardiology, ranging from cancer to a variety of inflammatory conditions. Challenges with the science are, however, less daunting to overcome than inertia, culture, habit and widespread marketing of unhealthy foods. Our goal must be to get data out to the medical community and the public where it can actually change lives—creating healthier and longer ones." (86)

How to cite this article: Rose S, Strombom A. Preventing stroke with a plant-based diet. Open Access J Neurol Neurosurg 2020; 14(2): 555882.
DOI: 10.19080/OAJNN.2020.14.555882

References

1. Mozaffarian D, Benjamin EJ, Go AS, Arnett DK, Blaha, MJ, et al. (2015) Heart disease and stroke statistics–2015 update: a report from the American Heart Association. *Circulation*. 131(4):e29-e322.
2. Allen CL, Bayraktutan U. (2008) Risk factors for ischaemic stroke. *Int J Stroke*. 3(2):105-116.
3. Boehme AK, Esenwa C, Elkind MSV. (2017) Stroke Risk Factors, Genetics, and Prevention. *Circ Res*. 120(3):472–495.
4. Adams Jr HP, Bendixen BH, Kappelle LJ, Biller J, Love B, et al. (1993) Classification of subtype of acute ischemic stroke. Definitions for use in a multicenter clinical trial. TOAST. Trial of Org 10172 in Acute Stroke Treatment. *Stroke*. 24(1):35-41.
5. Cheng NT, Kim AS. (2015) Intravenous thrombolysis for acute ischemic stroke within 3 hours versus between 3 and 4.5 hours of symptom onset. *Neurohospitalist*. 5(3):101-109.
6. Reeves MJ, Arora S, Broderick JP, Frankel M, Heinrich JP, et al. (2005) Acute stroke care in the US: results from 4 pilot prototypes of the Paul Coverdell National Acute Stroke Registry. *Stroke*. 36(6):1232-1240.
7. Powers WJ, Rabinstein AA, Ackerson T, Adeoye OM, Bambakidis NC, et al. (2018) 2018 guidelines for the early management of patients with acute ischemic stroke: a guideline for healthcare professionals from the American Heart Association/American Stroke Association. *Stroke*. 49(3):e46-e110.
8. Esenwa C, Gutierrez J. (2015) Secondary stroke prevention: challenges and solutions. *Vasc Health Risk Manag*. 11:437-450.
9. Morgenstern LB, Hemphill JC, Anderson C, Becker K, Broderick JP, et al. (2010) American Heart Association Stroke Council and Council on Cardiovascular Nursing Guidelines for the management of spontaneous intracerebral hemorrhage: a guideline for healthcare professionals from the American Heart Association/American Stroke Association. *Stroke*. 41(9):2108–2129.
10. Steiner T, Salman RAS, Beer R, Christensen H, Cordoniier C, et al. (2014) European Stroke Organization (ESO) guidelines for the management of spontaneous intracerebral hemorrhage. *Int. J. Stroke*. 9:840-855.
11. Hsieh FI, Chiou HY. (2014) Stroke: morbidity, risk factors, and care in Taiwan. *J Stroke*. 16(2):59–64.
12. O'Donnell MJ, Chin SL, Rangarajan S, Xavier D, Liu L, et al. (2016) Global and regional effects of potentially modifiable risk factors associated with acute stroke in 32 countries (INTERSTROKE): a case-control study. *Lancet*. 388(10046):761-775.
13. Kim W, Kim E. (2018) Heart Failure as a risk factor for stroke. *J Stroke*. 20(1):33-45.
14. Ma YH, Leng XY, Dong Y, Xu W, Cao X-P, et al. (2019) Risk factors for intracranial atherosclerosis: a systematic review and meta-analysis.. *Atherosclerosis*. 281: 71-77.
15. Okayama A, Okuda N, Miura K, Okamura T, Hayakawa T, et al. (2016) Dietary sodium-to-potassium ratio as a risk factor for stroke, cardiovascular disease and all-cause mortality in Japan: the NIPPON DATA80 cohort study. *BMJ Open*. 6:e011632.
16. Strombom A, Rose S. (2017) The prevention and treatment of Type II Diabetes Mellitus with a plant-based diet. *Endocrin Metab Int J*. 5(5):00138.
17. Rose S, Strombom A. (2018) A comprehensive review of the prevention and treatment of heart disease with a plant-based diet. *J Cardiol & Cardiovasc Ther*. 12(5):555847.
18. Hoevenaar-Blom MP, Nooyens ACJ, Kromhout D, Spijkerman A, Beulens, J, et al. (2012) Mediterranean style diet and 12-year incidence of cardiovascular diseases: the EPIC-NL cohort study. *PLoS One*. 7:e45458.
19. Kwok CS, Umar S, Myint PK, Mamas MA, Loke YK. (2014) Vegetarian diet, Seventh Day Adventists and risk of cardiovascular mortality:

How to cite this article: Rose S, Strombom A. Preventing stroke with a plant-based diet. Open Access J Neurol Neurosurg 2020; 14(2): 555882.
DOI: 10.19080/OAJNN.2020.14.555882

a systematic review and meta-analysis. *Int J Cardio*. 176(3):680-686.

20. Chiu THT, Chang HR, Wang LY, Chang CC, Lin MN, et al. (2020) Vegetarian diet and incidence of total, ischemic, and hemorrhagic stroke in 2 cohorts in Taiwan. *Neurology*. 94 (11):e1112-e1121.

21. Tong TYN, Appleby PN, Bradbury KE, Perez-Cornago A, Travis RC, et al. (2019) Risks of ischaemic heart disease and stroke in meat eaters, fish eaters, and vegetarians over 18 years of follow-up: results from the prospective EPIC-Oxford study. *BMJ*. 366:14897.

22. Ebrahim S, Sung J, Song YM, Ferrer RL, Lawlor DA, et al. (2006) Serum cholesterol, haemorrhagic stroke, ischaemic stroke, and myocardial infarction: Korean national health system prospective cohort study.. *BMJ*. 2006;333:22.

23. Gillman MW, Cupples LA, Gagnon D, Posner BM, Ellison RC. et al. (1995) Protective effects of fruits and vegetables on development of stroke in men. *JAMA*. 273(14):1113–1117.

24. Gey KF, Stähelin HB, Eichholzer M. (1993) Poor plasma status of carotene and vitamin C is associated with higher mortality from ischemic heart disease and stroke Basel Prospective Study. *Clin Invest Med*.71:3–6.

25. Khaw KT, Barrett-Connor E. (1987) Dietary potassium and stroke-associated mortality. *N Engl J Med*. 316:235–240.

26. Phillips RL, Lemon FR, Beeson WL, Kuzma JW. (1978) Coronary heart disease mortality among Seventh-Day Adventists with differing dietary habits: a preliminary report. *Am J Clin Nutr*. 31(10 Suppl):S191-S198.

27. De Biase S, Fernandes S, Gianini R, Duarte J. (2007) Vegetarian diet and cholesterol and triglycerides levels. *Arquivos Brasileiros de Cardiologia*. 88(1):35-9.

28. Thorogood M, Carter R, Benfield L, MCPherson K, Mann J. (1987) Plasma lipids and lipoprotein cholesterol concentrations in people with different diets in Britain. *British Medical Journal (Clin Res Ed)*. 295(6594):351–353.

29. Haddad E, Berk L, Kettering J, Hubbard R, Peters W. (1999) Dietary intake and biochemical, hematologic, and immune status of vegans compared with nonvegetarians. *Am J Clin Nutr*. 70(3 Suppl):586S-593S.

30. Bradbury KE, Crowe FL, Appleby PN, Schmidt JA, Travis RC, et al. (2014) Serum concentrations of cholesterol, apolipoprotein A-I and apolipoprotein B in a total of 1694 meat-eaters, fish-eaters, vegetarians and vegans. *Eur J Clin Nutr*. 68(2):178–183.

31. Kuchta A, Lebiedzińska A, Fijałkowski M, Gałąska R, Kreft E, et al. (2016) Impact of plant-based diet on lipid risk factors for atherosclerosis. *Cardiol J*. 23(2):141-148.

32. Glick-Bauer M, Yeh MC. (2014) The Health Advantage of a Vegan Diet: Exploring the Gut Microbiota Connection. *Nutrients*. 6(11):4822-38.

33. Moon AR, Choi DH, Jahng SY, Kim B-B, Seo H-J, et al. (2016) High-sensitivity C-reactive protein and mean platelet volume as predictive values after percutaneous coronary intervention for long-term clinical outcomes: a comparable and additive study. *Blood Coagul Fibrinolysis*. 27:70–76.

34. Jiménez MC, Rexrode KM, Glynn RJ, Ridker PM, Gaziano JM, et al. Association between high-sensitivity C-reactive protein and total stroke by hypertensive status among men. *J Am Heart Assoc*. 2015;4(9):e002073.

35. Zhou Y, Han W, Gong D, Man C, Fan Y. (2016) Hs-CRP in stroke: A meta-analysis.. *Clin Chim Acta*. 453:21–27.

36. Ridker PM. (2016) A test in context: high-sensitivity C-reactive protein. *J Am Coll Cardiol*. 67:712–723.

37. Huang X, Wang A, Liu X, Chen S, Zhu Y, et al. (2016) Association between high sensitivity C-Reactive protein and prevalence of asymptomatic carotid artery stenosis. *Atherosclerosis*. 246:44–49.

38. Rocco A, Ringleb PA, Grittner U, Nolte CH, Schneider A, et al. (2015) Follow-up C-reactive

How to cite this article: Rose S, Strombom A. Preventing stroke with a plant-based diet. Open Access J Neurol Neurosurg 2020; 14(2): 555882.
DOI: 10.19080/OAJNN.2020.14.555882

protein level is more strongly associated with outcome in stroke patients than admission levels. *Neurol Sci*. 36:2235–2241.

39. Szeto YT, Kwok TCY, Benzie IFF. (2004) Effects of long-term vegetarian diet on biomarkers of antioxidant status and cardiovascular disease risk. *Nutr*. 20(10):863-866.
40. Haghighatdoost F, Bellissimo N, deZepetnek JOT, Rouhani MH. (2017) Association of vegetarian diet with inflammatory biomarkers: a systematic review and meta-analysis of observational studies. *Public Health Nutr*. 20(15): 2713-2721.
41. Shah B, Newman JD, Woolf K, Ganguzza L, Guo Y, et al. (2018) Anti-inflammatory effects of a vegan diet versus the American Heart Association–recommended diet in coronary artery disease trial. *J Am Heart Assoc*. 7(23):e011367.
42. Fung TT, Chiuve SE, McCullough ML, Rexrode KM, Logroscino G, et al. (2008) Adherence to a DASH-style diet and risk of coronary heart disease and stroke in women. *Arch Intern Med*. 168(7):713-720.
43. Yokoyama Y, Nishimura K, Barnard ND, Takegami M, Watanabe M, et al. (2014) Vegetarian diets and blood pressure: a meta-analysis. *JAMA Intern Med*. 174:577–587.
44. Golzarand M, Bahadoran Z, Mirmiran P, Sadeghian-Sharif S, Azizi F. (2015) Dietary phytochemical index is inversely associated with the occurrence of hypertension in adults: a 3-year follow-up (the Tehran Lipid and Glucose Study). *Eur J Clin Nutr*. 69(3):392-398.
45. Chuang SY, Chiu T, Lee CY, Liu T-T, Tsao CK, et al. (2016) Vegetarian diet reduces the risk of hypertension independent of abdominal obesity and inflammation: a prospective study. *J Hypertens*. 34(11):2164-2171.
46. Fraser G, Katuli S, Anousheh R, Knutsen S, Herring P, et al. (2015) Vegetarian diets and cardiovascular risk factors in black members of the Adventist Health Study-2. *Public Health Nutr*. 18(3):537-545.
47. Chen R, Ovbiagele B, Feng W. (2016) Diabetes and stroke: epidemiology, pathophysiology, pharmaceuticals and outcomes. *Am J Med Sci*. 351(4):380-386.
48. Tonstad S, Butler T, Yan R, Fraser GE. (2009) Type of vegetarian diet, body weight, and prevalence of type 2 diabetes. *Diabetes Care*. 32(5):791-796.
49. Go A, Reynolds K, Yang J, Gupta N, Lenane J, et al. (2018) Association of burden of atrial fibrillation with risk of ischemic stroke in adults with paroxysmal atrial fibrillation: The KP-RHYTHM Study. *JAMA Cardiol*. 3(7):601-608.
50. Stoddard M, Dawkins P, Prince C, Ammash N. (1995) Left atrial appendage thrombus is not uncommon in patients with acute atrial fibrillation and a recent embolic event: a transesophageal echocardiographic study. *J Am Coll Cardiol*. 25(2):452-459.
51. Blackshear J, Odell J. (1996) Appendage obliteration to reduce stroke in cardiac surgical patients with atrial fibrillation. *Ann Thorac Surg*.61(2):755-759.
52. Brandes A, Smit MD, Nguyen BO, Rienstra M, Gelder ICV. (2018) Risk factor management in atrial fibrillation. *Arrhythm Electrophysiol Rev*. 7:118–127.
53. Wyse DG, Gelder ICV, Ellinor PT, Go AS, Kalman JM, et al. (2014) Lone atrial fibrillation: does it exist? *J Am Coll Cardiol*. 63:1715–1723.
54. Gallagher C, Hendriks JML, Mahajan R, Middeldorp ME, Elliott AD, et al. (2016) Lifestyle management to prevent and treat atrial fibrillation. *Expert Rev Cardiovasc Ther*. 14:799–809.
55. Vermond RA, Geelhoed B, Verweij N, Tieleman RG, Van der Harst P, et al. (2015) Incidence of atrial fibrillation and relationship with cardio-vascular events, heart failure, and mortality: a community-based study from the Netherlands. *J Am Coll Cardiol*. 66(9):1000–1007.

How to cite this article: Rose S, Strombom A. Preventing stroke with a plant-based diet. Open Access J Neurol Neurosurg 2020; 14(2): 555882.
DOI: 10.19080/OAJNN.2020.14.555882

56. Storz MA, Helle P. (2019) Atrial fibrillation risk factor management with a plant-based diet: A review. *J Arrhythm*. 35(6):781-788.

57. Joshi S, Ettinger L, Liebman SE. (2019) Plant-based diets and hypertension. *An J Lifestyle Med*. 14(4):397-405.

58. Alexander S, Ostfeld RJ, Allen K, Williams KA. (2017) A plant-based diet and hypertension. *J Geriatr Cardiol*. 14(5):327-330.

59. Rose S, Strombom A. (2020) Preventing thyroid diseases with a plant-based diet, while ensuring adequate iodine status. *Glob J Oto*. 21(4):556069.

60. Tonstad S, Nathan E, Oda K, Fraser GE. (2015) Prevalence of hyperthyroidism according to type of vegetarian diet. *Public Health Nutr*. 18(8):1482-1487.

61. Rose S, Strombom A. (2019) A plant-based diet prevents and treats chronic kidney disease. *JOJ Uro & Nephron*.6(3):555687.

62. Brouwer IA, Heeringa J, Geleijnse JM, Zock PL, Witteman JCM. (2006) Intake of very long-chain n-3 fatty acids from fish and incidence of atrial fibrillation. The Rotterdam Study. *Am Heart J*. 151:857–862.

63. Li FR, Chen GC, Qin J, Wu X. (2017) Dietary fish and long-chain n-3 polyunsaturated fatty acids intake and risk of atrial fibrillation: a meta-analysis. *Nutrients*. 9(9):955.

64. Velagaleti R, Vasan R. (2007) Heart Failure in the 21st Century: Is it a Coronary Artery Disease Problem or Hypertension Problem? *Cardiol Clin*.25(4):487-95.

65. Djoussé L, Driver J, Gaziano J. (2009) Relation between modifiable lifestyle factors and lifetime risk of heart failure. *JAMA*. 302(4):394-400.

66. Wang Y, Tuomilehto J, Jousilahti P, Antikainen R, Mähönen M, et al. (2011) Lifestyle factors in relation to heart failure among Finnish men and women. *Circ Heart Fail*. 4(5):607-12et al. (2011)

67. Pfister R, Sharp S, Luben R, Wareham N, Khaw K. (2011) Plasma vitamin C predicts incident heart failure in men and women in European Prospective Investigation into Cancer and Nutrition-Norfolk prospective study. *Am Heart J*. 162(2):246-53.

68. Rautiainen S, Levitan E, Mittleman M, Wolk A. (2015) Fruit and vegetable intake and rate of heart failure: a population-based prospective cohort of women. *Eur J Heart Fail*. 17(1):20-6.

69. Choi E, Allen K, McDonnough M, Massera D, Ostfeld R. (2017) A plant-based diet and heart failure: case report and literature review. *J Geriatr Cardiol*. 14(5):375-378.

70. Wirth J, di Giuseppe R, Boeing H, Weikert C. (2016) A Mediterranean style diet, its components and the risk of heart failure: a prospective population-based study in a non-Mediterranean country. *Eur J Clin Nutr*. 70(9):1015-21.

71. Nettleton J, Steffen L, Loehr L, Rosamond W, Folsom A. (2008) Incident heart failure is associated with lower whole-grain intake and greater high-fat dairy and egg intake in the Atherosclerosis Risk in Communities (ARIC) study. *J Am Diet Assoc*. 108(11):1881-7.

72. Ashaye A, Gaziano J, Djoussé L. (2011) Red meat consumption and risk of heart failure in male physicians. *Nutr Metab Cardiovasc Dis*. 21(12):941-6.

73. Kaluza J, Åkesson A, Wolk A. (2015) Long-term processed and unprocessed red meat consumption and risk of heart failure: a prospective cohort study of women. *Int J Cardiol*. 193:42-6.

74. Kerley CA. (2018) Review of Plant-based Diets to Prevent and Treat Heart Failure. *Card Fail Rev*. 4(1):54-61.

75. Djoussé L, Gaziano J. (2008) Egg consumption and risk of heart failure in the Physicians' Health Study. *Circulation*. 117(4):512-6.

76. Lara K, Levitan E, Guitterrez O, Shikany J, Safford MJS, et al. (2017) Dietary patterns and incident heart failure in adults with no known

coronary disease or heart failure: The REGARDS Cohort. *Circulation*. 136(Suppl 1).

77. Pischke C, Weidner G, Elliott-Eller M, Ornish D. (2007) Lifestyle changes and clinical profile in coronary heart disease patients with an ejection fraction of 40% in the Multicenter Lifestyle Demonstration Project.. *European Journal of Heart Failure*. 9(9):928-34.
78. Allen KE, Gumber D, Ostfeld RJ. (2019) Heart failure and a plant-based diet. A case-report and literature review. *Front Nutr*. 6:82.
79. Bloomer R, Kabir M, Canale R, Trepanowski J, Marshall K, et al. (2010) Effect of a 21 day Daniel Fast on metabolic and cardiovascular disease risk factors in men and women. *Lipids Health Dis*. 9:94.
80. Barnard N, Cohen J, Jenkins D, Turner-McGrievy G, Gloede L, et al. (2006) A low-fat vegan diet improves glycemic control and cardiovascular risk factors in a randomized clinical trial in individuals with type 2 diabetes. *Diabetes Care*. 29(8):1777-83.
81. Kahleova H, Matoulek M, Bratova M, Malinska H, Kazdova L, et.al. (2013) Vegetarian diet-induced increase in linoleic acid in serum phospholipids is associated with improved insulin sensitivity in subjects with type 2 diabetes. *Nutr Diabetes*. 3:e75.
82. Esselstyn CJ, Gendy G, Doyle J, Golubic M, Roizen M. (2014) A way to reverse CAD? *J Fam Pract*. 63(7):356-364b.
83. Drozek D, Diehl H, Nakazawa M, Kostohryz T, Morton D, et al. (2014) Short-term effectiveness of a lifestyle intervention program for reducing selected chronic disease risk factors in individuals living in rural appalachia: a pilot cohort study. *Advances in Preventive Medicine*. 2014:798184.
84. Jenkins D, Kendall C, Marchie A, Faulkner DW, Wong JMW, et al. (2005) Direct comparison of a dietary portfolio of cholesterol-lowering foods with a statin in hypercholesterolemic participants. *Am J Clin Nutr*. 2:380-387.
85. Ornish D, Scherwitz L, Billings J, Brown S, Gould KL et al. (1998) Intensive Lifestyle Changes for Reversal of Coronary Heart Disease. *JAMA*. 23:2001-7.
86. Williams K. (2017) Introduction to the "A plant-based diet and cardiovascular disease" special issue. *J Geriatr Cardiol*. 14(5):316.

How to cite this article: Rose S, Strombom A. Preventing stroke with a plant-based diet. Open Access J Neurol Neurosurg 2020; 14(2): 555882.
DOI: 10.19080/OAJNN.2020.14.555882

MedCrave
Step into the World of Research

Endocrinology & Metabolism International Journal

Review Article
Volume 5, Issue 5, 2017

DOI: 10.19080/OAJNN.2020.14.555882

The Prevention and Treatment of Type 2 Diabetes Mellitus with a Plant-Based Diet

Amanda Strombom and Stewart Rose*

Plant-Based Diets in Medicine, Bellevue, WA, USA

Received: October 23, 2017, **Published:** November 07, 2017

***Corresponding author:** Stewart Rose, Plant-Based Diets in Medicine, 12819 SE 38th St, #427, Bellevue, WA 98006, USA.

Abstract

Those following a plant-based diet have a 78% reduction risk of Type II diabetes mellitus (T2DM), as well as a 56% reduced risk of metabolic syndrome and a lower average BMI, 22.4 for men and 21.8 for women.

Vegetarians have less skeletal intramyocellular lipids, and better myocellular glucose disposal and mitochondrial function, and therefore have less peripheral insulin resistance. Vegetarians and vegans also have a much better inflammatory status, indicated by lower levels of inflammatory markers such as CRP and inflammatory adipocytokines such as IL-6, leptin, and higher levels of anti-inflammatory adipocytokines such as adiponectin.

Those following a plant-based diet consume much less persistent organic pollutant (POPs) which have been shown to cause beta-cell mitochondrial dysfunction. Finally, the gut microbiome of vegetarians has been shown to play a role in reducing insulin resistance and the level of inflammation in the body, and consequently their risk of T2DM.

Interventional studies show a reduction of HbA1C by as much as 2.4 percentage pts, which is more than is usually achieved with Metformin. Other clinical variables also show improvement such as reductions in BMI, total and LDL cholesterol and hsCRP.

Studies show compliance rates are good, ranging from 84% to 99%. Medications should be titrated as the patient shows improvements. Treatment with a plant-based diet has no contraindications or adverse reactions.

Keywords

Plant-based diets, Type II diabetes mellitus, insulin resistance, adipocytokines, persistent organic pollutants, vegetarian, vegan, metabolic syndrome, obesity.

Abbreviations

APOA1 – Apolipoprotein A1; APOB – Apolipoprotein B; ATP – Adenosine Triphosphate; BMI – Body Mass Index; CRP – Cardio-Reactive Protein; DAG – Diacylglycerol or Diglyceride; FACoA – Fatty acyl CoA; HbA1C – Hemoglobin A1c; HOMA-IR – Homeostatic Model Assessment of Insulin Resistance; HDL – High-Density Lipoprotein cholesterol; hsCRP – highly sensitive Cardio Reactive Protein; IL6 – Interleukin 6; Insig-1 – Insulin Induced gene-1; IRS-1 – Insulin Receptor Substrate 1; LDL – Low-Density Lipoprotein cholesterol; PCBs – Polychlorinated Biphenyls; PCDDs – Polychlorinated dibenzo-p-dioxins; PCDFs – Polychlorinated dibenzofurans; *PGC1α* – Peroxisome proliferator-activated receptor gamma-coactivator-1 alpha; POPs – Persistent Organic Pollutants; ROS – Reactive Oxygen Species; *SDHA* – Succinate dehydrogenase; SFRP5 – Secreted Frizzled-Related Protein 5; T2DM – Type 2 Diabetes Mellitus; TC- Total Cholesterol; TNF – Tumor necrosis factor;

1. Introduction

Today's physicians are only too aware of the prevalence of Type 2 Diabetes Mellitus (T2DM) currently in America, and of its complications such as diabetic peripheral neuropathy and diabetic nephropathy. The increased risk of coronary artery disease that type 2 diabetics face is on every physician's mind. Administrators and policy makers grapple with the dollar cost to the health care system from type 2 diabetes, and perhaps most worrisome of all, the rise in obesity and metabolic syndrome tells public health officials that the problem will likely get worse if nothing changes.

This article presents evidence of the safety and efficacy of plant-based diets for prophylaxis and treatment of type 2 diabetes mellitus. We have used "plant-based" to be synonymous with the term "vegan". The term "vegetarian" is used to define a plant-based diet that also may include dairy or eggs or both.

It has long been known and documented by a wide range of researchers that vegetarians in general, and vegans in particular, have much lower rates of type 2 diabetes. This fact has led researchers to investigate why those following a plant-based diet have a much lower risk of the disease. It has also led to the study of the efficacy of plant-based diets as a treatment for type 2 diabetes. The results of research are compelling. Plant-based diets both very substantially lower the risk of type 2 diabetes, and are quite efficacious in treating the disease.

Several reasons for this have emerged. Vegetarians have a much lower prevalence of type 2 diabetes mellitus risk factors such as obesity and metabolic syndrome. Those following a plant-based diet tend to consume more polyunsaturated fats and whole grain fibers, which have both been shown to reduce the risk of type 2 diabetes. They have less skeletal intramyocellular lipids, and better myocellular glucose disposal and mitochondrial function, and therefore have less peripheral insulin resistance. Vegetarians and vegans also have a much better inflammatory status, indicated by lower levels of inflammatory markers such as cardio-reactive protein and inflammatory adipocytokines such as IL-6, leptin, and higher levels of anti-inflammatory adipocytokines such as adiponectin. Since inflammation is now a known pathogenic factor, and since the adipocytokines have been shown to mediate insulin resistance and type 2 diabetes, vegetarians and vegans have a reduced risk of T2DM from these factors as well. Because persistent organic pollutants (POPs)

How to cite this article: Strombom A, Rose S (2017) The prevention and treatment of type 2 diabetes mellitus with a plant-based diet. Endocrinol Metab Int J 5(5): 00138.
DOI: 10.15406/emij.2017.05.00138

strongly bio-concentrate in animal fats, those following a plant-based diet consume much lower levels of POPs which have been shown to cause beta-cell mitochondrial dysfunction. Finally, the gut microbiome of vegetarians has also been shown to play a role in reducing insulin resistance and the level of inflammation in the body and consequently the risk of T2DM.

Vegetarians and vegan diets have been shown to be safe and efficacious treatments for type 2 diabetes, and their effects rival drugs such as Metformin. It should be noted that a full response usually takes a couple of months, but some initial effects may be noted after only two weeks. Patient compliance is good and the treatment is practically devoid of cost, contraindications and adverse effects. Clinical chemistry should be monitored frequently at first and medications should be titrated accordingly until the full effect of the dietary therapy is evident.

Plant- based nutritional medicine relies on evidence-based medicine and should form the basis of standard of care for patients with T2DM.

2. Epidemiology

Vegetarians have a 56% reduced risk of metabolic syndrome. (1) Vegetarian and vegans have a substantially lower risk of Type 2 Diabetes. The consumption of meat and the increase in risk of T2DM in a dose dependent manner has been established since at least 1985. (2) More recently, a large, well-regarded study showed that semi-vegetarians reduced their risk by 38%, pesco vegetarians by 51%, vegetarians by 61% and vegans by 78%. This indicates a dose response relationship between risk reduction and amount of plant foods in the diet. (3)

Many studies have been made of different demographic groups, showing substantial reductions in risk in those consuming a plant-based diet. Here are just a couple of examples. One study of the Taiwanese showed that vegetarian men had a decreased risk of T2DM of 51%, while pre-menopausal women had a decreased risk of 74%, and post-menopausal women a decreased risk of 75%. (4) These were considered notable findings, due to the increased genetic vulnerability to T2DM of this population, and that the average Taiwanese diet is already a relatively low-meat diet in the first place.

Among Blacks in the United States, those following a vegetarian diet reduced their risk of type 2 diabetes mellitus by 53% and those following a vegan diet by 70%. (5) This finding is notable, due to the increased prevalence of T2DM in this group.

2.1 Risk Factors

High body mass index (BMI) is a well-established risk factor for T2DM. Vegetarians and vegans have significantly lower BMI's on average. A study of American vegetarians and vegans found that that vegetarians had a mean BMI of 25.7 and vegans a mean BMI of 23.6. (6) A European study found the average BMI of vegetarians and vegans to be 23.3 and 22.4 respectively for men and 22.8 and 21.8 for women. (7) A study of German vegans found an average BMI of 22.3. (8) A study of vegetarian children found that they too had lower BMI's than their meat- eating counterparts with an average BMI of 17.3 in ages 6 to 11 and average of 20.0 ages 12-18. (9) One study found the risk of being overweight or obese is 65% less for vegans and 46% less for vegetarians. (10)

How to cite this article: Strombom A, Rose S (2017) The prevention and treatment of type 2 diabetes mellitus with a plant-based diet. Endocrinol Metab Int J 5(5): 00138.
DOI: 10.15406/emij.2017.05.00138

2.2 Dietary Components

When considering the different components in the diet, the consumption of n-6 (Omega 6) fats and whole grain foods stand out in the epidemiological research.

The evidence from research suggests that consuming polyunsaturated and or monounsaturated fats in preference to saturated fats and trans fatty acids, has beneficial effects on insulin sensitivity, and reduces the risk of T2DM. (11)

Among those consuming polyunsaturated fats, those who prefer linoleic acid from the n-6 series (Omega 6 fatty acids) show the best insulin sensitivity. (11) On the other hand, long-chain n-3 (Omega 3) fatty acids do not appear to improve insulin sensitivity or glucose metabolism. (11) Moreover, the research shows that high consumption of n-3 fatty acids may even impair insulin action in subjects with type 2 diabetes. (11, 12, 13, 14, 15, 16, 17, 18) While some believed that n-6 fatty acids are pro-inflammatory compared with n-3 fatty acids, this hypothesis is not supported by clinical or epidemiologic data in humans. (11) Rather, some data show that consumption of linoleic acid is inversely related to plasma C-reactive protein concentrations, and therefore is anti-inflammatory. (19, 20)

People who consume approximately 3 servings per day of whole grain foods are less likely to develop type 2 diabetes than low consumers (<3 servings per week) with a risk reduction in the order of 20-30%. (21)

3. Pathogenesis

3.1 Skeletal muscle insulin resistance

Skeletal muscle is the major site for disposal of ingested glucose in lean, healthy, normal-glucose-tolerant people. (22, 23, 24, 25, 26) Following a meal, approximately one third of ingested glucose is taken up by the liver and the rest by peripheral tissues, primarily skeletal muscle, via an insulin dependent mechanism. (22, 23, 24, 25, 26) The postprandial hyperglycemia stimulates insulin secretion from the pancreas, and the rise in plasma insulin concentration stimulates glucose uptake in skeletal muscle leading to the disposal of ingested glucose. (22, 23, 24, 25, 26)

In insulin resistant states, such as type 2 diabetes and obesity, insulin stimulated glucose disposal in skeletal muscle is markedly impaired. (22, 23, 24, 25, 26, 27, 28) The decreased insulin-stimulated glucose uptake is due to impaired insulin signaling, and multiple post receptor intracellular defects, including impaired glucose transport and glucose phosphorylation, and reduced glucose oxidation and glycogen synthesis. (29, 30, 31, 32)

There is growing evidence that mitochondrial dysfunction contributes to insulin resistance. (33, 34) Mitochondrial DNA content is frequently used as a marker for mitochondrial density in skeletal muscles. It has been shown to be lower in T2DM patients in comparison to lean controls. (35) Metabolic stresses imposed by obesity and hyperglycemia are often accompanied by increased rates of mitochondrial Reactive Oxygen Species (ROS) production. ROS affect mitochondrial structure and function and lead to Beta-cell failure. (36)

It can be concluded that both decreased mitochondrial fat oxidation and increased free fatty acid influx into skeletal muscle take place while in an insulin resistant state. Increased intramyocellular fat content and fatty acid metabolites, for

How to cite this article: Strombom A, Rose S (2017) The prevention and treatment of type 2 diabetes mellitus with a plant-based diet. Endocrinol Metab Int J 5(5): 00138.
DOI: 10.15406/emij.2017.05.00138

example, FACoA and DAG, are likely to play a pivotal role in the development of insulin resistance in skeletal muscle.

Through activation of serine/threonine kinases and serine phosphorylate, fatty acid metabolites impair IRS-1 phosphorylation by the insulin receptor and lead to the defect in insulin signaling in insulin resistant individuals. (22)

An increased intramyocellular fat content and fatty acid metabolites have been shown to play a pivotal role in the development of insulin resistance in skeletal muscle. Since the majority of fat oxidation takes place in the mitochondria, impaired fat oxidation in insulin resistant individuals suggests the presence of a mitochondrial defect, that contributes to the impaired muscle fat oxidation and increased intramyocellular fat content. Studies in humans, using molecular, biochemical, and MR spectroscopic techniques, have documented a defect in mitochondrial oxidative phosphorylation in a variety of insulin resistant states. While it is not usually possible to carry out these kinds of studies on humans, this study was able to use human skeletal muscle due to the accessibility of the tissue. (22)

The adipocytokine adiponectin, discussed in more detail in the next section, is found in lower levels in type 2 diabetic patients and the insulin resistant. Human studies show that low levels of adiponectin are also strongly correlated with high levels of intramyocellular lipids. (37) This is especially the case with the high molecular weight isoform. (38) As reported below, those following a plant-based, or vegan diet have higher levels of adiponectin. This adds to the lowered risk of insulin resistance that vegans experience.

Ex vivo human studies showed vegans to have an advantage with regard to skeletal muscle insulin sensitivity. One study showed that those following a plant based, or vegan diet, were shown to have lower intramyocellular lipid levels in their skeletal muscles. (39) Another study of those on a plant-based diet documented a lower intramyocellular lipid levels, a higher glucose disposal value, and a higher mitochondrial DNA content. (40)

These studies help explain the better skeletal muscle insulin sensitivity and much lower risk and prevalence of type 2 diabetes mellitus among vegans. The lower intramyocellular lipid levels, higher levels of adiponectin, better glucose disposal and increased mitochondrial DNA combine, in addition to the other factors addressed elsewhere in this report, to give those following a plant-based diet the advantages they experience with respect to type 2 diabetes.

3.2 Adipocytokines

Until recently, the adipose tissue was merely considered to support thermoregulation and provide the storage and release for free fatty acids. Within the last decade, it has become increasingly clear that adipose tissue is much more complex than was initially considered. The adipose tissue is an important endocrine organ that plays a key role in the integration of endocrine, metabolic, and inflammatory signals for the control of energy homeostasis (41). In addition to the dysregulation of its free fatty acid buffering capacity, (42) the adipocyte has been shown to secrete a variety of bioactive proteins into the circulation. These secretory proteins have been collectively named adipocytokines. (41)

Examples of adipocytokines include leptin, (43) tumor necrosis factor (TNF)-α, (44) plasminogen-activator inhibitor type 1 (PAI-1), (45) adipsin, (46) resistin, (47) adiponectin, (48) and interleukin (IL6) (48).

These interact with central as well as peripheral organs such as the brain, liver, pancreas, and skeletal muscle to control diverse processes, such as food intake, energy expenditure, carbohydrate and lipid metabolism, blood pressure, blood coagulation, and inflammation.

While many of these substances are adipocyte-derived and have a variety of endocrine functions, others are produced by resident macrophages and interact in a paracrine fashion to control adipocyte metabolism.

It is also abundantly clear that the dysregulation of adipocytokine secretion and action that occurs in obesity, plays a fundamental role in the development of a variety of cardiometabolic disorders, including the metabolic syndrome, type 2 diabetes, inflammatory disorders, and vascular disorders, that ultimately lead to coronary heart disease. (49, 50)

Adipocytokines can have pro- or anti-inflammatory properties according to their effects on inflammatory responses in adipose tissues. Most adipocytokines show pro-inflammatory activity with the noted exceptions of adiponectin, secreted frizzled-related protein 5 (SFRP5), visceral adipose tissue-derived serine protease inhibitor (Vaspin), and omentin-1. The pro-inflammatory adipocytokines are increased, whereas the anti-inflammatory adipocytokines are decreased, in obese rodents and humans with insulin resistance. (51)

The levels of some adipocytokines correlate with specific metabolic states and have the potential to impact directly upon the metabolic homeostasis of the system. Several of these adipocytokines mediate insulin resistance and diabetes (51, 52) While many adipocytokines have been discovered, this report will cover three with respect to insulin sensitivity and type 2 diabetes mellitus: leptin, adiponectin and IL 6. We refer you to other articles in the field that offer more extensive overviews of the entire secretome of adipocytes. (53, 54, 55)

3.2.1 Leptin

Leptin is an adipocyte-derived hormone and cytokine that regulates energy balance through a wide range of functions, including several that are important to cardiovascular health. Increased circulating leptin, a marker of leptin resistance, is common in obesity, and independently associated with insulin resistance and cardiovascular disease in humans. (56)

Evidence suggests that central leptin resistance causes obesity, and that obesity-induced leptin resistance injures numerous peripheral tissues, including liver, pancreas, platelets, vasculature, and myocardium. This metabolic and inflammatory mediated injury may result from either resistance to leptin's action in selective tissues, or excess leptin action from adiposity associated hyperleptinemia or both. (56)

In this sense, the term "leptin resistance" encompasses a complex pathophysiological phenomenon. The leptin axis has functional interactions with elements of metabolism, such as insulin, and inflammation, including mediators of innate immunity, such as interleukin 6. Leptin is even purported to physically interact with C-reactive protein, resulting in leptin resistance, which is particularly intriguing, given C-reactive protein's well-studied relationship to cardiovascular disease. (56)

How to cite this article: Strombom A, Rose S (2017) The prevention and treatment of type 2 diabetes mellitus with a plant-based diet. Endocrinol Metab Int J 5(5): 00138.
DOI: 10.15406/emij.2017.05.00138

Leptin plays a major role in the regulation of body weight. It circulates in both free and bound form. One of the leptin receptor isoforms exists in a circulating soluble form that can bind leptin. (57) Obesity in humans is associated with decreasing levels of the circulating soluble leptin receptor. The relationship of soluble leptin receptors with the degree of adiposity suggests that high soluble leptin receptor levels may enhance leptin action in lean subjects more than in obese subjects. (57)

Vegetarian diets reduce leptin levels in T2DM patients, as discussed in the Intervention section below.

3.2.2 Adiponectin

Adiponectin is the gene product of the adipose tissue's most abundant gene transcript 1 (apM1). (48) It is a collagen-like protein that is exclusively synthesized in white adipose tissue. It is induced during adipocyte differentiation, and circulates at relatively high (microgram/milliliter) concentrations in the serum. Adiponectin is highly expressed by adipocytes with potent anti-inflammatory properties. (51) Although adiponectin is secreted only from adipose tissue, its levels are paradoxically lower in obese than in lean humans. (52, 58)

A strong correlation between adiponectin and systemic insulin sensitivity has been well established both in vivo and in vitro in mice, other laboratory animals, and, most importantly, humans. (59, 41) In humans, plasma levels of adiponectin are significantly lower in insulin-resistant states including T2DM. (52, 58) Higher adiponectin levels are associated with a lower risk of T2DM across diverse populations, consistent with a dose-response relationship. (52, 60) As reported below, those placed or following a plant-based diet have higher levels of adiponectin.

3.2.3 Interleukin 6 and CRP

IL-6 is one of the major pro-inflammatory adipocytokines. Its expression level increases in the adipose tissue of obese patients. IL-6 secretion is increased in the adipocytes of obese subjects and may be important either as a circulating hormone or as a local regulator of insulin action. (61, 62) IL-6's mechanism of action is still not yet fully understood but is under active investigation. (63)

The primary source of circulating IL-6 is macrophages that have infiltrated white adipose tissue. It thus exerts its effect in a paracrine manner. (63) IL-6 has an important role in the regulation of whole body energy homeostasis and inflammation. Both in vitro and in vivo studies have confirmed that IL-6 is capable of suppressing lipoprotein lipase activity. IL-6 receptor is also expressed in several regions of the brain, such as the hypothalamus, which has a role in controlling appetite and energy intake. (64)

C-reactive protein (CRP) is an annular, pentameric protein found in blood plasma, the levels of which rise in response to inflammation. It is an acute phase protein of hepatic origin that increases following interleukin-6 secretion by macrophages and T cells.

Studies suggests that IL-6 may also be secreted in an endocrine manner in proportion to the expansion of fat mass particularly in the abdominal region, with a corresponding increase in hepatic production of CRP. (65)

Elevated CRP levels have been linked to an increased risk of later development of diabetes. (66, 67) Furthermore, CRP levels are higher in people with diabetes compared with those without diabetes, (68, 69, 70, 71) and the likelihood of elevated CRP concentrations were found to increase with increasing HbA1c levels. These findings suggest an association between glycemic control and systemic inflammation in people with established diabetes.

In patient studies, increased serum IL-6 correlates with obesity and insulin resistance. (72, 73, 74) Elevated levels of IL-6 and CRP resulted in a much higher risk of type 2 diabetes in a large cohort study P(<.001). The risk was 7.5 times higher for IL-6 and 15.7 times greater for CRP for highest versus lowest quartile in both. (66) Plasma IL-6 is also strongly correlated with obesity and insulin resistance. (61)

As reported below, intervention with a plant-based diet lowers the level of both IL-6 and CRP.

3.3 Persistent Organic Pollutants

Persistent organic pollutants (POPs) are synthetic organic chemicals that have an intrinsic resistance to natural degradation processes, and are therefore environmentally persistent and bio-accumulate through the food chain, increasing greatly in concentration at each subsequent trophic level. Examples of POPs include dioxins, furans, polychlorinated biphenyls (PCBs), and organochlorine pesticides – chemicals mainly created by industrial activities either intentionally or as by-products. (75) The introduction of POPs into the environment from anthropogenic activities resulted in their widespread dispersal and accumulation in soils and bodies of water, as well as in human and ecological food chains, where they are known to induce toxic effects.

Despite international agreements intended to limit the release of POPs such as organochlorine pesticides, polychlorinated biphenyls (PCBs), polychlorinated dibenzo-p-dioxins (PCDDs), and polychlorinated dibenzofurans (PCDFs), these POPs still persist in the environment and food chains. Regulations are often either not enforced or subscribed to. (76, 77, 78, 79, 80, 81)

There is evidence of long range transport of these substances to regions where they have never been used or produced, resulting in exposure of most human populations to POPs through consumption of fat-containing food such as fish, dairy products, and meat, (82, 83, 78) with the highest POP concentrations being commonly found in fatty fish. (75, 77, 82, 83, 84, 85, 86) Humans bioaccumulate these lipophilic pollutants in their adipose tissues for many years because POPs are highly resistant to metabolic degradation. (78, 87)

Persistent Organic Pollutants are widespread amongst the American public. A considerable number of POPs have been detected in the tissues of those studied. (88)

3.3.1 The Impact of POP exposure on laboratory animals

While human studies are always to be preferred, controlled experimentation of the impact of POPs must be limited to lab animals for ethical reasons. In the following study, the levels of POPs the rats were exposed to resulted in adipose concentrations typical of the average northern European adult, making the results obtained more realistic and therefore more relevant for human medical practice.

Adult male rats exposed to unrefined salmon oil, with its ordinarily occurring levels of POPs, developed insulin resistance, abdominal obesity, and hepatosteatosis. (89) The contribution of POPs to insulin resistance was also confirmed in cultured adipocytes where POPs, especially organochlorine pesticides, led to robust inhibition of insulin action. (89)

How to cite this article: Strombom A, Rose S (2017) The prevention and treatment of type 2 diabetes mellitus with a plant-based diet. Endocrinol Metab Int J 5(5): 00138.
DOI: 10.15406/emij.2017.05.00138

The rats exhibited profound dysregulation in hepatic lipid homeostasis accompanied by elevated levels of triacylglycerol, diacylglycerol, and total cholesterol. Altogether, these results demonstrate that POP exposure significantly affects the expression of critical genes involved in the regulation of lipid homeostasis. (89) Moreover, the POPs induced down-regulation of insulin-induced gene-1 (Insig-1) and Lpin1, (89) which are two master regulators of lipid homeostasis (and synthesis of triglyceride and cholesterol). (90, 91, 92, 93)

The effect of POPs on whole body insulin action was hyperinsulinemia and a greatly increased HOMA-IR. Moreover, intake of unrefined salmon oil led to impaired insulin-mediated glucose disposal in peripheral tissues, which mainly include skeletal muscles and adipose tissue.

As explained in the Skeletal Muscle Insulin Resistance section above, mitochondrial dysfunction contributes to insulin resistance, (33, 34) and mitochondria in type 2 diabetes Beta-cells exhibit both morphologic and functional abnormalities that are not observed in normal Beta-cells. (94) Together, these findings indicate that human Beta-cells exhibit abnormalities in glucose metabolism, and in mitochondrial structure and function, impairing both ATP production and glucose-stimulated insulin secretion. (95) Metabolic stresses imposed by obesity and hyperglycemia are often accompanied by increased rates of mitochondrial Reactive Oxygen Species (ROS) production. ROS affect mitochondrial structure and function and lead to Beta-cell failure. (36)

In this animal study, there was also significantly reduced expression of several genes related to mitochondrial function, such as *PGC1α* (peroxisome proliferator-activated receptor gamma-coactivator-1 alpha), citrate synthase, medium-chain acyl CoA dehydrogenase, and *SDHA* (succinate dehydrogenase), indicating the presence of alterations in mitochondrial function and oxidative capacities in the liver of the rats exposed to POPs. (89)

In vivo, chronic exposure to low doses of POPs commonly found in food chains induced severe impairment of whole body insulin action and contributed to the development of abdominal obesity and hepatosteatosis. Treatment in vitro of differentiated adipocytes, with nanomolar concentrations of POP mixtures at levels found in many foods, induced a significant inhibition of insulin dependent glucose uptake. (89)

These data taken together provide compelling evidence that exposure to POPs increases the risk of developing insulin resistance and metabolic disorders.

3.3.2 Epidemiological studies of POPs

Several epidemiological studies have reported an association between persistent organic pollutants and diabetes risk. Since 2005, at least 20 cross-sectional studies, conducted in about 12 countries, have been published documenting the association of POPs with diabetes risk. In addition, at least 7 longitudinal studies have been published from about 3 countries, showing the association of POPs with diabetes risk. (96) These findings have been supported by experimental studies both in humans and animals. Pathophysiological derangements, through which these pollutants exercise their harmful effect on diabetes risk, were studied. (97)

Several studies show a very strong association with several classes of POPs such organochlorine pesticides, PCBs (especially those with more than seven chlorines) and probably dioxins. Some specific congeners were associated with an increase in risk of over 30 times for those most exposed. Compared with subjects with serum concentrations below the limit of detection, after adjusting for age, sex, race and ethnicity, poverty income ratio, BMI, and waist circumference, diabetes prevalence was strongly positively associated with lipid-adjusted serum concentrations of all six POPs tested. (98)

When study participants were classified according to the sum of category numbers of the six POPs, adjusted odds ratios were 1.0, 14.0, 14.7, 38.3, and 37.7 (P for trend < 0.001). Surprisingly, in people with the lowest levels of POPs, being obese or overweight was not associated with an increased risk of diabetes. (98, 99) In an editorial published in The Lancet on the subject of Dr. Lee's findings, Dr. M. Porta writes, "This finding would imply that virtually all the risk of diabetes conferred by obesity is attributable to persistent organic pollutants, and that obesity is only a vehicle for such chemicals. This possibility is shocking." (100) Even low dose exposure to POPs conferred a very significant rise in the risk of type 2 diabetes. (101)

There is also a strong association between POPs and insulin resistance, often considered a pathogenic precursor of type 2 diabetes. The relationship strengthened with increasing HOMA-IR percentile: adjusted odds ratios comparing the highest versus lowest POPs quartile were 1.8 for being > or = 50th percentile of HOMA-IR, 4.4 for being > or = 75th percentile, and 7.5 for being > or = 90th percentile. (102) Other longitudinal studies have confirmed a significant association between POPs and insulin resistance. (103)

The role of POPs with endocrine disrupting activity, in the etiology of obesity and other metabolic dysfunctions, has been recently highlighted. Adipose tissue is a common site of POPs accumulation where they can induce adverse effects on human health. (104) Research strongly implicates Beta-cell mitochondrial dysfunction in the pathogenies of type 2 diabetes. (105, 106) Research shows an association between POPs and mitochondrial dysfunction in the Beta cells. (104, 107) One study showed a strong association, with a dose-response relationship with organochlorine POPs and diabetic peripheral neuropathy. Among five subclasses of POPs, organochlorine pesticides showed a strong dose-response relation with prevalence of peripheral neuropathy, adjusted odds ratios were 1.0, 3.6, and 7.3 (P for trend <0.01), respectively, across three categories of serum concentrations of organochlorine pesticides. (108) Studies show that diabetics with higher levels of POPs have several times the risk of diabetic nephropathy. (109, 110, 111, 112)

3.4 Microbiome Epidemiology

The gut microbiome has been suggested to play a role in type 2 diabetes. A small study in men, with and without type 2 diabetes, showed a lower abundance of Firmicutes and the class Clostridia, as well as a nonsignificant increase in Bacteroidetes and Proteobacteria in those with type 2 diabetes. (113) Furthermore, the ratio of Bacteroidetes to Firmicutes was positively associated with plasma glucose concentrations. A larger metagenome-wide association study in Chinese patients with T2DM reported differences in the gut microbiota relative to controls, with a decrease in the number of butyrate-producing bacteria, and an increase in the number of opportunistic pathogens. (114) Similarly,

How to cite this article: Strombom A, Rose S (2017) The prevention and treatment of type 2 diabetes mellitus with a plant-based diet. Endocrinol Metab Int J 5(5): 00138.
DOI: 10.15406/emij.2017.05.00138

this shift in the gut microbiota was also observed in a European cohort with type 2 diabetes. (115)

Plant-based dietary patterns may promote a more favorable gut microbial profile. Such diets are high in dietary fiber and fermentable substrate (i.e. non digestible or undigested carbohydrates), which are sources of metabolic fuel for gut microbial fermentation and, in turn, result in end products that may be used by the host (i.e. short chain fatty acids such as butyrate). These end products may have direct or indirect effects on modulating the health of their host. (116)

Over the past 10 years or so, data from different sources have established, to some degree, a causal link between the intestinal microbiota and obesity and insulin resistance. The lipopolysaccharide from intestinal flora bacteria can induce a chronic subclinical inflammatory process and obesity, leading to insulin resistance through activation of toll-like receptor 4. The reduction in circulating short-chain fatty acids may also have an essential role in the installation of reduced insulin sensitivity and obesity. Other mechanisms include the effects of bile acids, branched chain amino acids, and some other lesser known factors. (117) It is important to emphasize that diet-induced obesity promotes insulin resistance by mechanisms both independent and dependent on gut microbiota.

4. Interventional Studies

A number of studies have demonstrated that plant-based diets are safe and efficacious treatments of T2DM. These studies have demonstrated improvements across a broad range of clinical variables. We focus here mostly on those specifically related to type II diabetes. However, given the increased risk that type II diabetics have of coronary artery disease, concomitant improvement in cardiovascular parameters are very important and have been achieved by the studies noted below.

In one particularly successful study, which emphasized employing a plant-based diet and eliminating highly refined foods, good results were obtained in diabetic patients. After a median length on the diet of 7 months, the mean HbA1C dropped from 8.2% to 5.8% ($p = 0.002$), with sixty-two percent of participants reaching normoglycemic levels (HbA1C < 6.0%). (118)

A 3-month study of diabetic Koreans showed that a plant-based diet lowered their HbA1c levels by 0.9%, nearly triple the amount achieved with the Korean Diabetes Association diet. (119)

An Italian study using a vegan diet with Macrobiotic type menu items showed reductions in fasting glucose and insulin resistance (HOMA-IR) along with improvements in BMI and cardiovascular measurements. (120)

Here in the US, a 22-week study showed a drop of 1.23 Hba1c points on a vegan diet, while the standard American Diabetes Association diet resulted in only a 0.38 point drop. This study also showed a plant-based diet was about three times more effective. As in other studies, those on the plant-based diet had better reductions in BMI and cholesterol levels. (121)

Compare these results to the average effects of the most commonly prescribed drug for treatment of T2DM, Metformin. In a meta-analysis study of Metformin, the average change of glycosylated hemoglobin was 0.9% (95% CI -1.1 to -0.7), (122) so the effects of a plant-based diet rival, and in some cases, exceed the average effects of Metformin.

Looking more broadly at other variables, a 24-week study of diabetics placed on a vegetarian diet showed a wide range of effects including

How to cite this article: Strombom A, Rose S (2017) The prevention and treatment of type 2 diabetes mellitus with a plant-based diet. Endocrinol Metab Int J 5(5): 00138.
DOI: 10.15406/emij.2017.05.00138

changes in adipocytokines and inflammatory markers, BMI, fasting glucose, Hb1Ac as they have in other studies. However, this study also looked at additional variables. Highly Sensitive Cardio Reactive Protein (hsCRP) and homocysteine levels fell, a very desirable effect, indicating reduced inflammation and insulin resistance. In addition, adiponectin levels rose, which is also a desirable effect indicating improved insulin sensitivity. Resistin and leptin both were reduced, again indicating less insulin resistance. (123)

Linoleic acid is the most abundant polyunsaturated fat in the diet. One of the insulin-sensitizing components of a plant-based diet may be its n-6 polyunsaturated acid content. In a randomized trial by Summers et al., a diet rich in polyunsaturated n-6 (i.e. linoleic acid) improved insulin sensitivity when compared with a saturated-fat-rich diet after only 5 weeks. (124) A 24-week study of subjects placed on a n-6 strong plant-based diet showed that the insulin sensitizing effect experienced was related to the increased proportion of linoleic acid (n-6) in serum phospholipids. (125)

While the recommendation for most patients to increase exercise is sound, many are not compliant. It is therefore important to determine the benefit of dietary intervention independent of exercise. In a small 12-week pilot study, the use of a low fat, vegetarian diet in patients with non-insulin dependent diabetes was associated with significant reductions in fasting serum glucose concentration and body weight, in the absence of increased exercise. The mean fasting serum glucose of the experimental group, from 10.7 to 7.75 mmol/L (195 to 141 mg/dl) and the mean weight loss was 7.2 Kg and was significantly better than the control group ($P<0.05$). (126)

In a 7-month study by Jenkins et. al, a high-protein vegetarian diet, utilizing meat and dairy analogues, such as veggie burgers, veggie sausages (containing soy and wheat gluten proteins) and soy milk, along with tree nuts, was compared with a high carbohydrate vegetarian diet as a control. The experimental diet achieved the same significant reductions in HOMA-IR and fasting glucose as the control group. However, the experimental group achieved significantly greater weight loss, reduction in BMI, total cholesterol, LDL-C, TC:HDLC, and APOB and APOB:APOA1 and CHD 10-year risk on the experimental diet. There was also trend for lower hsCRP, though this was not quite significant. Given the popularity of meat and dairy analogues and tree nuts, patients preferring these foods may be able to achieve the same glycemic control while achieving even greater reduction in CHD risk. (127)

Generally, most patients require several weeks to several months to achieve a full therapeutic response. However, one study showed some results after only a week on a plant-based diet. Those with a fasting glucose above 126 mg/dL showed an average drop of 17mg/dL. (128)

Low grade inflammation of the intestine results in metabolic dysfunction, in which dysbiosis of the gut microbiota is intimately involved. Soluble dietary fiber induces prebiotic effects that may restore imbalances in the gut microbiota. In one study, obese subjects with type 2 diabetes were assigned to a vegetarian diet for 1 month, and blood biomarkers and fecal microbiota were monitored. The vegetarian diet reduced the Firmicutes to Bacteroidetes ratio in the gut microbiota. There was also notably a decrease in the pathobionts such as the Enterobacteriaceae, and an increase in commensal microbes such as Bacteroides fragilis and

How to cite this article: Strombom A, Rose S (2017) The prevention and treatment of type 2 diabetes mellitus with a plant-based diet. Endocrinol Metab Int J 5(5): 00138. DOI: 10.15406/emij.2017.05.00138

Clostridium species belonging to clusters XIVa and IV, resulting in reduced intestinal lipocalin-2 levels. (129)

Reduced Lipocalin-2 levels are associated with increased insulin sensitivity. (130) Lipocalin-2 is also an inflammatory marker. (130) This study underscores the benefits of soluble dietary fiber in the treatment of metabolic diseases, and shows that increased soluble fiber intake reduces gut inflammation by altering the gut microbiota. (129) The study also showed reduced body weight and concentrations of triglycerides, total cholesterol, low-density lipoprotein cholesterol and hemoglobin A1c, and improved fasting glucose and postprandial glucose levels.

5. Clinical Considerations

Patient compliance on plant-based diets has been good in almost all studies. The degree of compliance has often been very high. For instance, one study obtained a 99% compliance. (131) In a 22-week study 94% of subjects on a vegan diet were compliant. (121) In a somewhat longer study, 84% of the participants in each group completed all 24 weeks. (125) In studies of patients placed on plant-based diets for coronary artery disease, high compliance has been noted even over several years. For instance, one study of patients placed on a plant-based diet showed 89% compliance for 3.7 years. (132)

Compliance may be enhanced when the rationale for the treatment, and that the treatment is backed by research, is explained to the patient. (133) The doctor should prescribe the treatment by writing it down on a prescription form or other stationery with the physician's name on it. This written prescription is not only valuable to the patient, but can also be valuable in enlisting the support of family, friends and social contacts.

The effect of diet can be considerable. Treatment with a plant-based diet can be more effective than an anti-diabetic medication such as Metformin, combined with the recommended diet by the American Diabetes Association. While a patient using Metformin is transitioning to a plant-based diet, it is very important to reduce the risk of hypoglycemia, by monitoring clinical variables frequently in the early phase of treatment, until the full effect of a plant-based diet is evident. Medications should be titrated as the patient shows improvements. Severe cases will likely need continued medication albeit at reduced dosage.

As most clinicians are aware, several pathologies often cluster together. The same patient that presents with T2DM will often have one or more of the following diseases: obesity, hypertension, hypercholesterolemia/dyslipidemia and coronary artery disease. As plant-based diets are also effective treatments for those diseases as well, the physician will need to monitor clinical variables for those diseases and titrate the dosages of any medications prescribed for those conditions as well.

For patients with complications of type 2 diabetes such as diabetic peripheral neuropathy, a plant-based diet is also an efficacious treatment. Therefore, the symptoms associated diabetic peripheral should be monitored for improvement and any medications prescribed adjusted accordingly.

When starting the patient on a plant-based diet, foods with high levels of dietary fiber should be introduced slowly to avoid flatulence. From the point of view of treatment, soluble fiber is prebiotic for a therapeutic microbiome in type 2 diabetic

How to cite this article: Strombom A, Rose S (2017) The prevention and treatment of type 2 diabetes mellitus with a plant-based diet. Endocrinol Metab Int J 5(5): 00138.
DOI: 10.15406/emij.2017.05.00138

patients. However, from the point of view of prevention, the insoluble fiber of whole grain cereals is the most effective.

6. Discussion

The type 2 diabetic patient faces an increased risk of coronary artery disease and complications such diabetic peripheral neuropathy, diabetic nephropathy and diabetic retinopathy. The patient may already have comorbid conditions such as coronary artery disease, hypertension and obesity along with diabetic complications such as diabetic peripheral neuropathy. T2DM is a chronic disease that usually requires treatment for the rest of the patient's life.

The plant-based diet is not only a safe and efficacious treatment for T2DM, rivaling Metformin in effectiveness in many patients, but is also a safe and efficacious treatment for its most common comorbidities and complications. This treatment has no known contraindications or adverse effects. It obeys well the first rule of medicine: first do no harm. It is also much more cost effective. Plant-based nutritional medicine relies on evidence-based medicine and should form the basis of standard of care for patients with T2DM.

Prevention and treatment of T2DM with a plant-based diet operates on several levels at once. It reduces insulin resistance in the skeletal muscles. It reduces exposure to persistent organic pollutants, which cause mitochondrial cell dysfunction in the Beta cells and increased peripheral insulin resistance. It improves the profile of adipocytokines secreted. It also fosters a microbiome that helps prevent inflammation associated with type 2 diabetes. This multidimensional aspect of the treatment may account for its effectiveness. While some patients will still need medication, many others may no longer need medication. Even for those patients who still require medication to maintain a normoglycemic status, a substantial reduction in dosage may be possible.

While much research has been done on the prevention and treatment of T2DM with a plant-based diet, more research is needed to elucidate the relative benefits of the different foods that are included in the diet, beyond dietary fiber and polyunsaturated fats which have already been studied. While the therapeutic effect of a plant-based diet on complications, such as diabetic peripheral neuropathy, have been studied, there have been no studies on the risk reduction of diabetic retinopathy.

We live in an age of advanced medical technology. These advances have alleviated much suffering and saved countless lives. They have an unquestioned place in modern medicine. However, this can sometimes lead towards a kind of technological tunnel vision. Little notice is taken of treatments that, while lacking in technological sophistication, are nevertheless safe and quite efficacious. This indeed seems to be the case with treating T2DM with a plant-based diet.

Type 2 Diabetes Mellitus has a major impact on a patient's life, causing suffering and dollar costs to the patient as well. It is in the patient's interest to have this treatment presented to them. Many physicians are surprised to see how many patients would like to give it a try and patient compliance is usually quite good when the treatment is properly presented.

References

1. Rizzo N, Sabaté J, Jaceldo-Siegl K, Fraser G (2011). Vegetarian dietary patterns are associated with a lower risk of metabolic syndrome: the adventist health study 2. *Diabetes Care* 34(5):1225-7. Pubmed

How to cite this article: Strombom A, Rose S (2017) The prevention and treatment of type 2 diabetes mellitus with a plant-based diet. Endocrinol Metab Int J 5(5): 00138.
DOI: 10.15406/emij.2017.05.00138

2. Snowdon D, Phillips R (1985). Does a vegetarian diet reduce the occurrence of diabetes? *Am J Public Health* 75(5):507-12. Pubmed
3. Fraser GE (2009). Vegetarian diets:what do we know of their effects on common chronic diseases? *Am J Clin Nutr* 89(5):1607S-1612S. Pubmed
4. Chiu TH, Huang HY, Chiu YF, Pan WH, Chiu JP et.al (2014). Taiwanese Vegetarians and Omnivores: Dietary Composition, Prevalence of Diabetes and IFG. *PLoS ONE* 9(2):e88547. Pubmed
5. Tonstad S, Stewart K, Oda K, Batech M, Herring RP et.al (2013). Vegetarian diets and incidence of diabetes in the Adventist Health Study-2. *Nutr Metab Cardiovasc Dis.*23(4):292-9. Pubmed
6. Tonstad S, Butler T, Yan R, Fraser G (2009). Type of Vegetarian Diet, Body Weight, and Prevalence of Type 2 Diabetes. *Diabetes Care* 32(5):791–796. PMC
7. Bradbury K, Crowe F, Appleby P, Schmidt JA, Travis RC et.al (2014). Serum concentrations of cholesterol, apolipoprotein A-I, and apolipoprotein B in a total of 1 694 meat-eaters, fish-eaters, vegetarians, and vegans. *Eur J Clin Nutr* 68(2):178-183. Pubmed
8. Waldmann A, Koschizke J, Leitzmann C, Hahn A (2005). German vegan study: diet, life-style factors, and cardiovascular risk profile. *Ann Nutr Metab* 49(6):366-72. Pubmed
9. Haddad E, Tanzman J (2003). What do vegetarians in the United States eat? *Am J Clin Nutr* 78(3):626S-632S. Pubmed
10. Newby P, Tucker K, Wolk A (2005). Risk of overweight and obesity among semivegetarian, lactovegetarian, and vegan women. *Am J Clin Nutr* 81(6):1267-74. Pubmed
11. Risérus U, Willett W, Hu F (2009). Dietary fats and the prevention of type 2 diabetes. *Prog Lipid Res* 48(1):44-51. Pubmed
12. Mostad I, Bjerve K, Bjorgaas M, Lydersen S, Grill V (2006). Effects of n-3 fatty acids in subjects with type 2 diabetes: reduction of insulin sensitivity and time-dependent alteration from carbohydrate to fat oxidation. *Am J Clin Nutr* 84(3):540-550. Pubmed
13. Vessby B, Boberg M (1990). Dietary supplementation with n-3 fatty acids may impair glucose homeostasis in patients with non-insulin-dependent diabetes mellitus. *J Intern Med* 228(2):165-71. Pubmed
14. Boberg M, Pollare T, Siegbahn A, Vessby B (1992). Supplementation with n-3 fatty acids reduces triglycerides but increases PAI-1 in non-insulin-dependent diabetes mellitus. *Eur J Clin Invest* 22(10):645-50. Pubmed
15. Schectman G, Kaul S, Kissebah A (1998). Effect of fish oil concentrate on lipoprotein composition in NIDDM. *Diabetes* 37(11):1567-73. Pubmed
16. Borkman M, Chisholm D, Furler S, Storlien LH, Kraegen EW, et.al (1989). Effects of fish oil supplementation on glucose and lipid metabolism in NIDDM. *Diabetes* 38(10):1314-9. Pubmed
17. Axelrod L, Camuso J, Williams E, Kleinman K, Briones E, et.al (1994). Effects of a small quantity of omega-3 fatty acids on cardiovascular risk factors in NIDDM. A randomized, prospective, double-blind, controlled study. *Diabetes Care* 17(1):37-44. Pubmed
18. Hendra T, Britton M, Roper D, Wagaine-Twabwe D, Jeremy JY, et.al (1990). Effects of fish oil supplements in NIDDM subjects. Controlled study. *Diabetes Care* 13(8):821-9. Pubmed
19. Petersson H, Lind L, Hulthe J, Elmgren A, Cederholm T, et.al (2008). Serum fatty acid composition and indices of stearoyl-CoA desaturase activity are associated with systemic inflammation: longitudinal analyses in middle-aged men. *Brit J Nutr* 99(6):1186-1189. Pubmed
20. Petersson H, Lind L, Hulthe J, Elmgren A, Cederholm T, et.al (2009). Relationships between serum fatty acid composition and multiple markers of inflammation and

How to cite this article: Strombom A, Rose S (2017) The prevention and treatment of type 2 diabetes mellitus with a plant-based diet. Endocrinol Metab Int J 5(5): 00138.
DOI: 10.15406/emij.2017.05.00138

endothelial function in an elderly population. *Atherosclerosis* 203(1):298-303. Pubmed

21. Venn B, Mann J (2004). Cereal grains, legumes and diabetes. *Eur J Clin Nutr* 58(11):1443-61. Pubmed
22. Abdul-Ghani M, DeFronzo R (2010). Pathogenesis of Insulin Resistance in Skeletal Muscle. *J Biomed Biotechnol* 2010:19 pages. Pubmed
23. DeFronzo R (1988). The triumvirate: beta-cell, muscle, liver. A collusion responsible for NIDDM. *Diabetes* 37(6):667-87. Diabetes Journal
24. DeFronzo R (1997). Pathogenesis of type 2 diabetes: Metabolic and molecular implications for identifying diabetes genes. *Diabetes Reviews* 5(3):177-269. Influuent
25. DeFronzo R (2004). Pathogenesis of type 2 diabetes mellitus. *Med Clin North Am* 88(4):787-835. Pubmed
26. DeFronzo R (2009). From the Triumvirate to the Ominous Octet: A New Paradigm for the Treatment of Type 2 Diabetes Mellitus. *Diabetes* 58(4):773–795. PMC
27. DeFronzo R, Gunnarsson R, Björkman O, Olsson M, Wahren J (1985). Effects of insulin on peripheral and splanchnic glucose metabolism in noninsulin-dependent (type II) diabetes mellitus. *J Clin Invest* 76(1):149-55. PMC
28. Mitrakou A, Kelley D, Veneman T, Jenssen T, Pangburn T et.al (1990). Contribution of abnormal muscle and liver glucose metabolism to postprandial hyperglycemia in NIDDM. *Diabetes* 39(11):1381-90. Pubmed
29. Cusi K, Maezono K, Osman A, Pendergrass M, Patti ME et.al (2000). Insulin resistance differentially affects the PI 3-kinase- and MAP kinase-mediated signaling in human muscle. *J Clin Invest* 105(3):311-320. Pubmed
30. Bajaj M, Defronzo R (2003). Metabolic and molecular basis of insulin resistance. *J Nucl Cardiol* 10(3):311-23. Pubmed
31. Bouzakri K, Koistinen H, Zierath J (2005). Molecular mechanisms of skeletal muscle insulin resistance in type 2 diabetes. *Curr Diabetes Rev* 1(2):167-74. Pubmed
32. Karlsson H, Zierath J (2007). Insulin signaling and glucose transport in insulin resistant human skeletal muscle. *Cell Biochem Biophys.* 48(2):103-113. Pubmed
33. Lowell B, Shulman G (2005). Mitochondrial dysfunction and type 2 diabetes. *Science* 307(5708):384-7. Pubmed
34. Ma ZA, Zhao Z, Turk J (2012). Mitochondrial Dysfunction and β-Cell Failure in Type 2 Diabetes Mellitus. *Experimental Diabetes Research*. 2012:11 pages. Hindawi
35. Hoeks J, Schrauwen P (2012). Muscle mitochondria and insulin resistance: a human perspective. *Trends Endocrinol Metab* 23(9):444-450. Pubmed
36. Patanè G, Anello M, Piro S, Vigneri R, Purrello F, et.al (2002). Role of ATP production and uncoupling protein-2 in the insulin secretory defect induced by chronic exposure to high glucose or free fatty acids and effects of peroxisome proliferator-activated receptor-gamma inhibition. *Diabetes* 51(9):2749-56. Pubmed
37. Weiss R, Dufour S, Groszmann A, Petersen K, Dziura J, et.al (2003). Low Adiponectin Levels in Adolescent Obesity: A Marker of Increased Intramyocellular Lipid Accumulation. *J Clin Endocrinol* 88(5):2014–2018. Pubmed
38. Bredella M, Torriani M, Ghomi R, Thomas B, Brick D, et.al (2011). Adiponectin is inversely associated with intramyocellular and intrahepatic lipids in obese premenopausal women. *Obesity (Silver Spring)* 19(5):911-6. Pubmed
39. Goff L, Bell J, So P, Dornhorst A, Frost, G (2005). Veganism and its relationship with insulin resistance and intramyocellular lipid. *Eur J Clin Nutr* 59(2):291-8. Pubmed
40. Gojda J, Patková J, Jaček M, Potočková J, Trnka J, et.al (2013). Higher insulin sensitivity in vegans is not associated with higher mitochondrial density. *Eur J Clin Nutr* 67(12):1310-5. Pubmed

How to cite this article: Strombom A, Rose S (2017) The prevention and treatment of type 2 diabetes mellitus with a plant-based diet. Endocrinol Metab Int J 5(5): 00138. DOI: 10.15406/emij.2017.05.00138

41. Chandran M, Phillips S, Ciaraldi T, Henry R (2003). Adiponectin: More Than Just Another Fat Cell Hormone? *Diabetes Care* 26(8):2442-2450. Pubmed

42. Cantley J (2014). The control of insulin secretion by adipokines: current evidence for adipocyte-beta cell endocrine signalling in metabolic homeostasis. *Mammalian Genome* 25(9-10):442-54. Pubmed

43. Friedman J (2000). Obesity in the new millennium. *Nature* 404:632-634. Pubmed

44. Hotamisligil G (1999). The role of TNFalpha and TNF receptors in obesity and insulin resistance. *J Int Med* 245(6):621-5. Pubmed

45. Shimomura I, Funahasm T, Takahashi M, Maeda K, Kotani K, et.al (1996). Enhanced expression of PAI–1 in visceral fat: Possible contributor to vascular disease in obeisty. *Nature Medicine* 2:800 – 803. Pubmed

46. White R, Damm D, Hancock N, Rosen B, Lowell B, et.al (1992). Human adipsin is identical to complement factor D and is expressed at high levels in adipose tissue. *J Biol Chem* 267:9210-13. Pubmed

47. Steppan C, Bailey S, Bhat S, Brown E, Banerjee R, et.al (2001). The hormone resistin links obesity to diabetes. *Nature* 409(6818):307-12. Pubmed

48. Maeda K, Okubo K, Shimomura I, Funahashi T, Matsuzawa Y, et.al (1996). cDNA Cloning and Expression of a Novel Adipose Specific Collagen-like Factor, apM1 (AdiposeMost Abundant Gene Transcript 1). *Biochem Biophys Res Commun* 221(2):286-289. Pubmed

49. Harwood HJ (2012). The adipocyte as an endocrine organ in the regulation of metabolic homeostasis. *Neuropharmacology* 63(1):57-75. Pubmed

50. Deng Y, Scherer P (2010). Adipokines as novel biomarkers and regulators of the metabolic syndrome. *Ann N Y Acad Sci.* 1212:E1–E19. Pubmed

51. Kwon H, Pessin J (2013). Adipokines mediate inflammation and insulin resistance. *Front Endocrinol (Lausanne)* 4:71. Pubmed

52. Cao H (2014). Adipocytokines in obesity and metabolic disease. *J Endocrinol* 220(2):T47-T59. Pubmed

53. Halberg N, Wernstedt-Asterholm I, Scherer P (2008). The adipocyte as an endocrine cell. *Endocrinol Metab Clin North Am* 37(3):753-68, x-xi. Pubmed

54. Scherer P (2006). Adipose tissue: from lipid storage compartment to endocrine organ. *Diabetes* 55(6):1537-1545. Pubmed

55. Ahima R, Flier J (2000). Adipose tissue as an endocrine organ. *Trends Endocrinol Metab* 11(8):327-332. Pubmed

56. Martin S, Qasim A, Reilly M (2008). Leptin resistance: a possible interface of inflammation and metabolism in obesity-related cardiovascular disease. *J Am Coll Cardiol* 52(15):1201-1210. Pubmed

57. Ogier V, Ziegler O, Méjean L, Nicolas J, Stricker-Krongrad A (2002). Obesity is associated with decreasing levels of the circulating soluble leptin receptor in humans. *Int J Obes Relat Metab Disord* 26(4):496-503. Pubmed

58. Weyer C, Funahashi T, Tanaka S, Hotta K, Matsuzawa Y, et.al (2001). Hypoadiponectinemia in obesity and type 2 diabetes: close association with insulin resistance and hyperinsulinemia. *J Clin Endocrinol Metabol* 86(5):1930-35. Pubmed

59. Lu JY, Huang KC, Chang LC, Huang YS, Chi YC, et.al (2008). Adiponectin: a biomarker of obesity-induced insulin resistance in adipose tissue and beyond. *J Biomed Sci* 15(5):565-576. Springer

60. Li S, Shin H, Ding E, van Dam R (2009). Adiponectin levels and risk of type 2 diabetes: a systematic review and meta-analysis. *J Am Med Assoc.* 302(2):179-88. Pubmed

61. Kern P, Ranganathan S, Li C, Wood L, Ranganathan G (2001). Adipose tissue tumor necrosis factor and interleukin-6 expression in

human obesity and insulin resistance. *Am J Physiol Endocrinol Metab*. 280(5):E745-51. Pubmed

62. Mohamed-Ali V, Goodrick S, Rawesh A, Katz D, Miles J, et.al (1997). Subcutaneous adipose tissue releases interleukin-6, but not tumor necrosis factor-alpha, in vivo. *J Clin Endocrinol Metab* 82(12):4196-4200. Pubmed
63. Faloia E, Michetti G, De Robertis M, Luconi M, Furlani G, et.al (2012). Inflammation as a Link between Obesity and Metabolic Syndrome. *J Nutr Metabol* 2012:476380. Pubmed
64. Stenlöf K, Wernstedt I, Fjällman T, Wallenius V, Wallenius K, et.al (2003). Interleukin-6 levels in the central nervous system are negatively correlated with fat mass in overweight/obese subjects. *J Clin Endocrinol Metabol* 88(9):4379-83. Oxford
65. Khaodhiar L, Ling P, Blackburn G, Bistrian B (2004). Serum levels of interleukin-6 and C-reactive protein correlate with body mass index across the broad range of obesity. *JPEN J Parenter Enteral Nutr* 28(6):410-5. Pubmed
66. Pradhan A, Manson J, Rifai N, Buring J, Ridker P (2001). C-reactive protein, interleukin 6, and risk of developing type 2 diabetes mellitus. *J Am Med Assoc.*286(3):327-34. Pubmed
67. Barzilay J, Abraham L, Heckbert S, Cushman M, Kuller L, et.al (2001). The relation of markers of inflammation to the development of glucose disorders in the elderly: the Cardiovascular Health Study. *Diabetes* 50(10):2384-9. Pubmed
68. Ford E (1999). Body mass index, diabetes, and C-reactive protein among U.S. adults. *Diabetes Care* 22(12):1971-7. Pubmed
69. Grau A, Buggle F, Becher H, Werle E, Hacke W (1996). The association of leukocyte count, fibrinogen and C-reactive protein with vascular risk factors and ischemic vascular diseases. *Thromb Res* 82(3):245-55. Pubmed
70. Goldberg R (2000). Cardiovascular disease in diabetic patients. *Med Clin North Am* 84(1):81-93. Science Direct
71. King D, Mainous A, Buchanan T, Pearson W (2003). C-reactive protein and glycemic control in adults with diabetes. *Diabetes Care* 26(5):1535-9. Pubmed
72. Vozarova B, Weyer C, Hanson K, Tataranni P, Bogardus C, et.al (2001). Circulating interleukin-6 in relation to adiposity, insulin action, and insulin secretion. *Obes Res* 9(7):414-7. Pubmed
73. Bastard J, Maachi M, Van Nhieu J, Jardel C, Bruckert E, et.al (2002). Adipose tissue IL-6 content correlates with resistance to insulin activation of glucose uptake both in vivo and in vitro. *J Clin Endocrinol Metabol* 87(5):2084-9. Pubmed
74. Spranger J, Kroke A, Möhlig M, Hoffman K, Bergmann M, et.al (2003). Inflammatory cytokines and the risk to develop type 2 diabetes: results of the prospective population-based European Prospective Investigation into Cancer and Nutrition (EPIC)-Potsdam Study. *Diabetes* 52(3):812-7. Pubmed
75. Bergkvist C, Oberg M, Appelgren M, Becker W, Aune M, et.al (2008). Exposure to dioxin-like pollutants via different food commodities in Swedish children and young adults. *Food Chem Toxicol* 46(11):3360-7. Pubmed
76. Atlas E, Giam C (1981). Global transport of organic pollutants: ambient concentrations in the remote marine atmosphere. *Science* 11(4478):163-5. Pubmed
77. Dougherty C, Henricks Holtz S, Reinert J, Panyacosit L, Axelrad D, et.al (2000). Dietary exposures to food contaminants across the United States. *Environ Res* 84(2):170-85. Pubmed
78. Fisher B (1999). Most Unwanted. *Environ Health Persp* 107(1):A18-23. Europe PMC
79. Jorgenson J (2001). Aldrin and dieldrin: a review of research on their production, environmental deposition and fate, bioaccumulation, toxicology, and epidemiology in the United States. *Environ Health Persp* 109(Suppl 1):113-139. PMC

How to cite this article: Strombom A, Rose S (2017) The prevention and treatment of type 2 diabetes mellitus with a plant-based diet. Endocrinol Metab Int J 5(5): 00138. DOI: 10.15406/emij.2017.05.00138

80. Schafer K, Kegley S (2002). Persistent toxic chemicals in the US food supply. *J Epidemiol Community Health* 56(11):813-817. https://www.ncbi.nlm.nih.gov/pmc/articles/PMC1732058/

81. van den Berg H (2009). Global Status of DDT and Its Alternatives for Use in Vector Control to Prevent Disease. *Environ Health Persp* 117(11):1656-1663. https://www.ncbi.nlm.nih.gov/pubmed/20049114

82. Walker P, Rhubart-Berga P, McKenzie S, Kelling K, Lawrence R (2005). Public health implications of meat production and consumption. *Public Health Nutr* 8(4):348-356. https://www.ncbi.nlm.nih.gov/pubmed/15975179

83. Sasamoto T, Ushio F, Kikutani N, Saitoh Y, Yamaki Y, et.al (2006). Estimation of 1999-2004 dietary daily intake of PCDDs, PCDFs and dioxin-like PCBs by a total diet study in metropolitan Tokyo, Japan. *Chemosphere*. 64(4):634-41. https://www.ncbi.nlm.nih.gov/pubmed/16376969

84. Bocio A, Domingo J (2005). Daily intake of polychlorinated dibenzo-p-dioxins/polychlorinated dibenzofurans (PCDD/PCDFs) in foodstuffs consumed in Tarragona, Spain: a review of recent studies (2001-2003) on human PCDD/PCDF exposure through the diet. *Environ Res* 97(1):1-9. https://www.ncbi.nlm.nih.gov/pubmed/15476728

85. Schecter A, Colacino J, Haffner D, Patel K, Opel M, et.al (2010). Perfluorinated compounds, polychlorinated biphenyls, and organochlorine pesticide contamination in composite food samples from Dallas, Texas, USA. *Environ Health Persp* 118(6):796-802. https://www.ncbi.nlm.nih.gov/pubmed/20146964

86. Darnerud P, Atuma S, Aune M, Bierselius R, Glynn A, et.al (2006). Dietary intake estimations of organohalogen contaminants (dioxins, PCB, PBDE and chlorinated pesticides, e.g. DDT) based on Swedish market basket data. *Food Chem Toxicol* 44(9):1597-606. https://www.ncbi.nlm.nih.gov/pubmed/16730400

87. Kiviranta H, Tuomisto J, Tuomisto J, Tukiainen E, Vartiainen T (2005). Polychlorinated dibenzo-p-dioxins, dibenzofurans, and biphenyls in the general population in Finland. *Chemosphere* 60(7):854-69. https://www.ncbi.nlm.nih.gov/pubmed/15992592

88. Patterson D, Wong L, Turner W, Caudill S, Dipietro E, et.al (2009). Levels in the U.S. population of those persistent organic pollutants (2003-2004) included in the Stockholm Convention or in other long range transboundary air pollution agreements. *Environ Sci Technol* 43(4):1211-8. https://www.ncbi.nlm.nih.gov/pubmed/19320182

89. Ruzzin J, Petersen R, Meugnier E, Madsen L, Lock E, et.al (2010). Persistent organic pollutant exposure leads to insulin resistance syndrome. *Environ Health Persp* 118(4):465-71. https://www.ncbi.nlm.nih.gov/pubmed/20064776

90. Croce M, Eagon J, LaRiviere L, Korenblat K, Klein S, et.al (2007). Hepatic lipin 1beta expression is diminished in insulin-resistant obese subjects and is reactivated by marked weight loss. *Diabetes*. 56(9):2395-9. https://www.ncbi.nlm.nih.gov/pubmed/17563064

91. Engelking L, Kuriyama H, Hammer R, Horton J, Brown M, et.al (2004). Overexpression of Insig-1 in the livers of transgenic mice inhibits SREBP processing and reduces insulin-stimulated lipogenesis. *J Clin Invest* 113(8):1168-1175. https://www.ncbi.nlm.nih.gov/pmc/articles/PMC385408/

92. Finck B, Gropler M, Chen Z, Leone T, Croce M, et.al (2006). Lipin 1 is an inducible amplifier of the hepatic PGC-1alpha/PPARalpha regulatory pathway. *Cell Metabol* 4(3):199-210. https://www.ncbi.nlm.nih.gov/pubmed/16950137

93. Lee J, Ye J (2004). Proteolytic activation of sterol regulatory element-binding protein induced by cellular stress through depletion of Insig-1. *J Biol Chem* 279(43):45257-65. https://www.ncbi.nlm.nih.gov/pubmed/15304479

94. Marchetti P, Lupi R, Del Guerra S, Bugliani M, Marselli L, et.al (2010). The beta-cell in human

type 2 diabetes. *Adv Exp Med Biol* 654:501-14. https://www.ncbi.nlm.nih.gov/pubmed/20217512

95. Anello M, Lupi R, Spampinato D, Piro S, Masini M, et.al (2005). Functional and morphological alterations of mitochondria in pancreatic beta cells from type 2 diabetic patients. *Diabetologia* 48(2):282-9. https://www.ncbi.nlm.nih.gov/pubmed/15654602

96. Ngwa E, Kengne AP, Tiedeu-Atogho B, Mofo-Mato E, Sobngwi E (2015). Persistent organic pollutants as risk factors for type 2 diabetes. *Diabetol Metab Syndr* 7:41. https://www.ncbi.nlm.nih.gov/pubmed/25987904

97. Evangelou E, Ntritsos G, Chondrogiorgi M, Kavvoura F, Hernandez A, et.al (2016). Exposure to pesticides and diabetes: A systematic review and meta-analysis. *Environ Int.* 91:60-8. https://www.ncbi.nlm.nih.gov/pubmed/26909814

98. Lee D, Lee I, Song K, Steffes M, Toscano W, et.al (2006). A strong dose-response relation between serum concentrations of persistent organic pollutants and diabetes: results from the National Health and Examination Survey 1999-2002. *Diabetes Care* 29(7):1638-44. https://www.ncbi.nlm.nih.gov/pubmed/16801591

99. Longnecker M, Michalek J (2000). Serum dioxin level in relation to diabetes mellitus among Air Force veterans with background levels of exposure. *Epidemiology* 11(1):44-8. https://www.ncbi.nlm.nih.gov/pubmed/10615842

100. Lee D, Steffes M, Sjödin A, Jones R, Needham L, et.al (2010). Low dose of some persistent organic pollutants predicts type 2 diabetes: a nested case-control study. *Environ Health Perspect.* 118(9):1235-42. https://www.ncbi.nlm.nih.gov/pubmed/20444671

101. Lee D, Lee I, Jin S, Steffes M, Jacobs D (2007). Association between serum concentrations of persistent organic pollutants and insulin resistance among nondiabetic adults: results from the National Health and Nutrition Examination Survey 1999-2002. *Diabetes Care* 30(3):622-8. https://www.ncbi.nlm.nih.gov/pubmed/17327331

102. Suarez-Lopez J, Lee D, Porta M, Steffes M, Jacobs D (2015). Persistent organic pollutants in young adults and changes in glucose related metabolism over a 23-year follow-up. *Environ Res* 137:485-94. https://www.ncbi.nlm.nih.gov/pubmed/25706918

103. Pestana D, Faria G, Sá C, Fernandes V, Teixeira d, et.al (2014). Persistent organic pollutant levels in human visceral and subcutaneous adipose tissue in obese individuals–depot differences and dysmetabolism implications. *Environ Res* 133:170-7. https://www.ncbi.nlm.nih.gov/pubmed/24949816

104. De Tata V (2014). Association of dioxin and other persistent organic pollutants (POPs) with diabetes: epidemiological evidence and new mechanisms of beta cell dysfunction. *Int J Mol Sci.* 15(5):7787-811. https://www.ncbi.nlm.nih.gov/pmc/articles/PMC4057704/

105. Kwak S, Park K (2016). Role of mitochondrial DNA variation in the pathogenesis of diabetes mellitus. *Front Biosci (Landmark Ed).* 21:1151-67. https://www.ncbi.nlm.nih.gov/pubmed/27100497

106. Koliaki C, Roden M (2016). Alterations of Mitochondrial Function and Insulin Sensitivity in Human Obesity and Diabetes Mellitus. *Annu Rev Nutr* 36:337-67. https://www.ncbi.nlm.nih.gov/pubmed/27146012

107. Kim J, Lee H (2014). Metabolic syndrome and the environmental pollutants from mitochondrial perspectives. *Rev Endocr Metab Disord.* 15(4):253-62. https://www.ncbi.nlm.nih.gov/pubmed/25391628

108. Lee D, Jacobs DJ, Steffes M (2008). Association of organochlorine pesticides with peripheral neuropathy in patients with diabetes or impaired fasting glucose. *Diabetes* 57(11):3108-11. https://www.ncbi.nlm.nih.gov/pubmed/18647952

109. Sergeev A, Carpenter D (2010). Residential proximity to environmental sources of

How to cite this article: Strombom A, Rose S (2017) The prevention and treatment of type 2 diabetes mellitus with a plant-based diet. Endocrinol Metab Int J 5(5): 00138. DOI: 10.15406/emij.2017.05.00138

persistent organic pollutants and first-time hospitalizations for myocardial infarction with comorbid diabetes mellitus: a 12-year population-based study. *Int J Occup Med Environ Health* 23(1):5-13. https://www.ncbi.nlm.nih.gov/pubmed/20442057

110. Everett C, Thompson O (2014). Dioxins, furans and dioxin-like PCBs in human blood: causes or consequences of diabetic nephropathy? *Environ Res* 132:126-31. https://www.ncbi.nlm.nih.gov/pubmed/24769561

111. Pavlikova N, Smetana P, Halada P, Kovar J (2015). Effect of prolonged exposure to sublethal concentrations of DDT and DDE on protein expression in human pancreatic beta cells. *Environ Res* 142:257-63. https://www.ncbi.nlm.nih.gov/pubmed/26186133

112. Everett C, Thompson O (2015). Association of DDT and heptachlor epoxide in human blood with diabetic nephropathy. *Rev Environ Health* 30(2):93-7. https://www.ncbi.nlm.nih.gov/pubmed/25822320

113. Larsen N, Vogensen F, van den Berg F, Nielsen D, Andreasen A, et.al (2010). Gut microbiota in human adults with type 2 diabetes differs from non-diabetic adults. *PLoS One* 5(2):e9085. https://www.ncbi.nlm.nih.gov/pubmed/20140211

114. Qin J, Li R, Raes J, Arumugam M, Burgdorf KS, et.al (2010). A human gut microbial gene catalogue established by metagenomic sequencing. *Nature* 464(7285):59-65. https://www.ncbi.nlm.nih.gov/pmc/articles/PMC3779803/

115. Karlsson F, Tremaroli V, Nookaew I, Bergström G, Behre C, et.al (2013). Gut metagenome in European women with normal, impaired and diabetic glucose control. *Nature* 498(7452):99-103. https://www.ncbi.nlm.nih.gov/pubmed/23719380

116. Wong J (2014). Gut microbiota and cardiometabolic outcomes: influence of dietary patterns and their associated components. *Am J Clin Nutr* 100(Suppl 1):369S-77S. https://www.ncbi.nlm.nih.gov/pubmed/24898225

117. Saad M, Santos A, Prada P (2016). Linking Gut Microbiota and Inflammation to Obesity and Insulin Resistance. *Physiology (Bethesda)* 31(4):283-93. https://www.ncbi.nlm.nih.gov/pubmed/27252163

118. Dunaief D, Fuhrman J, Dunaief J, Ying G (2012). Glycemic and cardiovascular parameters improved in type 2 diabetes with the high nutrient density (HND) diet. *Open J Prevent Med* 2(3):364-371. http://journaldatabase.info/articles/glycemic_cardiovascular_parameters.html

119. Lee Y, Kim S, Lee I, Kim J, Park K, et.al (2016). Effect of a Brown Rice Based Vegan Diet and Conventional Diabetic Diet on Glycemic Control of Patients with Type 2 Diabetes: A 12-Week Randomized Clinical Trial. *PLoS One*. 11(6):e0155918. https://www.ncbi.nlm.nih.gov/pubmed/27253526

120. Soare A, Khazrai Y, Del Toro R, Roncella E, Fontana L, et.al (2014). The effect of the macrobiotic Ma-Pi 2 diet vs. the recommended diet in the management of type 2 diabetes: the randomized controlled MADIAB trial. *Nutr Metab* 11:39. https://nutritionandmetabolism.biomedcentral.com/articles/10.1186/1743-7075-11-39

121. Barnard N, Cohen J, Jenkins D, Turner-McGrievy G, Gloede L, et.al (2006). A low-fat vegan diet improves glycemic control and cardiovascular risk factors in a randomized clinical trial in individuals with type 2 diabetes. *Diabetes Care* 29(8):1777-83. https://www.ncbi.nlm.nih.gov/pubmed/16873779

122. Johansen K (1999). Efficacy of metformin in the treatment of NIDDM. Meta-analysis. *Diabetes Care* 22(1):33-37. https://www.ncbi.nlm.nih.gov/pubmed/10333900

123. Kahleova H, Matoulek M, Malinska H, Oliyarnik O, Kazdova L, et.al (2011). Vegetarian diet improves insulin resistance and oxidative stress markers more than conventional diet in subjects with Type 2 diabetes. *Diabet Med*. 28(5):549-59. https://www.ncbi.nlm.nih.gov/pubmed/21480966

124. Summers L, Fielding B, Bradshaw H, Ilic V, Beysen C, et.al (2002). Substituting dietary saturated fat with polyunsaturated fat changes abdominal fat distribution and improves insulin sensitivity. *Diabetologia* 45(3):369-77. https://www.ncbi.nlm.nih.gov/pubmed/11914742

125. Kahleova H, Matoulek M, Bratova M, Malinska H, Kazdova L, et.al (2013). Vegetarian diet-induced increase in linoleic acid in serum phospholipids is associated with improved insulin sensitivity in subjects with type 2 diabetes. *Nutr Diabetes*. 3:e75. https://www.ncbi.nlm.nih.gov/pubmed/23775014

126. Nicholson A, Sklar M, Barnard N, Gore S, Sullivan R, et.al (1999). Toward improved management of NIDDM: A randomized, controlled, pilot intervention using a lowfat, vegetarian diet. *Prev Med* 29(2):87-91. https://www.ncbi.nlm.nih.gov/pubmed/10446033

127. Jenkins D, Wong J, Kendall C, Esfahani A, Ng V, et.al (2014). Effect of a 6-month vegan low-carbohydrate ('Eco-Atkins') diet on cardiovascular risk factors and body weight in hyperlipidaemic adults: a randomised controlled trial. *BMJ Open*. 4:e003505. https://www.ncbi.nlm.nih.gov/pubmed/24500611

128. McDougall J, Thomas L, McDougall C, Moloney G, Saul B, et.al (2014). Effects of 7 days on an ad libitum low-fat vegan diet: the McDougall Program cohort. *Nutr J* 13:99. https://www.ncbi.nlm.nih.gov/pubmed/25311617

129. Kim M, Hwang S, Park E, Bae J (2013). Strict vegetarian diet improves the risk factors associated with metabolic diseases by modulating gut microbiota and reducing intestinal inflammation. *Environ Microbiol Rep*. 5(5):765-75. https://www.ncbi.nlm.nih.gov/pubmed/24115628

130. Wang Y, Lam K, Kraegen E, Sweeney G, Zhang J, et.al (2007). Lipocalin-2 is an inflammatory marker closely associated with obesity, insulin resistance, and hyperglycemia in humans. *Clin Chem* 53(1):34-41. https://www.ncbi.nlm.nih.gov/pubmed/17040956

131. Bloomer R, Kabir M, Canale R, Trepanowski JF, Marshall KE, et.al (2010). Effect of a 21 day Daniel Fast on metabolic and cardiovascular disease risk factors in men and women. *Lipids Health Dis*. 9:94. https://www.ncbi.nlm.nih.gov/pubmed/20815907

132. sselstyn CJ, Gendy G, Doyle J, Golubic M, Roizen MF (2014). A way to reverse CAD? *J Fam Pract*. 63(7):356-364b. https://www.ncbi.nlm.nih.gov/pubmed/25198208.

133. Drozek D, Diehl H, Nakazawa M, Kostohryz T, Morton D, et.al (2014). Short-term effectiveness of a lifestyle intervention program for reducing selected chronic disease risk factors in individuals living in rural appalachia: a pilot cohort study. *Adv Prev Med* 2014:798184. https://www.ncbi.nlm.nih.gov/pubmed/24527219

How to cite this article: Strombom A, Rose S (2017) The prevention and treatment of type 2 diabetes mellitus with a plant-based diet. Endocrinol Metab Int J 5(5): 00138. DOI: 10.15406/emij.2017.05.00138

Global Journal of
Otolaryngology
ISSN 2474-7556

Juniper
PUBLISHERS
key to the Researchers

Review Article
Glob J Otolaryngol
Volume 21 Issue 4 – February 2020
DOI: 10.19080/GJO.2020.21.556069

Preventing Thyroid Diseases with a Plant-Based Diet, While Ensuring Adequate Iodine Status

Stewart Rose and Amanda Strombom*

Plant-Based Diets in Medicine, USA

Submission: January 23, 2020; **Published:** February 04, 2020

***Corresponding author:** Amanda Strombom, Plant-Based Diets in Medicine, 12819 SE 38th St, #427, Bellevue, WA 98006, USA

Abstract

People with thyroid disorders in the US usually have an autoimmune disease, such as Hashimoto's thyroiditis or Grave's disease. Those following a plant-based diet are much less susceptible to auto-immune diseases in general. They also have a lower BMI on average. Since obesity is a significant risk factor for hypothyroidism, this contributes to the lower risk of hypothyroidism among vegans. However even after controlling for BMI and potential demographic confounders, vegans have been shown to experience a 22% lower risk of hypothyroidism, and a 51% risk of hyperthyroidism.

Given that they are unlikely to be consuming any seafood or dairy, iodine deficiency is a greater possibility for those following a plant-based diet. Studies show that many vegans have very adequate iodine status, but some are deficient. The median is mildly deficient, but the range can vary greatly.

Very low iodine intake can reduce thyroid hormone production even in the presence of elevated TSH levels. However, high intakes of iodine can cause some of the same symptoms as iodine deficiency—including goiter, elevated TSH levels, and hypothyroidism—because excess iodine in susceptible individuals inhibits thyroid hormone synthesis and thereby increases TSH stimulation, which can produce goiter. Laboratory tests that detect abnormal thyroid function may be more useful for diagnosing chronic iodine deficiency or excessive iodine intake and for monitoring the effects of iodine supplementation.

1. Introduction

1.1 Hypothyroidism

While the lack of iodine in the diet is the biggest risk factor for hypothyroidism worldwide, in the United States, obesity is a significant risk factor for hypothyroidism. (1) The relation between obesity and hypothyroidism appears to have several explanations. Obesity may result in raised Thyroid Stimulating Hormone (TSH) levels, partly due to a proinflammatory milieu and other endocrine derangements. (2) Persons with obesity are prone to develop autoimmune hypothyroidism, and even mild thyroid failure contributes to the progressive increase in body weight, which ultimately results in overt obesity. (3) So elevated TSH levels may be both the consequence and the cause of obesity. (2)

Vegans have a lower BMI on average (4) thus reducing their risk of hypothyroidism. However, the lower risk of hypothyroidism among vegans exists, even after controlling for BMI and potential demographic confounders. (5) One study showed that following a vegan diet tended to be associated with a 22% reduced risk of hypothyroidism, although statistical significance was not quite attained. (5)

1.2 Hyperthyroidism

Hyperthyroidism is a prevalent condition with many causes, of which the most common is Graves' disease (6). Graves' disease is an autoimmune disorder caused by antibodies directed against the thyrotropin receptor, resulting in excess synthesis and secretion of thyroid hormone. (7) The third National Health and Nutrition Examination Survey (NHANES III) showed the prevalence of hyperthyroidism in the United States to be 1.3% (8)

While the specifics of hyperthyroidism and diet have not been extensively studied, observations by Trowell five decades ago indicated that for rural sub-Saharan Africans consuming a near-vegan diet, a number of autoimmune disorders were rare, or virtually unknown, including thyrotoxicosis and Hashimoto's thyroiditis. (9) Data from the Adventist Health Study showed that a vegan diet reduced the risk of hyperthyroidism by 51% while a vegetarian diet reduced the risk by 28% showing a dose response relationship. (7)

This is to be expected since epidemiological studies have shown that vegetarians have lower risks of auto immune diseases in general. For instance, one study on Rheumatoid Arthritis (RA) showed that non-vegetarian women had a 57% increased risk of contracting RA, and semi-vegetarians an increased risk of 16%, when compared with vegetarian women. Non-vegetarian men showed an increased risk of 50% and semi-vegetarian men an increased risk of 14%. (10) An epidemiological study found that the risk of Crohn's disease reduced by 70% in females and 80% in males following a vegetarian diet. (11)

1.3 Iodine insufficiency

The most common cause of thyroid disorders worldwide is iodine deficiency, leading to goiter formation and hypothyroidism. In iodine-replete areas, most persons with thyroid disorders have an autoimmune disease, primarily Hashimoto's thyroiditis. (12)

Iodine deficiency can lead to a variety of medical problems at all ages in the humans. This is a special concern for pregnant women. Children of mothers having an iodine deficiency during pregnancy may have mental retardation, deaf mutism, spasticity and short stature. Congenital

How to cite this article: Rose S, Strombom A. Preventing Thyroid Diseases with a Plant-Based Diet, While Ensuring Adequate Iodine Status. Glob J Oto, 2020; 21(4): 556069.
DOI: 10.19080/GJO.2020.21.556069.

hypothyroidism due to iodine deficiency is the most common cause of preventable mental retardation in the world. (13) Despite ongoing public health efforts, iodine deficiency affects more than 2.2 billion individuals and remains the leading cause of preventable mental retardation worldwide. (14)

The earth's soils contain varying amounts of iodine, which in turn affects the iodine content of crops. In some regions of the world, iodine-deficient soils are common, increasing the risk of iodine deficiency among people who consume foods primarily from those areas. Worldwide, the soil in large geographic areas is deficient in iodine. 29% of the world's population is estimated to live in areas of deficiency. (15)

In the United States, before the 1920s and the introduction of iodized salt, iodine deficiency was common in the "goiter belt"—the Great Lakes, Appalachian, and the Pacific Northwest, and throughout most of Canada. (16) Programs to iodize salt have been implemented in many countries, significantly reducing the prevalence of iodine deficiency worldwide. (14, 17, 18)

In the United States table salt is available as iodized with potassium iodide, which is used by about 50%–60% of the U.S. population. However, the U.S. population receives only a small percentage of its salt from table salt because 70% of dietary salt is derived from processed food, which uses mostly noniodized salt. (19) A reduction in iodine intake can also be related to reduced salt intake for the treatment and prevention of essential hypertension. (13)

1.4 Iodine Status

Population iodine sufficiency is defined by median urinary iodine concentrations (14). Urinary iodine reflects dietary iodine intake directly because people excrete more than 90% of dietary iodine in the urine. (20) Iodine deficiency is diagnosed when the median iodine concentration is less than 50 ug/ml in a population. (18) Between 1971 and 2008, urinary iodine levels less than 50 µg/liter among U.S. women of child-bearing age rose from 4 to 15% (21)

Table 1: Iodine Status

Median Urinary Iodine concentration	Deficiency status (14)
100 µg/liter or greater in adults and 150 µg/liter or greater in pregnancy	Sufficient
50-99 µg/liter or greater in adults	Mild deficiency
20-49 µg/liter or greater in adults	Moderate deficiency
Less than 20 µg/liter or greater in adults	Severe deficiency

Under normal conditions, the body tightly controls thyroid hormone concentrations via Thyroid Stimulating Hormone (TSH) which is produced by the pituitary gland. The thyroid gland secretes the thyroid hormones triiodothyronine (T3) and thyroxine (T4) in response to TSH (also known as

How to cite this article: Rose S, Strombom A. Preventing Thyroid Diseases with a Plant-Based Diet, While Ensuring Adequate Iodine Status. Glob J Oto, 2020; 21(4): 556069.
DOI: 10.19080/GJO.2020.21.556069.

thyrotropin). The vast majority of T4 (99.97%) and T3 (99.70%) is tightly bound to thyroxine binding globulin (TBG) and other plasma proteins, and it is only the unbound or free thyroid hormones that are bioactive. Serum TSH is the most sensitive early indicator of thyroid dysfunction. (22) Typically, TSH secretion increases when iodine intake falls below about 100 mcg/day. (18) TSH increases thyroidal iodine uptake from the blood and the production of thyroid hormone.

TSH is regulated by circulating serum free thyroxine (FT4). Subclinical hypothyroidism is defined as elevated serum TSH in the setting of normal FT4. In overt hypothyroidism, serum TSH is elevated and serum FT4 is low. Serum free and total T3 concentrations usually do not decline until hypothyroidism is quite advanced, because elevated TSH stimulates the release of T3 from the thyroid. (23)

However, very low iodine intakes can reduce thyroid hormone production even in the presence of elevated TSH levels. If a person's iodine intake falls below approximately 10–20 mcg/day, hypothyroidism occurs (24), a condition that is frequently accompanied by goiter. Moderate to severe iodine deficiency may produce lower serum FT4 and consequent elevation of serum TSH. If the iodine deficiency is prolonged, goiter may develop and there may be an increase in circulating concentrations of thyroglobulin (Tg) (25) This possibility should be considered when reviewing lab results.

High intakes of iodine can cause some of the same symptoms as iodine deficiency—including goiter, elevated TSH levels, and hypothyroidism—because excess iodine in susceptible individuals inhibits thyroid hormone synthesis and thereby increases TSH stimulation, which can produce goiter. (17, 26) Excess iodine may induce hyperthyroidism in some patients, resulting in elevated FT4 and depressed TSH. (27)

1.5 Risk of fibrocystic breast disease

Fibrocystic breast disease is a benign condition characterized by lumpy, painful breasts and palpable fibrosis. It commonly affects women of reproductive age, but it can also occur during menopause, especially in women taking hormone replacement. (28) Breast tissue has a high concentration of iodine, especially during pregnancy and lactation. (20, 29) Some research suggests that iodine supplementation might be helpful for fibrocystic breast disease. (30)

In a double-blind study, researchers randomly assigned women with fibrocystic breast disease to receive daily supplements of iodine or placebo for 6 months. (28) At treatment completion, 65% of the women receiving iodine reported decreased pain compared with 33% of women in the placebo group. A more recent randomized, double-blind, placebo-controlled clinical trial had similar findings. (30) Women receiving supplemental iodine had a significant decrease in breast pain, tenderness, and nodularity compared with those receiving placebo. The researchers also reported a dose-dependent reduction in self-assessed pain. None of the doses was associated with major adverse events or changes in thyroid function test results though large doses of iodine were used.

Iodine deficiency has been proposed to play a causative role in the development of breast cancer. (31, 32) Dietary iodine has also been previously proposed to play a protective role in breast cancer. (33) The importance of iodine in breast cancer is further emphasized by the adjuvant effects of

How to cite this article: Rose S, Strombom A. Preventing Thyroid Diseases with a Plant-Based Diet, While Ensuring Adequate Iodine Status. Glob J Oto, 2020; 21(4): 556069.
DOI: 10.19080/GJO.2020.21.556069.

iodine (34) supplementation in combination with doxorubixin for breast cancer treatment. (35) In these studies, iodine treatment resulted in reduced tumor size and proliferating cell nuclear antigen (PCNA) expression.

Based on the importance of iodine in thyroid and breast health, fetal brain development, as well as deficits in nutritional trends among younger women, iodine testing and management may be considered as a potentially important aspect for clinical practice. (36)

1.6 Risk for those following a plant-based diet

Primary sources of iodine for a non-vegan are seafood and dairy products. Milk contains iodine due to the teat cleansers typically used in dairies. Since a plant-based diet does not include seafood or dairy, concern has been expressed that vegans may be more prone to iodine deficiency.

Studies show that many vegans have very adequate iodine status but some are deficient. (37) The median, however, is mildly deficient. In a study of vegans in the Boston area, median urinary iodine concentration of vegans were lower than for omnivores (78.5 μg/liter) but the range varied enormously (6.8 – 964.7 μg/liter). (37) However, it is reassuring that this was not associated with thyroid dysfunction.

Other studies of thyroid function in vegetarians and vegans are limited. Although serum TSH was generally normal in 101 British vegans, the geometric mean was 47% higher than for omnivores. (38) No thyroid function abnormalities were found in studies Swedish and Finnish vegans. (39, 40)

Although thyroid function is usually good, patients on a plant-based diet should be evaluated for iodine sufficiency if their diet seems to inadequate or if they eat foods grown in a region with low iodine content. A change in composition in the diet or supplements may be called for. Iodized salt can also be a good source of iodine.

2. Clinical considerations for ensuring adequate iodine intake

Although urinary iodine concentration is a sensitive indicator of recent iodine intake, laboratory tests that detect abnormal thyroid function may be more useful for diagnosing chronic iodine deficiency or excessive iodine intake, and for monitoring the effects of iodine supplementation. (41) Thyroid function testing includes measurement of serum concentrations of the following:

- Thyroid-stimulating hormone (TSH)
- Thyroxine (T4) as total T4 and free (ie, unbound) T4 (FT4)
- Thyroglobulin (Tg)
- Triiodothyronine (T3) as total T3 and free T3 (FT3)

Results from thyroid function studies are usually within the reference range in the presence of mild iodine insufficiency. However, in patients with euthyroidism and iodine deficiency, serum TSH levels may be normal to increased, T3 levels may be normal or slightly elevated, and T4 levels may be normal or decreased. Only in very extreme iodine deficiency does hypothyroidism develop, accompanied by an elevated serum TSH value and decreased T3 and T4 levels. (41)

How to cite this article: Rose S, Strombom A. Preventing Thyroid Diseases with a Plant-Based Diet, While Ensuring Adequate Iodine Status. Glob J Oto, 2020; 21(4): 556069.
DOI: 10.19080/GJO.2020.21.556069.

2.1 Dietary considerations

Table 2: Recommended Dietary Allowances for Iodine (17)

Age	Male	Female	Pregnancy	Lactation
Birth to 6 months	110 mcg*	110 mcg*		
7–12 months	130 mcg*	130 mcg*		
1–3 years	90 mcg	90 mcg		
4–8 years	90 mcg	90 mcg		
9–13 years	120 mcg	120 mcg		
14–18 years	150 mcg	150 mcg	220 mcg	290 mcg
19+ years	150 mcg	150 mcg	220 mcg	290 mcg

* Adequate Intake (AI)

Table 3: Typical Iodine content of some plant-based foods (42, 43)

Food	Serving size	Typical Iodine (mcg)
Legumes		
Black-eyed peas, cooked	175 ml (3/4 cup)	53
Green peas, cooked	125 ml (1/2 cup)	3-4
Kidney beans, cooked	175 ml (3/4 cup)	28
Lima beans, cooked	125 ml (1/2 cup)	8
Navy beans, cooked	175 ml (3/4 cup)	46
Pinto beans, cooked	175 ml (3/4 cup)	19
Soy nuts	60 ml (1/4 cup)	60

How to cite this article: Rose S, Strombom A. Preventing Thyroid Diseases with a Plant-Based Diet, While Ensuring Adequate Iodine Status. Glob J Oto, 2020; 21(4): 556069.
DOI: 10.19080/GJO.2020.21.556069.

Corn, cooked	125 ml (1/2 cup)	7
Prunes, dried	5 prunes	13
Commercial Cereals		
Crisped rice	30g	20
Oat o-shaped	30g	14
Shredded wheat	30g	8
Raisin bran	30g	6
Soda crackers	10 crackers	44
Bread (rye)	1 slice (35g)	17
Bread (whole wheat)	1 slice (35g)	32
Tortilla	½ tortilla (35g)	26
Rice, white cooked	125 ml (1/2 cup)	4
Macaroni, enriched boiled	1 cup	27

Cruciferous vegetables such as broccoli, cauliflower, and cabbage naturally release a compound called goitrin when they're hydrolyzed, or broken down. Goitrin can interfere with the synthesis of thyroid hormones. However, this is usually a concern only when coupled with an iodine deficiency. (17) Importantly, heating cruciferous vegetables denatures much or all of this potential goitrogenic effect. (44)

Soy is another potential goitrogen. However, numerous studies have found that consuming soy doesn't cause hypothyroidism in people with adequate iodine stores. (45, 46, 47)

Randomized controlled intervention trials in iodine- and iron-deficient populations have shown that providing iron along with iodine results in greater improvements in thyroid function and volume than providing iodine alone (48)

Seaweeds can be very high in iodine. It is possible some seaweed dishes may exceed the tolerable upper iodine intake level of 1100 microg/d. (49) One study showed the iodine content surveyed for nori was 29.3–45.8 mg/kg, for wakame 93.9–185.1 mg/kg, and for kombu 241–4921 mg/kg. Kombu has the highest average iodine content 2523.5 mg/kg, followed by wakame (139.7 mg/kg) and nori (36.9 mg/kg). (49) Patients who eat a lot of seaweed should counseled to consume them in moderation.

2.2 Supplements and medication interactions

Many multivitamin/mineral supplements contain iodine in the forms of potassium iodide or sodium iodide. Dietary supplements of iodine or iodine-containing kelp (a seaweed) are also available. One study found that potassium iodide is almost completely (96.4%) absorbed in humans. (50)

Currently, it is estimated that only 51% of the types of prenatal multivitamins marketed in the

United States contain iodine (51) and according to 2001–2006 NHANES data, 15% of lactating women and 20% of non-pregnant and pregnant women in the United States take a supplement containing iodine. (52)

Several medications can have drug interactions with iodine supplements. Angiotensin-converting enzyme (ACE) inhibitors, such as benazepril (Lotensin®), lisinopril (Prinivil® and Zestril®), and fosinopril (Monopril®). Taking potassium iodide with ACE inhibitors can increase the risk of hyperkalemia (elevated blood levels of potassium). (53)

Taking potassium iodide with potassium-sparing diuretics, such as spironolactone (Aldactone®) and amiloride (Midamor®), can increase the risk of hyperkalemia (53).

3. Discussion

Millions of people in America suffer from hyperthyroidism and hypothyroidism, most commonly in the form of Grave's disease or Hashimoto's Thyroiditis. While in some cases this may be due to lack of iodine, in the United States it is more likely due to obesity or an auto-immune disease. The risk of both of these is reduced with a plant-based diet.

Reducing the risk of hypothyroidism and hyperthyroidism with a plant-based diet would seem especially advantageous since a plant-based diet is safe, has no adverse reactions or contraindications, and can treat and prevent several common comorbidities such as rheumatoid arthritis, Crohn's disease, type II diabetes and coronary artery disease.

The preventative benefit of a plant-based diet might be stronger if the typical iodine intake were a bit higher. However, while those following a plant-based diet can be mildly deficient in iodine, the compensatory mechanism of increased production of TSH reduces the risk for vegans to experience thyroid dysfunction due to any lack of iodine.

References:

1. Sanyal D, Raychaudhuri M. (2016) Hypothyroidism and obesity: An intriguing link. *Indian J Endocrinol Metab*. 20(4):554–557.
2. Rotondi M, Magri F, Chiovato L. (2011) Thyroid and obesity: not a one-way interaction. *J Clin Endocrinol Metab*. 96(2):344-346.
3. Michalaki MA, Vagenakis AG, Leonardou AS, Argentou MN, Habeos IG, et al. (2006) Thyroid function in humans with morbid obesity. *Thyroid*. 16(1):73-78.
4. Strombom A, Rose S. (2017) The prevention and treatment of Type II Diabetes Mellitus with a plant-based diet. *Endocrin Metab Int J*. 5(5):00138.
5. Tonstad S, Nathan E, Oda K, Fraser G. (2013) Vegan diets and hypothyroidism. *Nutrients*. 5(11):4642–4652.
6. Cooper D. (2003) Hyperthyroidism. *Lancet*. 362(9382):459-468.
7. Tonstad S, Nathan E, Oda K, Fraser GE. (2015) Prevalence of hyperthyroidism according to type of vegetarian diet. *Public Health Nutr*. 18(8):1482-1487.
8. Hollowell JG, Staehling NW, Flanders WD, Hannon WH, Gunter EW, et al. (2002) Serum TSH, T(4), and thyroid antibodies in the United States population (1988 to 1994): National Health and Nutrition Examination Survey (NHANES III). *J Clin Endocrinol Metab*. 87(2):489-499.
9. McCarty MF. (2001) Upregulation of lymphocyte apoptosis as a strategy for preventing and treating autoimmune disorders: a role for whole-food vegan diets, fish oil and dopamine agonists. *Med Hypotheses*. 57(2):258-275.
10. Fraser G. (1999) Associations between diet and cancer, ischemic heart disease, and all-cause mortality in non-Hispanic white California

How to cite this article: Rose S, Strombom A. Preventing Thyroid Diseases with a Plant-Based Diet, While Ensuring Adequate Iodine Status. Glob J Oto, 2020; 21(4): 556069.
DOI: 10.19080/GJO.2020.21.556069.

Seventh-day Adventists. *Am J Clin Nutr.* 70(3):532s-538s.

11. D'Souza S, Levy E, Mack D, Israel D, Lambrette P, et al. (2008) Dietary patterns and risk for Crohn's disease in children. *Inflamm Bowel Dis.* 14(3):367-73.
12. Vanderpump MPJ. (2011) The epidemiology of thyroid disease. *Br Med Bull.* 99(1):39–51.
13. Srivastav A, Maisnam I, Dutta D, Ghosh S, Mukhopadhyay S, et al. (2012) Cretinism revisited. *Indian J Endocrinol Metab.* 16(Suppl 2):S336-S337.
14. World Health Organization, (2007) United Nations Children's Fund, International Council for the Control of Iodine Deficiency Disorders. *Assessment of iodine deficiency disorders and monitoring their elimination : a guide for programme managers.* Geneva: World Health Organization.
15. Pearce EN, Andersson M, Zimmermann MB. (2013) Global iodine nutrition: Where do we stand in 2013? *Thyroid.* 23(5):523-528.
16. UNICEF. (2006) *The state of the world's children.Women and Children: The double dividend of gender equality.* New York, UNICEF
17. Institute of Medicine, Food and Nutrition Board. (2001) *Dietary reference intakes for Vitamin A, Vitamin K, Arsenic, Boron, Chromium, Copper, Iodine, Iron, Manganese, Molybdenum, Nickel, Silicon, Vanadium, and Zinc.* Washington (DC): National Academies Press (US)
18. Zimmermann MB. (2009) Iodine deficiency. *Endocr Rev.* 30(4):376-408.
19. Dasgupta PK, Liu Y, Dyke JV. (2008) Iodine nutrition: iodine content of iodized salt in the United States. *Environ Sci Technol.* 42(4):1315-1323.
20. Patrick L. (2008) Iodine: deficiency and therapeutic considerations. *Altern Med Rev.* 13(2):116-127.
21. Caldwell KL, Makhmudov A, Ely E, Jones RL, Wang RY. (2011) Iodine status of the U.S. population, National Health and Nutrition Examination Survey, 2005–2006 and 2007–2008. *Thyroid.* 21(4):419-427.
22. Spencer C, LoPresti J, Patel A, Guttler RB, Eigen A, et al. (!999) Applications of a new chemiluminometric thyrotropin assay to subnormal measurement. *J Clin Endocrinol Metab.* 70(2):453-460.
23. Pearce E, Caldwell K. (2016) Urinary iodine, thyroid function, and thyroglobulin as biomarkers of iodine status. *Am J Clin Nutr.* 104 Suppl 3:898S-901S.
24. National Research Council. (2005) *Health Implications of Perchlorate Ingestion.* Washington, DC: The National Academies Press; 2005.
25. Zimmermann M. (2013) Iodine deficiency and endemic cretinism. In: Braverman LE, Cooper DS, eds. *Werner & Ingbar's the thyroid: a fundamental and clinical text.* 10th ed. Philadelphia: Lippincott
26. Pennington J. (!990) A review of iodine toxicity reports. *J Am Diet Assoc.* 90(11):1571-1581.
27. Roti E, Vagenakis A. (2013) Effect of excess iodide: clinical aspects. In: Braverman L, Cooper D, eds. *Werner & Ingbar's the thyroid: a fundamental and clinical text.* 10th ed. Philadelphia: Lippincott.
28. Ghent W, Eskin B, Low D, Hill L. (1993) Iodine replacement in fibrocystic disease of the breast. *Can J Surg.* 36(5):453-460.
29. Azizi F, Smyth P. (2009) Breastfeeding and maternal and infant iodine nutrition. *Clin Endocrinol (Oxf).* 70(5):803-809.
30. Kessler J. (2004) The effect of supraphysiologic levels of iodine on patients with cyclic mastalgia. *Breast J.* 10(4):328-336.
31. Eskin B. (1970) Iodine metabolism and breast cancer. *Trans NY Acad Sci.* 32(8):911-947.
32. Stadel B. (1976) Dietary iodine and risk of breast, endometrial, and ovarian cancer. *Lancet.* 1(7965):890-891.

33. Cann S, van Netten J, van Netten C. (2000) Hypothesis: iodine, selenium and the development of breast cancer. *Cancer Causes Control*. 11(2):121-127.
34. Aceves C, Anguiano B, Delgado G. (2005) Is iodine a gatekeeper of the integrity of the mammary gland? *J Mammary Gland Biol Neoplasia*. 10(2):189-196.
35. Alfaro Y, Delgado G, Cárabez A, Anguiano B, Aceves C. (2013) Iodine and doxorubicin, a good combination for mammary cancer treatment: antineoplastic adjuvancy, chemoresistance inhibition, and cardioprotection. *Mol Cancer*. 12:45.
36. Rappaport J. (2017) Changes in dietary iodine explains increasing incidence of breast cancer with distant involvement in young women. *J Cancer*. 8(2):174-177.
37. Leung AM, LaMar A, He X, Braverman LE, Pearce EN. (2011) Iodine status and thyroid function of Boston-area vegetarians and vegans. *J Clin Endocrinol Metab*. 96(8):E1303-E1307.
38. Key TJA, Thorogood M, Keenan J, Long A. (1992) Raised thyroid stimulating hormone associated with kelp intake in British vegan men. *J Hum Nutr*. 5(5):323–326.
39. Abdulla M, Andersson I, Asp NG, Berthelsen K, Birkhed D, et al. (1981) Nutrient intake and health status of vegans. Chemical analyses of diets using the duplicate portion sampling technique. *Am J Clin Nutr*.34(11):2464-2477.
40. Rauma AL, Törmälä ML, Nenonen M, Hänninen O. (!994) Iodine status in vegans consuming a living food diet. *Nutr Res*. 14(12):1789–1795.
41. Faix J, Miller W. (2016) Progress in standardizing and harmonizing thyroid function tests. *Am J Clin Nutr*. 104 Suppl 3:913S-917S.
42. Institute of Medicine. (2006)*Dietary reference intakes*. Washington: The National Academies Press.
43. Pennington J, Douglass JB. (2005) *Bowes and Church's food values of portions commonly used*: Lippincott Williams & Wilkins.
44. Rungapamestry V, Duncan AJ, Fuller Z, Ratcliffe B. (2007) Effect of cooking brassica vegetables on the subsequent hydrolysis and metabolic fate of glucosinolates. *Proc Nutr Soc*. 66(1):69-81.
45. Messina M, Redmond G. (2006) Effects of soy protein and soybean isoflavones on thyroid function in healthy adults and hypothyroid patients: a review of the relevant literature. *Thyroid*. 16(3):249-258.
46. Dillingham B, McVeigh B, Lampe J, Duncan A. (2007) Soy protein isolates of varied isoflavone content do not influence serum thyroid hormones in healthy young men. *Thyroid*. 17(2):131-137.
47. Otun J, Sahebkar A, Östlundh L, Atkin SL, Sathyapalan T. (2019) Systematic Review and Meta-analysis on the Effect of Soy on Thyroid Function. *Sci Rep*. 3964(2019)
48. Hess SY. (2010) The impact of common micronutrient deficiencies on iodine and thyroid metabolism: the evidence from human studies. *Best Pract Res Clin Endocrinol Metab*. 24(1):117-132.
49. Yeh TS, Hung NH, Lin TC. (2014) Analysis of iodine content in seaweed by GC-ECD and estimation of iodine intake. *J Food Drug Anal*. 22(2):189-196.
50. Aquaron R, Delange F, Marchal P, Lognoné V, Ninane L. Bioavailability of seaweed iodine in human beings. *Cell Mol Biol (Noisy-le-grand)*. 2002 ;48(5):563-569.
51. Leung AM, Pearce EN, Braverman LE. Iodine content of prenatal multivitamins in the United States. *N Engl J Med*. 2009;360(9):939-940.
52. Gregory CO, Serdula MK, Sullivan KM. Use of supplements with and without iodine in women of childbearing age in the United States.. *Thyroid*. 2009;19(9):1019-1020.
53. Hsu PP. Natural Medicines Comprehensive Database. J Med Libr Assoc. Jan 2002; 90(1):114.

How to cite this article: Rose S, Strombom A. Preventing Thyroid Diseases with a Plant-Based Diet, While Ensuring Adequate Iodine Status. Glob J Oto, 2020; 21(4): 556069.
DOI: 10.19080/GJO.2020.21.556069.

JOJ
Urology & Nephrology
ISSN: 2476-0552

Juniper Publishers
key to the Researchers

Review Article
Volume 6 Issue 3 – January 2019
DOI: 10.19080/JOJUN.2019.06.555687

JOJ uro & nephron

A Plant-Based Diet Prevents and Treats Chronic Kidney Disease

Stewart D Rose* **and Amanda J Strombom**

Plant-Based Diets in Medicine, USA

***Corresponding author:** Stewart D Rose, Plant-Based Diets in Medicine, 12819 SE 38th St, #427, Bellevue, WA 98006

Abstract

Interest in the dietary treatment of chronic kidney disease has been growing as its incidence has been increasing. Chronic Kidney Disease (CKD) is now the 8th leading cause of death in the United States and its treatment consumes substantial amounts of medical resources and money.

Several lines of epidemiological research have shown a lower risk of chronic kidney disease among vegetarians. It also shows a substantially increased risk among omnivores, especially those who eat red and processed meats.

Although the practice started long ago, research on the use of a low-protein plant-based diet to treat chronic kidney disease diet has intensified in recent years. This research has shown that a low-protein vegetarian diet is safe and efficacious at both treating and slowing the progression of chronic kidney disease.

Treatment with a low-protein vegetarian diet, often supplemented with keto analogues, has been shown to reduce acidosis, phosphotemia, uremia, proteinuria and to slow progression. Research shows that this treatment does not result in malnutrition. Research has also shown that larger amounts of plant protein than animal protein can be consumed, without deleterious effects.

Treatment with a low protein vegetarian diet also has the advantage of preventing and treating common comorbidities such as type 2 diabetes and coronary artery disease.

1. Introduction

Chronic kidney disease is a major health care problem, and slowing its progression to end-stage renal disease (ESRD) has obvious clinical and economic benefits. (1, 2, 3) Diet is the largest risk factor for CKD patients for death and disability. (4, 5)

A low-protein diet (LPD) as a therapeutic measure in chronic kidney disease (CKD) was suggested by Beale as early as 1869, (6) and the first attempt to experimentally evaluate a LPD in humans was done by Smith in 1926. (7)

For at least a century, chronic uraemia has been considered an example of "protein intoxication." Thus, in the history of renal medicine, low protein diets have been attempted as a way to correct the metabolic alterations caused by kidney failure as much as possible. (8, 9) Indeed, the first systematic studies on low-protein diets in uraemia patients started with the observation that a protein-restricted diet was effective in reducing the symptoms of "uraemic toxicity" and that it was even able to prolong life. (10, 11, 12, 13) In the mid 1960s, Giordano and Giovannetti were the first to show that a low-protein diet was able to reduce almost all uraemic signs and symptoms. (14)

By lowering blood urea and other nitrogenous waste products, a low-protein diet has favorable effects on secondary hyperparathyroidism, (15) peripheral resistance to insulin, (16) hyperlipidaemia, (17) hypertension and acid–base disorders. (18)

Four meta-analyses of studies on the effects of a low-protein diet on CKD progression in diabetic and non-diabetic patients, have been performed since the early 1990s, all showing a beneficial effect. (19, 20, 21, 22, 13)

Today, the main nutrition-related goals for people with chronic kidney disease involve the slowing of kidney failure progression rate, minimizing uremic toxicity and metabolic disorders of kidney failure, diminishing proteinuria, maintaining good nutritional status, and lowering the risk of complications including cardiovascular disease, bone disease, and disturbed blood pressure control. (23) A low-protein plant-based diet has been shown to help accomplish all of these treatment goals.

Plant-based diets lend themselves well to low-protein diets suitable for CKD patients. They are a safe and efficacious treatment and still supply adequate protein while helping to prevent and treat common comorbidities. (24, 25)

2. Epidemiological studies

Several epidemiological studies consistently show that vegans (those who follow a plant-based diet) have a decidedly lower risk of chronic kidney disease than those who consume animal derived foods. These studies also indicate that as a group those following a plant-based diet have better renal function than those following an omnivorous diet. Furthermore, epidemiological studies show that vegans also have much lower levels of risk factors for chronic kidney disease such as type 2 diabetes and hypertension.

Epidemiological studies have been able to show which foods raise and which foods lower the risk of chronic kidney disease. These studies show that while eating red meat and other sources of saturated fat raise the risk of chronic kidney disease, consuming tree nuts, legumes, fruits and vegetables lowers it. Studies comparing those who consume animal protein with those who consume equal amounts of plant protein show that those who consume plant protein have a lower risk of chronic kidney disease, indicating a significant advantage for those following a plant-based diet. The vegan diet is associated with glomerular and systemic hemodynamic changes which may be beneficial in the prevention of glomerular sclerotic changes in health and disease. Details of these studies are provided below:

One study showed that vegans had a lower glomerular filtration rate (GFR). Early elevation of the GFR plays a central role in the pathogenesis and

How to cite this article: Stewart D Rose, Amanda J Strombom. A plant-based diet prevents and treats chronic kidney disease. JOJ uro & nephron. 2019; 6(3): 555687.
DOI: 10.19080/JOJUN.2019.06.555687

progression of renal disease. (26) Since those following a plant-based diet have a lower GFR they are at reduced risk of incipient or early stage kidney disease. In this study omnivores were found to have a GFR of 113 ml/min/1.73 m^2, the vegetarians 105 ml/min/1.73 m^2 and the vegans 100 ml/min/1.73 m^2. (27) Omnivores also had a significantly higher mean urinary albumin excretion rate than vegans, and higher mean diastolic blood pressure than both vegans and lactovegetarians.

Vegans have been found to have a 75% decreased risk of hypertension and a 78% reduced risk of type II diabetes. (28) Since type 2 diabetes and hypertension are both risk factors for CKD, (29, 30) these contribute to their lower risk of CKD. An uncontrolled diabetic and/or hypertensive patient can easily and quickly progress to an end-stage kidney disease patient. (30)

A study was designed to investigate the effect of protein intake on glomerular filtration rate, and to demonstrate and evaluate the functional reserve of the kidney. Normal subjects ingesting a meat-centered diet had a significantly higher creatinine clearance than a comparable group of normal subjects ingesting a vegetarian diet. (31)

An epidemiological study with a 23-year follow up period showed that diets with different dietary protein sources have different risks of incident CKD: red and processed meat are adversely associated with CKD risk, while nuts and legumes are protective against the development of CKD. Red and processed meat increased the risk of CKD by 23% (Q5:Q1) whereas a higher dietary intake (Q5:Q1) of nuts and legumes resulted in a 19% and 17% decreased risk respectively. (32)

In a study of adults aged 45-74 years old, red meat intake was strongly associated with an increased risk of the eventual development of End Stage Renal Disease (ESRD) in previously healthy people in a dose-dependent manner, with the highest quartile having a 40% increased risk over the lowest. In substitution analysis, replacing one serving of red meat with other food sources of protein was associated with a maximum relative risk reduction of 62.4%. This study shows that red meat intake may increase the risk of ESRD in the general population, and that substituting alternative sources of protein may reduce the incidence of ESRD. (33)

Female participants in the Nurses' Health Study who had followed a western dietary pattern (higher intake of red and processed meats, saturated fats, and sweets) had 2.17 times the risk of microalbuminuria, and a 77% greater risk of rapid estimated Glomerular Filtration Rate (eGFR) decline, compared with those following a prudent diet high in fruits, vegetables, legumes and whole grains. (34)

The Western-style diet is high in animal fat with high levels of saturated fats. A cross-sectional study (Reasons for Geographic and Racial Differences in Stroke Study; REGARDS), including more than 19,000 adults over 45 years of age, found a significant association between saturated fat intake and hyperalbuminuria. (35, 36) Several studies showed that the use of animal proteins compared to plant proteins induced a worsening of hard outcomes such as mortality and CKD progression. (37, 38)

In a meta-study that included six studies, healthy dietary patterns high in fruits, vegetables, legumes and whole grains were consistently associated with lower mortality or ESRD among adults with CKD, with a risk reduction of 30%. (39) Substituting soy and other legumes for red meat resulted in a reduced risk for ESRD by about 50%-62% (39)

Looking at soy protein specifically, one study showed that independent of the quantity of protein, soy protein has significantly different renal effects from animal protein in normal humans, which could be partly explained by differences in glucagon and renal vasodilatory prostaglandin secretion. (40) This study also showed that among normal healthy subjects, the GFR, RPF (Renal Plasma Flow) and fractional clearance of albumin and IgG were significantly higher when following the animal protein diet, compared to the soy protein diet, even though the quantity of protein were the same in both groups. (40)

3. Intervention and Pathophysiology

Mounting evidence indicates that dietary intervention with plant-based, alkali-inducing diets is kidney protective. The National Kidney Foundation recommends a vegetarian diet as being beneficial to CKD patients. (25)

Dietary intervention was the mainstay approach for kidney failure in the first half of the 20th century, and diet manipulation was tried in its last decades. (41, 42) Different dietary protein regimens have been proposed: conventional low-protein diets (LPDs; 0.6 g/kg per day), very low-protein diets (VLPDs; 0.3–0.4 g/kg per day), and practically vegetarian diets supplemented with either essential amino acids or a mixture of essential amino acids and nitrogen-free ketoanalogues (keto diet or KD). (41, 42, 43)

Dietary proteins are the source of nitrogen, phosphate, and acid load. A reduction in protein consumption has been shown to result in better control of blood pressure and a decrease in proteinuria, which are major determinants of the progression of CKD. (44) Moreover, certain complications of advanced CKD, such as mineral metabolism disorders, acidosis, and oxidative stress, also involved in accelerating its progression, (45) were favorably influenced by low-protein diets. (4, 45) In a meta-study of low-protein diets, reducing protein intake in patients with chronic kidney disease reduces the occurrence of renal death by 32% as compared with higher or unrestricted protein intake. (21)

Research data indicates that the underlying renal disease and the type of diet used considerably influence the rate of progression of chronic renal failure. In relative terms, the course of the renal disease is mostly changed in patients suffering from glomerulonephritis, while in absolute terms patients suffering from polycystic kidney disease exhibit the slowest rate of progression. The comparison suggests that a low-protein diet purely based on vegetarian food might considerably slow down the overall rate of progression of chronic renal failure. (46)

Diets in developed societies are largely acid producing, in part because of the proportionately greater amount of animal-sourced proteins (which are acid producing) than plant-sourced proteins (which are largely base producing). (4) The two changes in dietary protein quality therefore receiving the most attention currently are substituting plant-sourced for animal-sourced protein and substituting non-nitrogen ketoanalogue proteins in place of animal proteins.

3.1 Substituting plant-sourced protein

Studies show that the introduction of plant-derived protein in place of animal-derived protein improves metabolic acidosis, reduces kidney injury, and slows nephropathy progression, (4, 18, 47) and that plant-based diets can delay the

How to cite this article: Stewart D Rose, Amanda J Strombom. A plant-based diet prevents and treats chronic kidney disease. JOJ uro & nephron. 2019; 6(3): 555687.
DOI: 10.19080/JOJUN.2019.06.555687

progression of chronic kidney disease, provide endothelial protection, help control hypertension, and decrease proteinuria, phosphotemia, acidosis, uremia, FGF 23 and hyperparathyroidism. (48, 49, 50, 51, 40, 52, 53, 54)

Fruits and vegetables can be used to treat CKD without producing hyperkalemia. A one-year study of fruits and vegetables in the diet in individuals with stage 4 CKD was associated with lower than baseline urine indices of kidney injury. The results indicate that fruits and vegetables improve metabolic acidosis and reduce kidney injury in stage 4 CKD without producing hyperkalemia. (37)

Higher initial glomerular filtration rates (GFRs), associated with higher risk of CKD, have been demonstrated in patients without CKD on an animal-protein diet, in comparison to persons on a vegetable-based diet. (55, 56) A study of patients without CKD on a high protein diet (1 g/kg/day) of either soy, animal protein, or animal protein diet supplemented with fiber, revealed significantly higher renal plasma flow, GFR, and proteinuria in those on the animal protein diet compared to individuals on the soy diet. (40) The transition from mixed animal–vegetable diet (1.0 to 1.3 g/kg/day) to a plant-based diet (0.7 g/kg/day) was demonstrated to be associated with a significant decrease in GFR and proteinuria in patients with non-diabetic nephrosis. (57)

In another study, a diet supplying only foods of plant origin in definite proportions was used to give an essential amino acid supply satisfying the recommended dietary allowance. This was possible using an appropriate cereal legume mixture. Additional positive features of this special plant-based diet were the high ratio of unsaturated to saturated fatty acids, the absence of cholesterol, and the lower net acid production in comparison with a mixed diet. Improvements were noted in several clinical variables. (57)

A study investigated the impact of a vegetarian diet on the nutritional status of hemodialysis (HD) patients. This study revealed that HD patients on vegetarian diets might have a smaller BMI, but subjective global assessment and function of daily activities were similar to those of the non vegetarians. The haematocrit of vegetarians can be maintained with a higher erythropoietin dose. (58)

A predominantly vegetarian diet may also have important beneficial effects on diabetic nephropathy without the need for a heavily restricted total protein intake. (59) This is because plant protein does not create a lower GFR the way that meat protein does. In addition, a plant-based diet can lower glycated hemoglobin even more than metformin. (60)

Studies on animal models suggest that a vegetarian diet is suitable and nutritionally adequate in CKD. (61, 62, 63) Human studies confirm this. (64) Barsotti et al. showed that a vegan diet is fully sufficient for a low-protein diet for CKD patients. (57)

3.2 Supplementing with ketoanalogues

Naturally occurring amino acids contain nitrogen, which when metabolized yield nitrogenous wastes that increase BUN and cause untoward effects on kidney function. (4) Substituting non-nitrogen ketoanalogues can allow patients to realize the benefit of dietary protein while avoiding possible untoward effects of nitrogenous wastes. (45) Furthermore, adding base-producing plant proteins lowers levels of the pathogenic substances which induce the interstitial fibrosis that promotes nephropathy progression. (4, 65) Favorable

How to cite this article: Stewart D Rose, Amanda J Strombom. A plant-based diet prevents and treats chronic kidney disease. JOJ uro & nephron. 2019; 6(3): 555687.
DOI: 10.19080/JOJUN.2019.06.555687

metabolic effects of a ketoanalogue-supplemented diet were shown in many observational studies. (43, 44, 66, 67, 68)

In one study by Garneata et al, patients receiving a vegetarian, ketoanalogue-supplemented diet experienced an improvement of metabolic abnormalities. The authors concluded that a vegetarian ketoanalogue-supplemented diet is nutritionally safe, and may defer dialysis initiation in patients with eGFR<20 ml/min by ameliorating CKD–associated metabolic disturbances. (24) This study brings forth useful insights into strategies using low-protein diets that can be aimed at slowing nephropathy progression. (4)

A CKD study by Aparicio et al. demonstrated that in regularly and carefully monitored CKD patients, vegetarian diets with low or even a very low-protein content supplemented with keto-analogues, provided a satisfactory nutritional status. Improvements in the albumin excretion rate were noted. (68)

In another study, twenty steroid-resistant, nephrotic patients were treated with a vegan, low-protein diet, supplemented with essential amino acids and ketoanalogues (supplemented vegan diet), for almost 5 months. Before the study, these patients followed an unrestricted protein, low sodium diet. Proteinuria, daily urea nitrogen excretion and creatinine clearance decreased significantly on the ketoanalogue-supplemented vegan diet without inducing clinical or laboratory signs of malnutrition. (69)

A very low-protein, ketoanalogue-supplemented, vegetarian diet was also demonstrated to be safe for predialysis patients, since it exerted no detrimental effect on the short- and long-term outcomes of patients, even those already on renal replacement therapy. (70) A prospective, randomized, controlled trial of the safety and efficacy of a ketoanalogue-supplemented, vegetarian, very low-protein diet (KD; 0.3 g/kg vegetable proteins and 1 cps/5 kg ketoanalogues per day) revealed the correction of metabolic abnormalities, no changes in nutritional parameters, and no adverse reactions in non-diabetic adults with stable eGFR <30 mL/min per 1.73 m^2. (70)

The largest study addressing CKD, the Modification of Diet in Renal Disease (MDRD) Study, provided minimal results. (71) However, in this long term study, compliance and therefore protein intake was problematic. (72) Follow up protein measurements were not taken, greatly reducing confidence in the outcome.

3.3 Type I Diabetes – Diabetic Nephropathy

Interventional studies show that a low protein vegetarian diet can slow the progression of chronic kidney disease in Type 1 diabetics and improve their clinical laboratory test results.

According to a meta-analysis of five studies including a total of 108 patients, dietary protein restriction slowed the progression of diabetic nephropathy in patients with type 1 diabetes. (19) More recently, a 4-year randomized controlled trial with 82 patients, who had type 1 diabetes with progressive diabetic nephropathy, showed that a moderately low-protein diet (0.9 g/kg/ day) reduced the risk of end-stage renal disease or death by 76%, although no effect on GFR decline was observed. (73) The mechanisms by which a low-protein diet may reduce progression of diabetic nephropathy are still unknown, but might be related to improved lipid profile and/or glomerular hemodynamics.

How to cite this article: Stewart D Rose, Amanda J Strombom. A plant-based diet prevents and treats chronic kidney disease. JOJ uro & nephron. 2019; 6(3): 555687.
DOI: 10.19080/JOJUN.2019.06.555687

Another study specifically looked at the effect of a vegetarian low-protein, low phosphorous diet on patients with diabetic nephropathy secondary to type I diabetes. The diet used provided 0.3gm/Kg/day protein, no more than 3.5mg /Kg/day phosphorus, and 60% of the calories were from carbohydrate. The sodium and potassium contents were 0.3 and 1.1 mmol/Kg/day respectively. The diet was also supplemented with a mixture of keto amino acid analogues and essential amino acids 126mg/Kg/day, $CaCO_3$ 3-6gm/day, and a multivitamin with iron. (74)

This study showed that a supplemented vegetarian diet in type I diabetes patients with overt nephropathy resulted in a slowing or even arrest of the progression of renal failure. Despite the increased carbohydrate, there was no need to increase the dose of insulin and in some patients the dose was decreased. The diet also reduced proteinuria and serum urea. (74)

3.4 CKD in Pregnancy

Using the most recent classification system, 3% of women of childbearing age are affected by CKD. (75, 76) For these women, the risk of an adverse pregnancy rises very significantly, even in stage 1. (77) Despite vast improvements in fetal outcomes, pregnancy in women with CKD is fraught with hazards; worsening renal function and complications such as preeclampsia and premature delivery are common. (78)

During the pregnancy of a patient with CKD, the amount of protein in the diet must be balanced between the goal of diminishing hyperfiltration and increasing metabolic needs of pregnancy. (25) Due to the fact that pregnancy induces hyperfiltration, diets with restricted amount of protein should be beneficial in this group of patients. (79, 80) Vegan or vegetarian supplemented low-protein diets in pregnant women with stages 3–5 CKD reduce the risk of small-for-gestational-age babies, without detrimental effects on kidney function or proteinuria in the mother. (81)

CKD during pregnancy presents a clinical challenge, especially considering the paucity of therapeutic tools available in pregnant women. One study investigated the feasibility of supplemented vegetarian low-protein diets in pregnancy, as a "rescue treatment" for severe CKD and or proteinuria. (79) None of the 11 patients needed renal replacement therapy within the 6 months before delivery. No patient complained of side effects, nor developed hyperkalemia or hypercalcaemia. All babies were well at 1 month post delivery, and 7.5 years later. (79) A supplemented vegetarian low-protein diet (0.6–0.7 g/kg per day) turned out to be sufficient for the maintenance of satisfactory nutritional status during the pregnancy and after delivery, even in breast-feeding women. (48)

For pregnant women with focal segmental glomerulosclerosis, a study showed that a moderately protein restricted, keto analogue supplemented, plant-based diet helped control proteinuria. (82)

Another study reviewed the results obtained over 15 years of treating pregnant women with CKD on moderately restricted plant-based low-protein diets. It confirms that such a diet is a safe option in the management of pregnant CKD patients. (83) A trend towards better preserved fetal growth was observed.

These results indicate that the treatment of pregnant CKD women on moderately restricted plant-based low-protein diet is a safe option in the management of pregnant CKD.

How to cite this article: Stewart D Rose, Amanda J Strombom. A plant-based diet prevents and treats chronic kidney disease. JOJ uro & nephron. 2019; 6(3): 555687.
DOI: 10.19080/JOJUN.2019.06.555687

3.5 Acidosis

Metabolic acidosis is a common complication of chronic kidney disease. The frequency of metabolic acidosis increases along with the decrease of renal function, especially when the glomerular filtration rate falls below 30–40 mL/min/1.73 m^2. (84, 85, 86) The most common negative consequences are as follows: bone demineralization, (87) tubulointerstitial fibrosis, (88, 89) inflammation, (90) the stimulation of the renin-angiotensin system (91) and adrenocortiocotrophic hormone. (92) According to studies, metabolic acidosis is also associated with increased cardiovascular risk. (93, 94, 95, 96, 97)

Mechanisms by which metabolic acidosis may stimulate nephropathy progression in CKD involve sustained, high levels of mediators of increased distal nephron acidification in response to GFR reduction, such as endothelin and aldosterone. (98) In CKD patients, low bicarbonate reflects primary metabolic acidosis, (99) and it is considered to be a risk factor for mortality and CKD progression. (100, 101, 96, 97, 102, 103)

Growing evidence suggests that the source of protein (plant or animal) may be more important than the quantity of protein consumed. Meat produces more of a dietary acid load (DAL) than plant foods. A typical diet in industrialized countries produces acid of about 1 mEq/kg/day. However, it is reduced by more than one third among vegetarians and is close to neutrality among vegans. (104) Another study showed that higher levels of DAL were associated with 3.04 times higher risk of ESRD in the highest versus lowest tertile. (105)

The fact that the acid load linked to animal proteins is higher than that linked to plant proteins is already known in the scientific community. (105, 106, 38) Moe et al. showed that the use of only plant proteins, compared to animal proteins, was able to reduce daily serum and urinary phosphate levels in eight subjects, the load of sodium, calcium and phosphorus being equal. (14, 49)

One reason for this is the tendency for excess meat intake to disrupt the acid base balance, since protein derived from animal sources contains acid-forming substances such as sulfur-containing amino acids and phosphorus, in addition to the excessive protein load. Sulfur-containing amino acids, when oxidized, generate sulphate, a non-metabolizable anion that contributes to total body acid load. (107, 97, 37)

Protein from plant sources contains higher levels of glutamate, an anionic amino acid that upon metabolism consumes hydrogen ions to remain neutral, thereby reducing acidity levels. (107, 97, 37) Plant foods are also generally higher in anionic potassium salts, which also result in the consumption of hydrogen ions upon metabolism and thus reducing acid load. (107, 97, 37)

In response to an increase in acid load, the kidney adapts by increasing ammonium ion excretion in order to expel excess hydrogen ions, therefore increasing the demand for ammonia production. (108) This stimulates the breakdown of glutamine and other amino acids, promoting protein catabolism and muscle wasting (109) while also leading to renal hypertrophy. (110)

Metabolic acidosis also promotes protein muscle wasting via the activation of the ATP-dependent ubiquitin proteasome system. (111) In response to a high acid load, the kidney also undergoes functional changes, including promotion of glomerular hyperfiltration and renal vasodilation, features typical of early diabetic kidney disease. (107, 97, 37)

How to cite this article: Stewart D Rose, Amanda J Strombom. A plant-based diet prevents and treats chronic kidney disease. JOJ uro & nephron. 2019; 6(3): 555687.
DOI: 10.19080/JOJUN.2019.06.555687

Current guidelines recommend treatment with alkali when bicarbonate levels are lower than 22 mMol/L, (84) to prevent complications, such as insulin resistance, (112, 113) cardiovascular diseases and progression of CKD, among others. (114, 96) The Kidney Disease Outcomes Quality Initiative (KDOQI) recommends Na+ citrate or $NaHCO_3$ in the treatment of metabolic acidosis in CKD. (115) However, Na+, Na+ citrate and $NaHCO_3$ may aggravate volume retention and/or hypertension in CKD. (107)

A correction of metabolic acidosis can also be achieved with a diet rich in fruit and vegetables, (47, 116, 117, 118, 37, 4, 119, 120, 121, 122) as well as with a very low-protein vegetarian diet. (107) A plant-based diet was shown to influence survival through its effect on metabolic acidosis. (118) Results from the Chronic Renal Insufficiency Cohort Study suggest that consumption of a greater proportion of protein from plant sources is associated with higher bicarbonate levels, as well as an improved phosphorous balance in patients with CKD. (123)

A case-control study by Di Iorio et al. (107) clearly demonstrated that a very low-protein diet (VLPD) containing a high quantity of fruit and vegetables, with a very low amount of protein, supplemented with essential amino acids and ketoanalogs of non essential amino acids, reduced net endogenous acid production (NEAP) by 53% after six months and 67% after 12 months, and potential renal acid load (PRAL) by 120% after six months and 138% after 12 months. Also, the correction of hyperpotassemia, as a consequence of a physiological correction of metabolic acidosis, was observed after 12 months on the VLPD diet. (107)

A study by Bellasi et al. (93) indicated the relationship between metabolic acidosis and insulin resistance in diabetic patients with chronic kidney disease. They also showed that oral sodium bicarbonate administration or a low-protein vegetarian diet rich in fruit and vegetables, prescribed to avoid or correct metabolic acidosis, improved insulin sensitivity in the CKD plus diabetes mellitus (DM) population. (93)

A study of stage 3 CKD patients showed an increase of bicarbonate levels by increasing the amount fruits and vegetables in their diet. (47)

A one year study of either added fruits and vegetables or sodium bicarbonate in individuals with stage 4 CKD, yielded an equal eGFR (estimated glomerular filtration rate) in both cases. It was associated with higher-than-baseline plasma total, and lower-than-baseline urine indices of kidney injury. The data indicated that fruits and vegetables improved metabolic acidosis and reduced kidney injury in stage 4 CKD without producing hyperkalemia. (37)

3.6 Omega-6 Fatty Acids

Recent studies suggest additional potential benefits of healthy eating on CKD progression. Individuals consuming too much saturated fat are more likely to progress to CKD. (124) Growing evidence suggests the potential benefit of dietary fat modification strategies in CKD patients, including increasing the amount of linoleic acid (n-6 PUFA) from vegetable oils and thus reducing the amount of saturated fat ingested. (125, 126)

The best way to do this is to reduce the consumption of animal products which are high in saturated fat, and to increase the amount of nuts and seeds which are rich in linoleic acid. No studies

How to cite this article: Stewart D Rose, Amanda J Strombom. A plant-based diet prevents and treats chronic kidney disease. JOJ uro & nephron. 2019; 6(3): 555687.
DOI: 10.19080/JOJUN.2019.06.555687

have yet shown a benefit from increasing Omega-3 fatty acids for CKD patients.

3.7 The Nephrotoxic Effects of Persistent Organic Pollutants

The impact of environmental chemicals on public health and clinical well-being has long been recognized, with a historical focus on heavy metals and molecules that are produced in the work place. Increasing data have, however, indicated that the general public is exposed to a wide range of chemicals as a consequence of normal consumer activities. These activities include dietary intake of food. (127, 128) Numerous reports have documented toxicity that occurs in response to graded exposure to a wide range of environmental chemicals.

Persistent organic pollutants (POPs) are synthetic organic chemicals such as dioxins, furans, polychlorinated biphenyls (PCBs), and organochlorine pesticides – chemicals mainly created by industrial and agrichemical activities either intentionally or as by-products – that have an intrinsic resistance to natural degradation processes, and are therefore environmentally persistent and bio-accumulate through the food chain, increasing greatly in concentration at each subsequent trophic level. (129) POPs accumulate in adipose tissue of animals as well as humans. Thus the majority of human exposure to persistent organic pollutants occurs as a result of eating foods containing meat, milk, eggs and fish due to accumulation of POPs in animal fat. (130, 131)

Polychlorinated dibenzo-p-dioxins (PCDDs), dibenzofurans (PCDFs), and polychlorinated biphenyls (PCBs) are lipophilic and can persist in the body for years. (132) An individual's body burden is a product of multiple years of exposure and a lifetime of varying elimination rates. Different congeners of PCDDs, PCDFs, and PCBs each have different levels of persistence in the human body, reflected in their different reported half-lives. In human adipose tissue, they may represent a pool of toxicants with diverse health effects including carcinogenesis and renal damage. (133)

The kidney, because of its high rate of perfusion, active transport capabilities, and concentrating functions, is often exposed to much higher concentrations of chemicals than are other organs. These high concentrations may cause toxic effects to the kidney. (134) Emerging data suggest that the kidney is an important site of injury after chemical exposure with POPs. (130, 131)

Prolonged cumulative lifetime exposure to certain POPs, in conjunction with age-associated decline in kidney function and other comorbid conditions, may accelerate the rate of deterioration in kidney function and progression to CKD. (130, 131)

Exposure to persistent organic pollutants are a very strong risk factor for type 2 diabetes. (60) Since the kidneys function to remove waste products from the blood, diabetic nephropathy could partly be either the cause or the consequence (or both) of exposure to dioxins, furans and dioxin-like PCBs. (131)

One study examined the association of agricultural persistent organic pollutants including six organochlorine pesticides and pesticide metabolites in human blood. When p,p'-DDT and heptachlor epoxide were both elevated, the odds ratio for diabetic nephropathy was 2.76 times the average. When six of six organochlorine pesticides and pesticide metabolites, were elevated, the odds ratio for diabetic nephropathy was 3.00. (135)

How to cite this article: Stewart D Rose, Amanda J Strombom. A plant-based diet prevents and treats chronic kidney disease. JOJ uro & nephron. 2019; 6(3): 555687.
DOI: 10.19080/JOJUN.2019.06.555687

Another study assessed the association of persistent organic pollutants from industrial processes including 6 chlorinated dibenzo-p-dioxins, 9 chlorinated dibenzofurans and 8 polychlorinated biphenyls (PCBs) in blood with diabetic nephropathy (defined as urinary albumin to creatinine ratio >30 mg/g) in diabetics as defined by a glycated hemoglobin of >6.5%. When 4 or more of the 23 chemicals were elevated the risk for diabetic nephropathy was 7 times higher than otherwise. (131)

PCDDs and PCDFs are readily absorbed through the digestive tract, which is enhanced through the ingestion of fatty foods. The lipophilic characteristics of PCDDs and PCDFs allows for slow excretion in bile and urine, (136, 131) thus prolonging the exposure of kidney and colon cells to these toxins.

PCB metabolism primarily occurs in the liver, where it must first be hydroxylated to increase the polarity of the molecule, before it is excreted in the bile. (137) The rate of metabolism varies depending on the degree of chlorination of the congener. (138) Metabolism of PCBs can also produce toxicologically active agents, such as arene oxides that must be enzymatically detoxified and excreted, and/or can form toxic adducts which can damage the kidney cells' DNA. (139)

Dioxins metabolism also takes place in the liver. Metabolites are excreted through the biliary fecal route. The half-life of dioxins can be up to several decades, due to enterohepatic recirculation. The effects of dioxins are chiefly mediated by the aryl hydrocarbon receptor (AHR), a ligand-activated transcription factor that regulates gene expression. (136)

Studies have shown that those exposed to the greatest amount of toxins have reduced renal function. Compared to the lowest quartile, the highest quartile of toxin exposure resulted in a 14.8 ml/min/1.73 m^2 and a 21.5 ml/min/1.73 m^2 reduction in estimated GFR in men and women, respectively. (136, 131) This decrease in GFR must be distinguished from the lower GFRs that healthy vegans have, that are a consequence of healthy kidneys.

The risk of hyperuricemia was higher for higher serum concentrations of organochlorine pesticides, PCDDs, and dioxin-like substances raising the risk of uremia by 1.4, 1.3, and 2.4 respectively. (136, 131, 140)

Even adults with only low level exposure to dioxins are also still at heightened risk of hyperuricaemia. The increase in risk of hyperuricemia ranged from 2.3 to 3.0, depending upon the specific dioxin congener exposure. (136, 131, 140)

3.8 Bacterial Toxicology

Uremic retention molecules (URMs), contributing to the syndrome of uremia, may be classified according to their site of origin, that is, endogenous metabolism, microbial metabolism, or exogenous intake. It is increasingly recognized that bacterial metabolites, such as phenols, indoles, and amines, may contribute to uremic toxicity. In vitro studies have implicated bacterial URMs in CKD progression, cardiovascular disease, and bone and mineral disorders. Furthermore, several observational studies have demonstrated a link between serum levels of bacterial URMs and clinical outcomes. Bacterial metabolism may therefore be an important therapeutic target in CKD. There is evidence that reduced renal clearance, increased colonic generation and absorption explain the high levels of bacterial URMs in CKD. (141)

How to cite this article: Stewart D Rose, Amanda J Strombom. A plant-based diet prevents and treats chronic kidney disease. JOJ uro & nephron. 2019; 6(3): 555687.
DOI: 10.19080/JOJUN.2019.06.555687

The microbial metabolism of protein also produces a number of metabolites that may negatively affect the kidneys. (142, 143) Indoxyl sulfate (IS) and p-cresyl sulfate (PCS) are uremic toxins derived solely from colonic bacterial fermentation of protein. (142, 143, 144)

Circulating indoxyl sulphate can increase oxidative stress in the renal tubular cells and the glomeruli. (145, 143) Also, in-vitro indoxyl sulphate has been observed to activate inflammatory pathways resulting in an increase in the expression of monocyte chemoattractant protein-1 (MCP-1) and intracellular adhesion molecule-1 (ICAM-1). (146) P-cresyl sulfate has similarly been linked to CKD and CVD mortality, although the mechanism is not yet as well defined. (147, 148)

Interestingly, it has been noted that vegetarians have lower levels of these nephrotoxic compounds compared with omnivores, in both healthy (149) and CKD populations. (150) Vegetarians tend to have higher fiber intakes, (147) which could be metabolized by the colonic microbiota instead of amino acids, leading to a reduction in indoxyl sulphate and p-cresyl sulfate. This provides another mechanism to explain why vegetarian protein sources appear less detrimental than animal protein sources.

Furthermore, carnitine and lecithin present in red meat are metabolized by the microbiota to form trimethylamine-N-oxide, (151) which has been linked to cardiovascular events. The interaction between animal sources of protein and gut bacteria in CKD warrants further investigation.

Determining an optimum protein to fiber ratio could allow for appropriate protein intake to prevent protein energy wasting, without adverse effects on renal outcomes. (143) Not only do vegetarian proteins carry an advantage, but vegetarians themselves produce less sulphate and p-cresyl sulfate. In one study comparing healthy vegetarian to non-vegetarians, the average PCS excretion was 62% lower and average IS excretion was 58% lower in vegetarians, compared to participants consuming an unrestricted diet. (150) In the same study vegetarian patients undergoing hemodiafiltration also had lower levels of Indoxyl sulfate and p-cresyl sulfate. (150)

Treatment of ESRD is now focused on removing uremic solutes by dialysis. In theory, treatments that reduce solute production could also reduce solute levels and ameliorate uremic illness. (149) Over the long term, vegetarian and unrestricted diets may influence PCS and IS production by altering the colon microbial flora, or microbiome, as well as by providing different nutrients to colon microbes on a day-to-day basis. (149)

Dietary fiber was considered as a treatment for chronic renal failure more than 30 years ago, where it was found to reduce plasma urea. (152) Interventions that have focused on increasing total dietary fiber intake in patients with pre dialysis CKD have reported reductions in serum creatinine levels (153) and plasma p-cresol. (154) A four-week study in which patients with chronic renal failure consumed 50 grams per day of acacia gum, a highly fermentable fiber, led to a mean reduction in plasma urea of 12%. (155) In another study, supplementation with acacia gum for three months led to decreases in serum urea, creatinine and phosphate by 31%, 10% and 22%, respectively. (156)

Recently, several short term studies have been undertaken using non digestible carbohydrates in patients receiving dialysis. A four-week Belgian study in haemodialysis patients showed that plasma

How to cite this article: Stewart D Rose, Amanda J Strombom. A plant-based diet prevents and treats chronic kidney disease. JOJ uro & nephron. 2019; 6(3): 555687.
DOI: 10.19080/JOJUN.2019.06.555687

p-cresyl sulfate decreased by 20% when supplemented with oligofructose-enriched inulin. (157) This result has been echoed in a similar study that combined galacto-oligosaccharides with probiotics. (158) While neither of these studies showed a reduction in indoxyl sulphate, a recent six-week dietary intervention with resistant starch in haemodialysis patients led to a mean reduction of plasma indoxyl sulphate and p-cresyl sulfate by 29% and 28%, respectively. (159)

Some guidelines for the management of CKD make no mention to the role of non-digestible carbohydrates, which some researchers feel should be rectified on the basis of emerging evidence. (160) Dietary fiber intake is about 20%–30% lower in haemodialysis patients compared to control subjects, (161, 162) with dialysis patients consuming approximately 11 g/day dietary fiber, significantly less than the recommendation of 25 g/day. (163) These data suggest that non-digestible carbohydrates are effective at improving biochemical markers in haemodialysis patients, and that dietary interventions involving these compounds may be particularly relevant given the low intakes seen in this population. The use of dietary fiber supplementation is a simple, non-invasive option that does not negatively impact patients' quality of life. (164, 143, 25)

3.9 Phosphorus

In patients with chronic kidney disease, high dietary phosphorus burden may worsen hyperparathyroidism and renal osteodystrophy, promote vascular calcification and cardiovascular events, and increase mortality. In addition to the absolute amount of dietary phosphorus, its type (organic versus inorganic), source (animal- versus plant-derived), and ratio to dietary protein may be important. Organic phosphorous in plant foods such as seeds and legumes is less bioavailable because of limited gastrointestinal absorption. (165)

Disturbances in mineral metabolism are common complications of chronic kidney disease (CKD), beginning at approximately CKD stage 3 and 4. Patients with advanced chronic kidney disease maintain a positive phosphorus balance through phosphaturia. The damaged kidney is unable to fully excrete a phosphorus load, which leads to compensatory secondary hyperparathyroidism and elevations in fibroblast growth factor 23 (FGF23) in an attempt to increase urinary phosphorus excretion to maintain phosphorus balance. (166, 165) This provides the rationale for recommendations to restrict dietary phosphate intake to 800 mg/d.

Protein-rich foods such as legumes, meat, poultry, fish, eggs and dairy products are the main sources of organic phosphate. A strong positive correlation between dietary protein from animals and phosphorous intake is responsible for the frequent association of high protein intake in the diet with excessive ingestion of phosphorous, and the resulting hyperphosphatemia in people with CKD. (65, 152)

However, the protein source of the phosphate is important, as a high protein (and high phosphorus) diet does not always translate to increased serum phosphate levels. (167) The bioavailability of organic phosphate varies depending on the food source:

Food Source	Bioavailability of Phosphorus	References
Plant Sources	20-40%	(168, 169, 170)
Dairy products	30-60%	
Meat products	Up to 80%	(165, 167, 168)
Inorganic Phosphate additives	90-100%	(171)
Phosphoric acid in cola drinks	100%	(158)

The difference in phosphorus bioavailability between meat and plant protein sources may partially explain the benefits of consuming a greater proportion of protein from plants sources, as described above. Phosphate absorption is linearly related to phosphate intake, with bioavailability being the major determining factor in phosphate uptake from the diet. (172) Thus, for organic phosphate, food choices can make a significant difference in the amount of phosphate that is absorbed from the diet.

Inorganic phosphorous may be added to foods in the form of additives, which are typically used to improve taste, texture, shelf life or processing time. (173) These additives are primarily inorganic phosphate salts that require no enzymatic digestion and dissociate rapidly in the low pH environment of the stomach. The phosphoric acid in cola drinks has a bioavailability of 100%. (158) These foods should therefore be avoided.

In one inpatient study, the results indicated that 1 week on a vegetarian diet led to lower serum phosphorus levels and decreased FGF23 levels. (166)

3.10 The use of soy protein

The type of protein consumed affects alterations in kidney-related biomarkers in CKD patients. One study sought to assess the effects of soy protein consumption on renal related markers among type 2 diabetic patients with nephropathy. A randomized clinical trial was conducted with one diet containing 0.8 g/kg protein (70% animal and 30% vegetable proteins), and a similar diet contained the same amount of protein with 35% animal protein, 35% soy protein, and 30% other vegetable proteins. Consumption of soy protein reduced urinary urea nitrogen, proteinuria, blood sodium), and serum phosphorus compared with animal protein consumption. (174)

A meta study of 12 CKD studies showed that dietary soy resulted in a significant decrease in serum creatinine, phosphorous, CRP and proteinuria in predialytic patients. The study also found that soy protein intake could maintain the nutritional status in dialysis patients, though no significant change in CRP, BUN, and serum phosphorus was detected. (175)

Another study found that a diet with a higher proportion of protein from plant sources, primarily soy, is associated with lower mortality in those with eGFR < 60 mL/min/1.73 m2 of 23% Therefore, at a given total protein intake, a higher proportion of dietary protein from plant sources such as soy is associated with lower mortality risk in chronic kidney disease. (176)

How to cite this article: Stewart D Rose, Amanda J Strombom. A plant-based diet prevents and treats chronic kidney disease. JOJ uro & nephron. 2019; 6(3): 555687.
DOI: 10.19080/JOJUN.2019.06.555687

These studies show that soy, a popular and readily available source of plant-based protein, is an effective choice for treating CKD patients.

3.11 Cardiovascular Disease and Hypertension

Cardiovascular disease remains a major cause of morbidity and mortality in patients with chronic kidney disease (CKD), accounting for approximately 50% of all deaths in patients on dialysis and in recipients of renal transplants. (177) Recent studies have demonstrated that modification of the dietary pattern by reducing animal protein intake and increasing consumption of plant-based foods could influence cardiovascular risk profile and mortality rate. Moreover, phosphate bioavailability from plant proteins is reduced. These effects lead to some benefits for chronic kidney disease (CKD) patients. (178)

The vegan diet, known for its better lipoprotein profile and antioxidant content, can protect against CVD. One study compared patients with advanced chronic kidney disease on a conventional low-protein diet with those on a ketoanalogue supplemented vegan diet. Patients on a vegan diet showed increased HDL cholesterol levels with a reduction of LDL cholesterol and an increase of apoA1/apoB ratio. A significant reduction of total homocysteine, Lp(a) and CRP levels were also observed in vegan patients. (179)

Dialysis patients have both traditional and non-traditional risk factors for cardiovascular disease, including the retention of advanced glycation end products (AGE). In one study, skin auto fluorescence (SAF), a marker of tissue AGE deposition, was reduced in vegetarian hemodialysis patients compared to patients on a conventional chronic kidney disease diet. This study showed that a vegetarian diet may reduce exposure to preformed dietary AGE thus reducing their risk of CVD. (180)

A study comparing a vegan diet to the more conventional low and very low-protein diet found that vitamin K1, fiber content, and the alkalizing potential were all better on a vegan diet than the other diets. The net endogenous acid production decreased the most, and the same finding occurred for the potential renal acid load (PRAL). These features may have favorable effects on Vitamin K1 status, intestinal microbiota and acid-base balance. Thus the vegan diet also has beneficial effects on vascular calcification and bone disease, on protein metabolism, on colonic environment and circulating levels of microbial derived uremic toxins. (181)

The low-protein and phosphorus intake has a crucial role for reducing proteinuria and preventing and reversing hyperphosphatemia and secondary hyperparathyroidism, which are major causes of the vascular calcifications, cardiac damage, and mortality risk of uremic patients. The reduction of nitrogenous waste products and lowering of serum PTH levels may also help ameliorate insulin sensitivity and metabolic control in diabetic patients, as well as increase the responsiveness to erythropoietin therapy, thus allowing greater control of anemia. Vegetarian diets may have also anti-inflammatory and antioxidant properties. Proper nutritional treatment early in the course of renal disease may be useful to reduce the cardiovascular risk in the renal patient. (182)

In one study patients were examined for triglycerides (TG), total cholesterol, HDL and LDL cholesterol, and apolipoproteins Apo A1, Apo B, and Lp(a). Lipid peroxidation (LP) has recently been suggested to trigger the atherosclerotic process as well as to worsen the progression of renal disease. Autoantibodies against oxidized low-density lipoproteins (Ox-LDLAb) were considered to provide a sensitive marker to detect LDL oxidation in vivo. This study shows that the vegan diet, by reducing LP, total cholesterol, TG, and Lp(a), decreases the risk of cardiovascular disease and is worth being considered as an alternative effective therapeutic tool in patients with advanced CKD. (183)

In another study of CKD patients, Lp(a) concentrations increased with the progression of renal failure, and a significant correlation was observed with serum creatinine (sCr). Despite the elevated sCr levels, patients on a keto analogue supplemented vegetarian diet had an almost normal Lp(a) concentration while only 15% of the reference group had. (184)

Elevated blood pressure (BP) is one of the most frequent complications of chronic kidney disease. (185) Its correction is an important intervention because uncontrolled hypertension is a recognized determinant of progression of renal damage. (186, 187, 188, 189) It also represents a major cause for the elevated cardiovascular morbidity and mortality detected in these patients. (190, 191, 192, 193) Accordingly, current clinical practice guidelines strongly suggest reducing BP to less than 130/80 mm Hg. (194)

One study of stage 4 and 5 patients on a very low-protein ketoanalogue supplemented diet, where the protein was mostly plant protein, showed an average decrease in blood pressure from 143/84 to 128/78. The benefit of the mostly vegetable protein diet was observed, even in patients who started with inadequate BP control at baseline in spite of multidrug antihypertensive therapy. (195) Other studies have shown that vegetarian diets are associated with lower blood pressure. (196, 197, 198, 199)

A recent study showed that a vegan diet was associated with lower blood pressure in asymptomatic participants with proteinuria. (200) This diet could be a nonpharmacologic method to reduce blood pressure and help prevent chronic kidney disease.

4. Clinical Considerations

Several studies have determined the nutritional safety of plant-based diets in CKD patients, despite dietary protein restriction. Plant- based diets are associated with a reduced risk of all-cause mortality in CKD patients. Studies confirm a kidney protective effect of plant-based diets in the primary prevention of CKD and the secondary prevention of CKD progression. (201)

Dietary therapy has to be deeply analyzed, and nutritional prescription has to be focused not only on reduction of protein content but also on proteins' quality. (105, 106, 38, 37, 4, 107)

Adherence to diet, fluids and dialysis are the cornerstone of renal failure treatment. (202) Extensive changes to food and lifestyle are required for patients with CKD. Many diet components must be monitored such as calories, protein, sodium, potassium, calcium, phosphorus, and fluid. (203) No single educational or clinical strategy has been shown to be consistently effective across CKD populations. Highest adherence has been observed when both diet and education efforts are individualized to each patient and adapted over time to changing lifestyle and CKD variables. (204) Factors such as taste, convenience and the impact of the diet on social eating occasions are also important in enhancing dietary adherence. (205) The education focus may be more

How to cite this article: Stewart D Rose, Amanda J Strombom. A plant-based diet prevents and treats chronic kidney disease. JOJ uro & nephron. 2019; 6(3): 555687.
DOI: 10.19080/JOJUN.2019.06.555687

effective by addressing one opportunity at a time, rather than a broad long term diet planning strategy. (204)

Social support is especially important for both hemodialysis and peritoneal dialysis patients in terms of greater satisfaction and quality of life and fewer hospitalizations. Intervention studies to possibly improve these outcomes are warranted. (206)

A regimen with 0.6 g/kg/day of proteins is often difficult for a patient to maintain unless a vegan diet (usually supplemented with keto acids) has been recommended. To take the protein level even lower, 'non-proteic' (commercially available) carbohydrates can be added. The combination of both approaches allows protein intakes as low as 0.3 g/kg/day. (3)

In a 4-year study by Piccoli, implementation was aimed at testing a simplified approach to a plant-based low-protein diet (protein intake of 0.6 g/kg/day) in patients with severe or progressive CKD, who had been referred to a new nephrology unit. In this study, flexibility started from the prescription, as the diet was simply based on allowed and forbidden foods, without the need to weigh all foods. Occasional free choice meals were allowed to reduce the psychological burden. (3) This method achieved positive results, while providing a simpler regimen for patients.

Supplementation of a VLPD with ketoanalogues seems to have some advantages above and beyond the protein restriction. If enough energy is provided, ketoanalogues could be converted to essential amino acids by urea recycling, allowing for a nutritionally safe, more severe reduction in protein intake. (41, 43) Furthermore, the calcium content of ketoanalogue preparations and their phosphate binder capabilities allow for even better correction of mineral metabolic abnormalities. (41, 44)

It is noteworthy that educational level (often associated with higher compliance), diabetes, overall comorbidity (often associated with poor dietary compliance) and old age (frequently considered to impair efficient modulation of the diet) were not confirmed as strong relevant factors in attaining the medium term follow up goals of this diet. (3)

In this study, the diet was initially prescribed as a one-month trial and was prescribed and managed by the nephrologist in the context of the routine clinical follow up. Interestingly, in stable patients with at least 6 months of follow up, compliance was impressive, with a median protein intake of 0.5 g/kg/day. This supports the hypothesis that subtle personal preferences, as well as clear motivations, are fundamental in the relationship with food and diet. Therefore, the authors conclude, this diet should be proposed to all patients without preclusion. (3)

The CKD patient often presents with other chronic diseases such as hypercholesterolemia, (207) coronary artery disease, (208, 209) and type 2 diabetes. (60) The plant-based diet is useful for treating these comorbid diseases as well. Clinical parameters should be monitored and medications adjusted as the treatment effect becomes evident.

5. Discussion

The overall prevalence of chronic kidney disease in the general population is approximately 14 percent. Medicare spending for patients with CKD ages 65 and older exceeded $50 billion in 2013 and represented 20 percent of all Medicare spending in this age group. Given that the plant-based diet reduces the risk of chronic kidney disease in the first place, it would seem to be a very valuable prophylaxis. At least three main reasons suggest that the time is ripe for a systematic integration of a vegetarian diet into the clinical treatment of CKD: the cost of dialysis, the clinical advantages and the failure of early dialysis to prolong survival. (3)

CKD is a challenging disease to treat for both patient and physician. There are many clinical variables to be simultaneously managed. Complicating treatment even further is that treatment often needs to be modified as the disease progresses. The plant-based diet can treat phosphotemia, uremia, acidosis, proteinuria, acidosis and intestinal dysbiosis, and can help prevent chronic kidney disease from advancing to end stage renal disease.

Almost half of individuals with CKD also have diabetes and/or self-reported cardiovascular disease. CKD often occurs in the context of multiple comorbidities and has been termed a "disease multiplier." (210) The plant-based diet helps prevent type 2 diabetes, as well as treat it even more effectively than the leading medication, Metformin. It can also help prevent and treat coronary artery disease, the leading cause of mortality in chronic kidney disease. The plant-based diet has no contraindications or adverse reactions. It reduces health care costs for both the patient and society.

Low-protein plant-based diets do not result in malnutrition or hyperkalemia, and are even safe in pregnancy. It may also be possible to raise the amount of protein in the diet, if the protein is plant-derived. Supplementation with ketoanalogues make the treatment more efficacious.

Plant-based diets are no longer very unusual as they have become more popular in the general population in recent years. Given all of the benefits, the plant-based diet deserves a place among the physician's treatment options for CKD.

References

1. Berger A, Edelsberg J, Inglese G, Bhattacharyya S, Oster G. (2009) Cost comparison of peritoneal dialysis versus hemodialysis in end-stage renal disease. *Am J Manag Care* 15(8):509-18.
2. Meguid El Nahas A, Bello A. (2005) Chronic kidney disease: the global challenge. *Lancet* 365(9456):331-40.
3. Piccoli G, Ferraresi M, Deagostini M, et al. (2013) Vegetarian low-protein diets supplemented with keto analogues: a niche for the few or an option for many? *Nephrol Dial Transplant* 28(9):2295-305.
4. Goraya N, Wesson D. (2016) Dietary Protein as Kidney Protection: Quality or Quantity? *J Am Soc Nephrol* 27(7):1877-9.
5. Murray C, Atkinson C, Bhalla K, et al. (2013) The State of US Health, 1990-2010 Burden of Diseases, Injuries, and Risk Factors. *JAMA* 310(6):591-606.
6. Beale LS. (1869) *Kidney Diseases, Urinary Deposits and Calculous Disorders, Their Nature and Treatment*. Third Edition ed. London: John Churchill and Sons.
7. Giordano C, Madias M. (1982) Protein restriction in chronic renal failure. *Kidney International* 22(4):401-408.
8. Lewis D. (1921) On the Influence of a Diet with High Protein Content on the Kidney. *Can Med Assoc J* 11(9):682-683.
9. Addis T, Lew W. (1939) Diet and death in acute uremia. *J Clin Invest.* 18(6):773-5.
10. Addis T. (1949) *Glomerular nephritis: Diagnosis and treatment*. London, UK: Macmillan.
11. Piccoli G. (2010) Patient-based continuum of care in nephrology: why read Thomas Addis'

How to cite this article: Stewart D Rose, Amanda J Strombom. A plant-based diet prevents and treats chronic kidney disease. JOJ uro & nephron. 2019; 6(3): 555687.
DOI: 10.19080/JOJUN.2019.06.555687

"Glomerular Nephritis" in 2010? *J Nephrol* 23(2):164-7.

12. Borst J. (1948) Protein katabolism in uraemia; effects of protein-free diet, infections, and blood-transfusions. *Lancet* 1(6509):824-9.
13. Thilly N. (2013) Low-protein diet in chronic kidney disease: from questions of effectiveness to those of feasibility. *Nephrol Dial Transplant* 28(9):2203-5.
14. Giovannetti S, Maggiore Q. (1964) A low-nitrogen diet with proteins of high biological value for severe chronic uraemia. *Lancet* 1(7341):1000-3.
15. Lafage M, Combe C, Fournier A, Aparicio M. (1992) Ketodiet, physiological calcium intake and native vitamin D improve renal osteodystrophy. *Kidney Int* 42(5):1217-25.
16. Rigalleau V, Combe C, Blanchetier V, Aubertin J, Aparicio M, et al. (1997) Low protein diet in uremia: effects on glucose metabolism and energy production rate. *Kidney Int* 51(4):1222-7.
17. Bernard S, Fouque D, Laville M, Zech P. (1996) Effects of low-protein diet supplemented with ketoacids on plasma lipids in adult chronic renal failure. *Miner Electrolyte Metab* 22(1-3):143-6.
18. Goraya N, Simoni J, Jo C, Wesson D. (2012) Dietary acid reduction with fruits and vegetables or bicarbonate attenuates kidney injury in patients with a moderately reduced glomerular filtration rate due to hypertensive nephropathy. *Kidney Int*. 81(1):86-93.
19. Pedrini M, Levey A, Lau J, Chalmers T, Wang P. (1996) The Effect of Dietary Protein Restriction on the Progression of Diabetic and Nondiabetic Renal Diseases: A Meta-Analysis. *Ann Intern Med* 124(7):627-32.
20. Fouque D, Laville M, Boissel J, Chifflet R, Labeeuw M, et al. (1992) Controlled low protein diets in chronic renal insufficiency: meta-analysis. *BMJ* 304(6821):216-220.
21. Fouque D, Laville M. (2009) Low protein diets for chronic kidney disease in non diabetic adults. *Cochrane Database Syst Rev*. (3):CD001892.
22. Kasiske B, Lakatua J, Ma J, Louis T. (1998) A meta-analysis of the effects of dietary protein restriction on the rate of decline in renal function. *Am J Kidney Dis* 31(6):954-61.
23. Renal Dietitians Dietetic Practice Group. (2002) *National Renal Diet: Professional Guide*. 2nd Ed ed. Chicago, Ill: The American Dietetic Association.
24. Garneata L, Stancu A, Dragomir D, Stefan G, Mircescu G. (2016) Ketoanalogue-Supplemented Vegetarian Very Low–Protein Diet and CKD Progression. *J Am Soc Nephrol* 27(7):2164-76.
25. Gluba-Brzózka A, Franczyk B, Rysz J. (2017) Vegetarian Diet in Chronic Kidney Disease—A Friend or Foe. *Nutrients* 9(4):E374.
26. Trevisan R, Dodesini A. (2017) The hyperfiltering kidney in diabetes. *Nephron* 136(4):277-280.
27. Wiseman M, Hunt R, Goodwin A, Gross J, Keen H, et al. (1987) Dietary Composition and Renal Function in healthy subjects. *Nephron* 46(1):37-42.
28. Fraser GE. (2009) Vegetarian diets:what do we know of their effects on common chronic diseases? *American Journal of Clinical Nutrition*. 89(5):1607S-1612S.
29. Burrows N, Hora I, Geiss L, Gregg E, Albright A. (2017) Incidence of End-Stage Renal Disease Attributed to Diabetes Among Persons with Diagnosed Diabetes — United States and Puerto Rico, 2000–2014. *MMWR Morb Mortal Wkly Rep*. 66(43):1165-1170.
30. Kazancioğlu R. (2013) Risk factors for chronic kidney disease: an update. *Kidney Int Suppl (2011)*. 3(4):368-371.

How to cite this article: Stewart D Rose, Amanda J Strombom. A plant-based diet prevents and treats chronic kidney disease. JOJ uro & nephron. 2019; 6(3): 555687.
DOI: 10.19080/JOJUN.2019.06.555687

31. Bosch J, Saccaggi A, Lauer A, Ronco C, Belledonne M, et al. (1983) Renal function reserve in humans. Effect of protein intake on glomerular filtration. *Am J Med* 75(6):943-50.
32. Haring B, Selvin E, Liang M, Coresh J, Grams M, et al. (2017) Dietary Protein Sources and Risk for Incident Chronic Kidney Disease: Results From the Atherosclerosis Risk in Communities (ARIC) Study. *J Ren Nutr* 27(4):233-242.
33. ew Q, Jafar T, Koh H, Jin A, Chow K, et al. (2017) Red Meat Intake and Risk of ESRD. *J Am Soc Nephrol*. 28(1):304-312.
34. Lin J, Fung T, Hu F, Curhan G. (2011) Association of dietary patterns with albuminuria and kidney function decline in older white women: a subgroup analysis from the Nurses' Health Study. *Am J Kidney Dis*. 57(2):245-54.
35. Lin J, Judd S, Le A, Ard J, Newsome B, et al. (2010) Associations of dietary fat with albuminuria and kidney dysfunction. *Am J Clin Nutr* 92(4):897-904.
36. Odermatt A. (2011) The Western-style diet: a major risk factor for impaired kidney function and chronic kidney disease. *Am J Physiol Renal Physiol* 301(5):F919-31.
37. Goraya N, Simoni J, Jo C, Wesson D. (2013) A Comparison of Treating Metabolic Acidosis in CKD Stage 4 Hypertensive Kidney Disease with Fruits and Vegetables or Sodium Bicarbonate. *Clin J Am Soc Nephrol* 8(3):371-81.
38. Gutiérrez O, Muntner P, Rizk D, et al. (2014) Dietary patterns and risk of death and progression to ESRD in individuals with CKD: A cohort study. *Am J Kidney Dis* 64(2):204-13.
39. Kelly J, Palmer S, Wai S, Ruospo M, Carrero J, et al. (2017) Healthy Dietary Patterns and Risk of Mortality and ESRD in CKD: A Meta-Analysis of Cohort Studies. *Clin J Am Soc Nephrol* 12(2):272-279.
40. Kontessis P, Jones S, Dodds R, Trevisan R, Nosadini R, et al. (1990) Renal, metabolic and hormonal responses to ingestion of animal and vegetable protein. *Kidney Int* 38(1):136-44.
41. Chauveau P, Combe C, Rigalleau V, Vendrely B, Aparicio M. (2007) Restricted protein diet is associated with decrease in proteinuria: Consequences on the progression of renal failure. *J Ren Nutr*. 17(4):250-7.
42. Ikizler T. (2009) Dietary protein restriction in CKD: The debate continues. *Am J Kidney Dis* 53(2):189-91.
43. KDIGO (2013) 2012 clinical practice guideline for the evaluation and management of chronic kidney disease. *Kidney Int Suppl* 3(1):5-10.
44. Mitch W. (!991) Dietary protein restriction in chronic renal failure: Nutritional efficacy, compliance, and progression of renal insufficiency. *J Am Soc Nephrol* 2(4):823-31.
45. Malvy D, Maingourd C, Pengloan J, Bagros P, Nivet H. (1999) Effects of severe protein restriction with ketoanalogues in advanced renal failure. *J Am Coll Nutr* 18(5):481-6.
46. Gretz N, Meisinger E, Strauch M. (1987) Influence of diet and underlying renal disease on the rate of progression of chronic renal failure. *Infusionstherapie* 14(Suppl 5):21-25.
47. Goraya N, Simoni J, Jo C, Wesson D. (2014) Treatment of metabolic acidosis in patients with stage 3 chronic kidney disease with fruits and vegetables or oral bicarbonate reduces urine angiotensinogen and preserves glomerular filtration rate. *Kidney Int* 86(5):1031-8.
48. Zaldivar M, Peixoto A. (2003) CKD series: cardiovascular risk reduction in patients with chronic kidney disease. *Hosp Physician* 39:29-35, 50.
49. Anderson J. (2008) Beneficial effects of soy protein consumption for renal function. *Asia Pac J Clin Nutr* 17(Suppl 1):324-8.
50. Bernstein A, Treyzon L, Li Z. (2007) Are high-protein, vegetable based diets safe for

How to cite this article: Stewart D Rose, Amanda J Strombom. A plant-based diet prevents and treats chronic kidney disease. JOJ uro & nephron. 2019; 6(3): 555687.
DOI: 10.19080/JOJUN.2019.06.555687

kidney function: a review of the literature. *J Am Diet Assoc* 107(4):644-50.

51. Ahmed F. (1991) Effect of diet on progression of chronic renal disease. *J Am Diet Assoc* 91(10):1266-70.
52. Cupisti A, Ghiadoni L, D'Alessandro C, et al. (2007) Soy protein diet improves endothelial dysfunction in renal transplant patients. *Nephrol Dial Transplant* 22(1):229-34.
53. Elliott P, Stamler J, Dyer A, et al. (2006) Association between protein intake and blood pressure: the INTERMAP Study. *Arch Intern Med* 166(1):79-87.
54. Azadbakht L, Atabak S, Esmaillzadeh A. (2008) Soy protein intake, cardiorenal indices, and C reactive protein in type II diabetes with nephropathy; a longitudinal randomized clinical trial. *Diabetes Care* 31(4):648-54.
55. Anderson J, Blake J, Turner J, Smith B. (1998) Effects of soy protein on renal function and proteinuria in patients with type 2 diabetes. *Am J Clin Nutr* 68(6 Suppl):1347S-1353S.
56. Lohsiriwat S. (2013) Protein diet and estimated glomerular filtration rate. *Open J Nephrol* 3(2):97-100.
57. Barsotti G, Morelli E, Cupisti A, Meola M, Dani L, Giovannetti S. (1996) A low-nitrogen low-phosphorus Vegan diet for patients with chronic renal failure. *Nephron* 74(2):390-4.
58. Wu T, Chang C, Hsu W, et al. (2011) Nutritional status of vegetarians on maintenance haemodialysis. *Nephrology (Carlton)* 16(6):582-7.
59. Jibani M, Bloodworth L, Foden E, Griffiths K, Galpin O. (1991) Predominantly vegetarian diet in patients with incipient and early clinical diabetic nephropathy: Effects of albumin excretion rate and nutritional status. *Diabet Med* 8(10):949-53.
60. Strombom A, Rose S. (2017) The prevention and treatment of Type II Diabetes Mellitus with a plant-based diet. *Endocrin Metab Int J* 5(5):00138.
61. Ogborn M, Bankovic-Calic N, Shoesmith C, Buist R, Peeling J. (1998) Soy protein modification of rat polycystic kidney disease. *Am J Physiol* 274(3 Pt 2):F541-9.
62. Trujillo J, Ramírez V, Pérez J, et al. (2005) Renal protection by a soy diet in obese Zucker rats is associated with restoration of nitric oxide generation. *Am J Physiol Renal Physiol* 288(1):F108-16.
63. Moe S, Chen N, Seifert M, et al. (2009) A rat model of chronic kidney disease-mineral bone disorder. *Kidney Int* 75(2):176-84.
64. Mitch W, Remuzzi G. (2016) Diets for patients with chronic kidney disease, should we reconsider? *BMC Nephrol* 17:80.
65. Wesson D, Jo C, Simoni J. (2015) Angiotensin II-mediated GFR decline in subtotal nephrectomy is due to acid retention associated with reduced GFR. *Nephrol Dial Transplant* 30(5):762-70.
66. Mitch W. (2000) Are supplements of ketoacids and amino acids useful in treating patients with chronic renal failure? *Wien Klin Wochenschr* 112(20):863-4.
67. Combe C, Deforges-Lasseur C, Caix J, Pommereau A, Marot D, Aparicio M. (1993) Compliance and effects of nutritional treatment on progression and metabolic disorders of chronic renal failure. *Nephrol Dial Transplant* 8(5):412-8.
68. Aparicio M, Fouque D, Chauveau P. (2009) Effect of a very low-protein diet on long-term outcomes. *Am J Kidney Dis* 54(1):183.
69. Barsotti G, Morelli E, Cupisti A, Bertoncini P, Giovannetti S. (1991) A special, supplemented 'vegan' diet for nephrotic patients. *Am J Nephrol* 11(5):380-5.
70. Chauveau P, Couzi L, Vendrely B, et al. (2009) Long-term outcome on renal replacement

therapy in patients who previously received a keto acid-supplemented very-low-protein diet. *Am J Clin Nutr* 90(4):969-74.

71. Levey A, Adler S, Caggiula A, et al. (1996) Effects of dietary protein restriction on the progression of advanced renal disease in the Modification of Diet in Renal Disease Study. *Am J Kidney Dis* 27(5):652-63.
72. Menon V, Kopple J, Wang X, et al. (2009) Effect of a very low-protein diet on outcomes: Long-term follow-up of the Modification of Diet in Renal Disease (MDRD) Study. *Am J Kidney Dis* 53(2):208-17.
73. Hansen H, Tauber-Lassen E, Jensen B, Parving H. (2002) Effect of dietary protein restriction on prognosis in patients with diabetic nephropathy. *Kidney Int* 62(1):220-8.
74. Barsotti G, Navalesi R, Giampetro O, et al. (1988) Effects of a vegetarian, supplemented diet on renal function, proteinuria and glucose metabolism in patients with overt diabetic nephropathy and renal insufficiency. In: Schmicker R, Kokot F, Gretz N, eds. *Contributions to Nephrology, Metabolic Disturbances in the Predialytic Phase of Chronic Renal Failure*. Vol 65: Karger.
75. Piccoli G, Attini R, Vasario E, et al. (2010) Pregnancy and chronic kidney disease: a challenge in all CKD stages. *Clin J Am Soc Nephrol* 5(5):844-55.
76. Cabiddu G, Castellino S, Gernone G, et al. (2016) A best practice position statement on pregnancy in chronic kidney disease: the Italian Study Group on Kidney and Pregnancy. *J Nephrol* 29(3):277-303.
77. Piccoli G, Fassio F, Attini R, et al. (2012) Pregnancy in CKD: whom should we follow and why? *Nephrol Dial Transplant* 27(Suppl 3):iii111-8.
78. Vellanki K. (2013) Pregnancy in chronic kidney disease. *Adv Chronic Kidney* 20(3):223-228.
79. Piccoli G, Attini R, Vasario E, et al. (2011) Vegetarian supplemented low-protein diets. A safe option for pregnant CKD patients: Report of 12 pregnancies in 11 patients. *Nephrol Dial Transplant* 26(1):196-205.
80. Brenner B, Lawler E, Mackenzie H. (1996) The hyperfiltration theory: a paradigm shift in nephrology. *Kidney Int* 49(6):1774-7.
81. Piccoli G, Leone F, Attini R, et al. (2014) Association of Low-Protein Supplemented Diets with Fetal Growth in Pregnant Women with CKD. *Clin J Am Soc Nephrol* 9(5):864-73.
82. Attini R, Leone F, Montersino B, et al. (2017) Pregnancy, Proteinuria, Plant-Based Supplemented Diets and Focal Segmental Glomerulosclerosis: A Report on Three Cases and Critical Appraisal of the Literature. *Nutrients* 9(7):E770.
83. Attini R, Leone F, Parisi S, et al. (2016) Vegan-vegetarian low-protein supplemented diets in pregnant CKD patients: fifteen years of experience. *BMC Nephrol* 17(1):132.
84. Kopple J. (2001) National kidney foundation K/DOQI clinical practice guidelines for nutrition in chronic renal failure. *Am J Kidney Dis* 37(1 Suppl 2):S66-70.
85. Chen W, Abramowitz M. (2014) Metabolic acidosis and the progression of chronic kidney disease. *BMC Nephrol* 15:55.
86. Huston H, Abramowitz M, Zhang Y, Greene T, Raphael K. (2015) Net endogenous acid production and mortality in NHANES III. *Nephrology (Carlton)* 20(3):209-15.
87. Bushinsky D, Chabala J, Gavrilov K, Levi-Setti R. (1999) Effects of in vivo metabolic acidosis on midcortical bone ion composition. *Am J Physiol* 277(5 Pt 2):F813-9.
88. Wesson D, Dolson G. (1997) Endothelin-1 increases rat distal tubule acidification in vivo. *Am J Physiol* 273(4 Pt 2):F586-94.

How to cite this article: Stewart D Rose, Amanda J Strombom. A plant-based diet prevents and treats chronic kidney disease. JOJ uro & nephron. 2019; 6(3): 555687.
DOI: 10.19080/JOJUN.2019.06.555687

89. Wesson D, Simoni J. (2009) Increased tissue acid mediates a progressive decline in the glomerular filtration rate of animals with reduced nephron mass. *Kidney Int* 75(9):929-35.

90. Bellocq A, Suberville S, Philippe C, et al. (1998) Low environmental pH is responsible for the induction of nitric-oxide synthase in macrophages. Evidence for involvement of nuclear factor-kappaB activation. *J Biol Chem* 273(9):5086-92.

91. Ng H, Chen H, Tsai Y, Yang Y, Lee C. (2011) Activation of intrarenal renin-angiotensin system during metabolic acidosis. *Am J Nephrol* 34(1):55-63.

92. Wood C, Isa A. (1991) Intravenous acid infusion stimulates ACTH secretion in sheep. *Am J Physiol* 260(1 Pt 1):E154-61.

93. Bellasi A, Di Micco L, Santoro D, et al. (2016) Correction of metabolic acidosis improves insulin resistance in chronic kidney disease. *BMC Nephrol* 17:158.

94. Simon E, Hamm L. (2010) A basic approach to CKD. *Kidney Int* 77(7):567-9.

95. Teta D. (2015) Insulin resistance as a therapeutic target for chronic kidney disease. *J Ren Nutr* 25(2):226-9.

96. de Brito-Ashurst I, Varagunam M, Raftery M, Yaqoob M. (2009) Bicarbonate supplementation slows progression of CKD and improves nutritional status. *J Am Soc Nephrol* 20(9):2075-84.

97. Rysz J, Franczyk B, Ciałkowska-Rysz A, Gluba-Brzózka A. (2017) The Effect of Diet on the Survival of Patients with Chronic Kidney Disease. *Nutrients* 9(5):pii: E495.

98. Wesson D, Simoni J. (2010) Acid retention during kidney failure induces endothelin and aldosterone production which lead to progressive GFR decline, a situation ameliorated by alkali diet. *Kidney Int* 78(11):1128-35.

99. Raphael K, Murphy R, Shlipak M, et al. (2016) Bicarbonate Concentration, Acid-Base Status, and Mortality in the Health, Aging, and Body Composition Study. *Clin J Am Soc Nephrol* 11(2):308-16.

100. Kovesdy C, Anderson J, Kalantar-Zadeh K. (2009) Association of serum bicarbonate levels with mortality in patients with non-dialysis-dependent CKD. *Nephrol Dial Transplant* 24(4):1232-7.

101. Navaneethan S, Schold J, Arrigain S, et al. (2011) Serum bicarbonate and mortality in stage 3 and stage 4 chronic kidney disease. *Clin J Am Soc Nephrol* 6(10):2395-402.

102. Dobre M, Yang W, Chen J, et al. (2013) Association of Serum Bicarbonate With Risk of Renal and Cardiovascular Outcomes in CKD: A Report From the Chronic Renal Insufficiency Cohort (CRIC) Study. *Am J Kidney Dis* 62(4):670-8.

103. Shah S, Abramowitz M, Hostetter T, Melamed M. (2009) Serum Bicarbonate Levels and the Progression of Kidney Disease: A Cohort Study. *Am J Kidney Dis* 54(2):270-7.

104. Chauveau P, Lasseur C, Nodimar C, et al. (2018) [Dietary acid load: A novel target for the nephrologist?] [Article in French]. *Nephrol Ther* 14(4):240-246.

105. Banerjee T, Crews D, Wesson D, Tilea A, Saran R, et al. (2015) High Dietary Acid Load Predicts ESRD among Adults with CKD. *J Am Soc Nephrol* 26(7):1693-700.

106. Wesson D, Nathan T, Rose T, Simoni J, Tran R. (2007) Dietary protein induces endothelin-mediated kidney injury through enhanced intrinsic acid production. *Kidney Int* 71(3):210-7.

107. Di Iorio B, Di Micco L, Marzocco S, et al. (2017) Very Low-Protein Diet (VLPD) Reduces Metabolic Acidosis in Subjects with Chronic Kidney Disease: The “Nutritional Light Signal” of the Renal Acid Load. *Nutrients* 9(1):pii: E69.

108. Adeva M, Souto G. (2011) Diet-induced metabolic acidosis. *Clin Nutr* 30(4):416-21.

109. Alpern R, Sakhaee K. (1997) The clinical spectrum of chronic metabolic acidosis: Homeostatic mechanisms produce significant morbidity. *Am J Kidney Dis* 29(2):291-302.

110. Kurtz I. (1991) Role of Ammonia in the Induction of Renal Hypertrophy. *Am J Kidney Dis* 17(6):650-3.

111. Mitch W, Medina R, Grieber S, et al. (1994) Metabolic acidosis stimulates muscle protein degradation by activating the adenosine triphosphate-dependent pathway involving ubiquitin and proteasomes. *J Clin Invest* 93(5):2127-33.

112. Kobayashi S, Maesato K, Moriya H, Ohtake T, Ikeda T. (2005) Insulin resistance in patients with chronic kidney disease. *Am J Kidney Dis* 45(2):275-80.

113. Mak R. (1998) Effect of metabolic acidosis on insulin action and secretion in uremia. *Kidney Int* 54(2):603-7.

114. Kurella M, Lo J, Chertow G. (2005) Metabolic syndrome and the risk for chronic kidney disease among nondiabetic adults. *J Am Soc Nephrol* 16(7):2134-40.

115. 115. Tyson C, Lin P, Corsino L, et al. (2016) Short-term effects of the DASH diet in adults with moderate chronic kidney disease: A pilot feeding study. *Clin Kidney J* 9(4):592-8.

116. Wesson D, Jo C, Simoni J. (2012) Angiotensin II receptors mediate increased distal nephron acidification caused by acid retention. *Kidney Int* 82(11):1184-94.

117. Goraya N, Wesson D. (2014) Is dietary acid a modifiable risk factor for nephropathy progression? *Am J Nephrol* 39(2):142-4.

118. Goraya N, Wesson D. (2015) Dietary interventions to improve outcomes in chronic kidney disease. *Curr Opin Nephrol Hypertens* 24(6):505-10.

119. Phisitkul S, Khanna A, Simoni J, et al. (2010) Amelioration of metabolic acidosis in patients with low GFR reduced kidney endothelin production and kidney injury, and better preserved GFR. *Kidney Int* 77(7):617-23.

120. Goraya N, Wesson D. (2013) Does correction of metabolic acidosis slow chronic kidney disease progression? *Curr Opin Nephrol Hypertens* 22(2):193-7.

121. Goraya N, Wesson D. (2012) Acid-base status and progression of chronic kidney disease. *Curr Opin Nephrol Hypertens* 21(5):552-6.

122. Phisitkul S, Hacker C, Simoni J, Tran R, Wesson D. (2008) Dietary protein causes a decline in the glomerular filtration rate of the remnant kidney mediated by metabolic acidosis and endothelin receptors. *Kidney Int* 73(2):192-9.

123. Scialla J, Appel L, Wolf M, et al. (2012) Plant Protein Intake Is Associated with Fibroblast Growth Factor 23 and Serum Bicarbonate in Patients with CKD: The Chronic Renal Insufficiency Cohort Study. *J Ren Nutr* 22(4):379-388.

124. Lin J, Hu F, Curhan G. (2010) Associations of diet with albuminuria and kidney function decline. *Clin J Am Soc Nephrol* 5(5):836-43.

125. Huang X, Stenvinkel P, Qureshi A, et al. (2013) Clinical determinants and mortality predictability of stearoyl-CoA desaturase-1 activity indices in dialysis patients. *J Intern Med* 273(3):263-72.

126. Huang X, Stenvinkel P, Qureshi A, et al. (2012) Essential polyunsaturated fatty acids, inflammation and mortality in dialysis patients. *Nephrol Dial Transplant* 27(9):3615-20.

127. Kataria A, Trasande L, Trachtman H. (2015) The effects of environmental chemicals on renal function. *Nat Rev Nephrol* 11(10):610-25.

How to cite this article: Stewart D Rose, Amanda J Strombom. A plant-based diet prevents and treats chronic kidney disease. JOJ uro & nephron. 2019; 6(3): 555687.
DOI: 10.19080/JOJUN.2019.06.555687

128. Sears M, Genuis S. (2012) Environmental Determinants of Chronic Disease and Medical Approaches: Recognition, Avoidance, Supportive Therapy, and Detoxification. *J Environ Public Health* 2012:356798.

129. Bergkvist C, Oberg M, Appelgren M, Becker W, Aune M, et al. (2008) Exposure to dioxin-like pollutants via different food commodities in Swedish children and young adults. *Food and Chemical Toxicology* 46(11):3360-7.

130. IARC Working Group on the Evaluation of Carcinogenic Risk to Humans. (2012) 2, 3, 7, 8 tetrachlorodibenzo-para-dioxin, 2, 3, 4, 7, 8-pentachlorodibenzofuran, and 3, 3, 4, 4'5-pentachlorobiphenyl. *Chemical agents and related occupations*. Vol IARC Monographs on the Evaluation of Carcinogenic Risks to Humans, No.100F. Lyon (France): International Agency for Research on Cancer.

131. Everett C, Thompson O. (2014) Dioxins, furans and dioxin-like PCBs in human blood: causes or consequences of diabetic nephropathy? *Environ Res* 132:126-31.

132. Milbrath M, Wenger Y, Chang C, Emond C, Garabrant D, et al. (2009) Apparent Half-Lives of Dioxins, Furans, and Polychlorinated Biphenyls as a Function of Age, Body Fat, Smoking Status, and Breast-Feeding. *Environ Health Perspect* 117(3):417-25.

133. Patanè G, Anello M, Piro S, Vigneri R, Purrello F, et al. (2002) Role of ATP production and uncoupling protein-2 in the insulin secretory defect induced by chronic exposure to high glucose or free fatty acids and effects of peroxisome proliferator-activated receptor-gamma inhibition. *Diabetes* 51(9):2749-56.

134. Kluwe W, Hook J. (1980) Effects of environmental chemicals on kidney metabolism and function. *Kidney Int* 18(5):648-55.

135. Everett C, Thompson O. (2015) Association of DDT and heptachlor epoxide in human blood with diabetic nephropathy. *Rev Environ Health* 30(2):93-7.

136. Kitamura K, Nagao M, Yamada T, Sunaga M, Hata J, Watanabe S. (2001) Dioxins in bile in relation to those in the human liver and blood. *J Toxicol Sci* 26(5):327-36.

137. Tremaine L, Quebbemann A. (1985) The renal handling of terephthalic acid. *Toxicol Appl Pharmacol* 77(1):165-74.

138. Frederiksen H, Skakkebaek N, Andersson A. (2007) Metabolism of phthalates in humans. *Mol Nutr Food Res* 51(7):899-911.

139. Hauser R, Meeker J, Park S, Silva M, Calafat A. (2004) Temporal variability of urinary phthalate metabolite levels in men of reproductive age. *Environ Health Perspect* 112(17):1734-40.

140. Lee Y, Bae S, Lee S, Jacobs DJ, Lee D. (2013) Persistent organic pollutants and hyperuricemia in the U.S. general population. *Atherosclerosis* 230(1):1-5.

141. Evenepoel P, Meijers B, Bammens B, Verbeke K. (2009) Uremic toxins originating from colonic microbial metabolism. *Kidney Int Suppl* (114):S12-9.

142. Rossi M, Johnson D, Xu H, et al. (2015) Dietary protein-fiber ratio associates with circulating levels of indoxyl sulfate and p-cresyl sulfate in chronic kidney disease patients. *Nutr Metab Cardiovasc Dis*. 25(9):860-5.

143. Snelson M, Clarke R, Coughlan M. (2017) Stirring the Pot: Can Dietary Modification Alleviate the Burden of CKD? *Nutrients* 9(3):E265.

144. Meijers B, Evenepoel P. (2011) The gut–kidney axis: Indoxyl sulfate, p-cresyl sulfate and CKD progression. *Nephrol Dial Transplant* 26(3):759-61.

145. Niwa T. (2010) Indoxyl sulfate is a nephro-vascular toxin. *J Ren Nutr* 20(5 Suppl):S2-6.

146. Tumur Z, Shimizu H, Enomoto A, Miyazaki H, Niwa T. (2010) Indoxyl sulfate upregulates

expression of ICAM-1 and MCP-1 by oxidative stress-induced NF-kappaB activation. *Am J Nephrol* 31(5):435-41.

147. Bammens B, Evenepoel P, Keuleers H, Verbeke K, Vanrenterghem Y. (2006) Free serum concentrations of the protein-bound retention solute p-cresol predict mortality in hemodialysis patients. *Kidney Int* 69(6):1081-7.
148. Liabeuf S, Barreto D, Barreto F, et al. (2010) Free p-cresylsulphate is a predictor of mortality in patients at different stages of chronic kidney disease. *Nephrol Dial Transplant* 25(4):1183-91.
149. Patel K, Luo F, Plummer N, Hostetter T, Meyer T. (2012) The Production of p-Cresol Sulfate and Indoxyl Sulfate in Vegetarians versus Omnivores. *Clin J Am Soc Nephrol* 7(6):982-8.
150. Kandouz S, Mohamed A, Zheng Y, Sandeman S, Davenport A. (2016) Reduced protein bound uraemic toxins in vegetarian kidney failure patients treated by haemodiafiltration. *Hemodial Int* 20(4):610-617.
151. Koeth R, Wang Z, Levison B, et al. (2013) Intestinal microbiota metabolism of L-carnitine, a nutrient in red meat, promotes atherosclerosis. *Nat Med* 19(5):576-585.
152. Rampton D, Cohen S, Crammond V, et al. (1984) Treatment of chronic renal failure with dietary fiber. *Clin Nephrol* 21(3):159-63.
153. Salmean Y, Segal M, Langkamp-Henken B, Canales M, Zello G, Dahl W. (2013) Foods With Added Fiber Lower Serum Creatinine Levels in Patients With Chronic Kidney Disease. *J Ren Nutr* 23(2):e29-32.
154. Salmean Y, Segal M, Palii S, Dahl W. (2015) Fiber supplementation lowers plasma p-Cresol in chronic kidney disease patients. *J Ren Nutr* 25(3):316-20.
155. Bliss D, Stein T, Schleifer C, Settle R. (1996) Supplementation with gum arabic fiber increases fecal nitrogen excretion and lowers serum urea nitrogen concentration in chronic renal failure patients consuming a low-protein diet. *Am J Clin Nutr* 63(3):392-8.
156. Ali A, Ali K, Fadlalla A, Khalid K. (2008) The effects of gum arabic oral treatment on the metabolic profile of chronic renal failure patients under regular haemodialysis in Central Sudan. *Nat Prod Res* 22(1):12-21.
157. Meijers B, De Preter V, Verbeke K, Vanrenterghem Y, Evenepoel P. (2010) p-Cresyl sulfate serum concentrations in haemodialysis patients are reduced by the prebiotic oligofructose-enriched inulin. *Nephrol Dial Transplant* 25(1):219-24.
158. Sirich T, Plummer N, Gardner C, Hostetter T, Meyer T. (2014) Effect of Increasing Dietary Fiber on Plasma Levels of Colon-Derived Solutes in Hemodialysis Patients. *Clin J Am Soc Nephrol.* 9(9):1603-10.
159. Fernandez-Prado R, Esteras R, Perez-Gomez M, et al. (2017) Nutrients turned into toxins: microbiota modulation of nutrient properties in chronic kidney disease. *Nutrients* 9(5):E489.
160. Evenepoel P, Meijers B. (2012) Dietary fiber and protein: Nutritional therapy in chronic kidney disease and beyond. *Kidney Int* 81(3):227-9.
161. Cupisti A, D'Alessandro C, Valeri A, et al. (2010) Food Intake and Nutritional Status in Stable Hemodialysis Patients. *Ren Fail* 32(1):47-54.
162. Kalantar-Zadeh K, Kopple J, Deepak S, Block D, Block G. (2002) Food intake characteristics of hemodialysis patients as obtained by food frequency questionnaire. *J Ren Nutr* 12(1):17-31.
163. Khoueiry G, Waked A, Goldman M, et al. (2011) Dietary Intake in Hemodialysis Patients Does Not Reflect a Heart Healthy Diet. *J Ren Nutr* 21(6):438-47.
164. Lu L, Huang Y, Wang M, et al. (2017) Dietary fiber intake is associated with chronic kidney disease (CKD) progression and cardiovascular

How to cite this article: Stewart D Rose, Amanda J Strombom. A plant-based diet prevents and treats chronic kidney disease. JOJ uro & nephron. 2019; 6(3): 555687.
DOI: 10.19080/JOJUN.2019.06.555687

risk, but not protein nutritional status, in adults with CKD. *Asia Pac J Clin Nutr* 26(4):598-605.

165. Kalantar-Zadeh K, Gutekunst L, Mehrotra R, et al. (2010) Understanding sources of dietary phosphorus in the treatment of patients with chronic kidney disease. *Clin J Am Soc Nephrol* 5(3):519-30.
166. Moe S, Zidehsarai M, Chambers M, et al. (2011) Vegetarian compared with meat dietary protein source and phosphorus homeostasis in chronic kidney disease. *Clin J Am Soc Nephrol* 6(2):257-64.
167. Kloppenburg W, Stegeman C, Hovinga T, et al. (2004) Effect of prescribing a high protein diet and increasing the dose of dialysis on nutrition in stable chronic haemodialysis patients: A randomized, controlled trial. *Nephrol Dial Transplant* 19(5):1212-23.
168. Cupisti A, Kalantar-Zadeh K. (2013) Management of Natural and Added Dietary Phosphorus Burden in Kidney Disease. *Semin Nephrol* 33(2):180-90.
169. Uribarri J. (2007) Phosphorus homeostasis in normal health and in chronic kidney disease patients with special emphasis on dietary phosphorus intake. *Semin Dial* 20(4):295-301.
170. Lynch K, Lynch R, Curhan G, Brunelli S. (2011) Prescribed Dietary Phosphate Restriction and Survival among Hemodialysis Patients. *Clin J Am Soc Nephrol* 6(3):620-9.
171. Bover J, Andrés E, Lloret M, Aguilar A, Ballarín J. Dietary and pharmacological control of calcium and phosphate metabolism in dialysis patients. *Blood Purif.* 2009;27:369-386.
172. Uribarri J, Calvo M. (2003) Hidden sources of phosphorus in the typical American diet: does it matter in nephrology? *Semin Dial* 16(3):186-8.
173. Calvo M, Moshfegh A, Tucker K. (2014) Assessing the Health Impact of Phosphorus in the Food Supply: Issues and Considerations. *Adv Nutr* 5(1):104-113.
174. 174. Azadbakht L, Esmaillzadeh A. (2009) Soy protein consumption and kidney related biomarkers among type 2 diabetics: a cross-over, randomized clinical trial. *J Ren Nutr* 19(6):479-86.
175. Jing Z, Wei-Jie Y. (2016) Effects of soy protein containing isoflavones in patients with chronic kidney disease: A systematic review and meta-analysis. *Clin Nutr* 35(1):117-24.
176. Chen X, Wei G, Jalili T, et al. (2016) The associations of plant protein intake with all-cause mortality in CKD. *Am J Kidney Dis* 67(3):423-30.
177. Neven E, D'Haese P. (2011) Vascular calcification in chronic renal failure: what have we learned from animal studies? *Circ Res* 108(2):249-64.
178. Chauveau P, Combe C, Fouque D, Aparicio M. (2013) Vegetarianism: advantages and drawbacks in patients with chronic kidney diseases. *J Ren Nutr* 23(6):399-405.
179. Bergesio F, Monzani G, Guasparini A, et al. (2005) Cardiovascular risk factors in severe chronic renal failure: the role of dietary treatment. *Clin Nephrol* 64(2):103-12.
180. Nongnuch A, Davenport A. (2015) The effect of vegetarian diet on skin autofluorescence measurements in haemodialysis patients. *Br J Nutr* 113(7):1040-3.
181. Cupisti A, D'Alessandro C, Gesualdo L, et al. (2017) Non-traditional aspects of renal diets: focus on fiber, alkali and vitamin K1 intake. *Nutrients* 9(5):E444.
182. Cupisti A, Aparicio M, Barsotti G. (2007) Potential benefits of renal diets on cardiovascular risk factors in chronic kidney disease patients. *Ren Fail* 29(5):529-34.
183. Bergesio F, Monzani G, Ciuti R, et al. (2001) Autoantibodies against oxidized LDL in chronic

renal failure: role of renal function, diet, and lipids. *Nephron* 87(2):127-33.

184. Monzani G, Bergesio F, Ciuti R, et al. (1997) Lp(a) levels: effects of progressive chronic renal failure and dietary manipulation. *J Nephrol* 10(1):41-5.
185. De Nicola L, Minutolo R, Chiodini P, Zoccali C, Castellino P, et al. (2006) Global approach to cardiovascular risk in chronic kidney disease: reality and opportunities for intervention. *Kidney Int* 69(3):538-45.
186. Bakris G, Weir M, Shanifar S, et al. (2003) Effects of blood pressure level on progression of diabetic nephropathy. Results from the RENAAL Study. *Arch Intern Med* 163(13):1555-65.
187. Jafar T, Stark P, Schmid C, et al. (2003) Progression of chronic kidney disease: the role of blood pressure control, proteinuria, and angiotensin-converting enzyme inhibition. *Ann Intern Med* 139(4):244-52.
188. Bakris G, Williams M, Dworkin L, et al. (2000) Preserving renal function in adults with hypertension and diabetes: a consensus approach: National Kidney Foundation Hypertension and Diabetes Executive Committees Working Group. *Am J Kidney Dis* 36(3):646-61.
189. De Nicola L, Minutolo R, Bellizzi V, et al. (2004) Achievement of target blood pressure levels in chronic kidney disease: a salty question? *Am J Kidney Dis* 43(5):782-95.
190. Sarnak M, Levey A, Schoolwerth A, et al. (2003) Kidney disease as a risk factor for development of cardiovascular disease. A statement from the American Heart Association Councils on kidney in cardiovascular disease, high blood pressure research, clinical cardiology, and epidemiology and prevention. *Hypertension* 42(5):1050-65.
191. Keith D, Nichols G, Gullion C, Brown J, Smith D. (2004) Longitudinal follow-up and outcomes among a population with chronic kidney disease in a large managed care organization. *Arch Intern Med* 164(6):659-63.
192. Go A, Chertow G, Fan D, McCulloch C, Hsu C. (2004) Chronic kidney disease and the risks of death, cardiovascular events and hospitalization. *N Engl J Med* 351(13):1296-305.
193. Sarnak M, Greene T, Wang X, et al. (2005) The effect of a lower target blood pressure on the progression of kidney disease: long-term follow-up of the modification of diet in renal disease study. *Ann Intern Med* 142(5):342-51.
194. Kidney Disease Outcomes Quality Initiative (K/DOQI). (2004) K/DOQI clinical practice guidelines on hypertension and antihypertensive agents in chronic kidney disease. *Am J Kidney Dis* 43(5 Suppl 1):S1-290.
195. Bellizzi V, Di Iorio B, De Nicola L, et al. (2007) Very low protein diet supplemented with ketoanalogs improves blood pressure control in chronic kidney disease. *Kidney Int* 71(3):245-51.
196. Sacks F, Kass E. (1988) Low blood pressure in vegetarians: effects of specific foods and nutrients. *Am J Clin Nutr* 48(3 Suppl):795-800.
197. Chuang S, Chiu T, Lee C, et al. (2016) Vegetarian diet reduces the risk of hypertension independent of abdominal obesity and inflammation: a prospective study. *J Hypertens* 34(11):2164-71.
198. Beilin L, Rouse I, Armstrong B, Margetts B, Vandongen R. (1988) Vegetarian diet and blood pressure levels: incidental or causal association? *Am J Clin Nutr* 48(3 Suppl):806-10.
199. Lindahl O, Lindwall L, Spångberg A, Stenram A, Ockerman P. (1984) A vegan regimen with reduced medication in the treatment of hypertension. *Br J Nutr* 52(1):11-20.

How to cite this article: Stewart D Rose, Amanda J Strombom. A plant-based diet prevents and treats chronic kidney disease. JOJ uro & nephron. 2019; 6(3): 555687.
DOI: 10.19080/JOJUN.2019.06.555687

200. Liu H, Liu J, Kuo K. (2018) Vegetarian diet and blood pressure in a hospital-based study. *Tzu Chi Medical Journal* 30(3):176-180.
201. Chauveau P, Koppe L, Combe C, Lasseur C, Trolonge S, Aparicio M. (2019) Vegetarian diets and chronic kidney disease. *Nephrol Dial Transplant* 34(2):199-207
202. Ahrari S, Moshki M, Bahrami M. (2014) The relationship between social support and adherence of dietary and fluids restrictions among hemodialysis patients in Iran. *J Caring Sci* 3(1):11-19.
203. Beto J, Schury K, Bansal V. (2016) Strategies to promote adherence to nutritional advice in patients with chronic kidney disease: a narrative review and commentary. *Int J Nephrol Renovasc Dis* 9:21-33.
204. Beto J, Ramirez W, Bansal V. (2014) Medical nutrition therapy in adults with chronic kidney disease: integrating evidence and consensus into practice for the generalist registered dietitian nutritionist. *J Acad Nutr Diet* 114(7):1077-87.
205. Lambert K, Mullan J, Mansfield K. (2017) An integrative review of the methodology and findings regarding dietary adherence in end stage kidney disease. *BMC Nephrol* 18(1):318.
206. Plantinga L, Fink N, Harrington-Levey R, et al. (2010) Association of social support with outcomes in incident dialysis patients. *Clin J Am Soc Nephrol* 5(8):1480-8.
207. Jenkins D, Kendall C, Marchie A, et al. (2005) Direct comparison of a dietary portfolio of cholesterol-lowering foods with a statin in hypercholesterolemic participants. *American Journal of Clinical Nutrition* 81(2):380-7.
208. Ornish D, Scherwitz L, Billings J, et al. (1998) Intensive Lifestyle Changes for Reversal of Coronary Heart Disease. *JAMA* 280(23):2001-7.
209. Ornish D, Brown S, Scherwitz L, et al. (1990) Can lifestyle changes reverse coronary heart disease? The Lifestyle Heart Trial. *Lancet* 336(8708):129-33.
210. Kidney Disease Statistics for the United States. (2015) *National Institute of Diabetes and Digestive and Kidney Diseases*. Available at: https://www.niddk.nih.gov/health-information/health-statistics/kidney-disease. Accessed Jan 3, 2018.

How to cite this article: Stewart D Rose, Amanda J Strombom. A plant-based diet prevents and treats chronic kidney disease. JOJ uro & nephron. 2019; 6(3): 555687.
DOI: 10.19080/JOJUN.2019.06.555687

Cancer Therapy & Oncology
International Journal
ISSN: 2473-554X

Juniper Publishers
key to the Researchers

Review Article
Volume 11 Issue 3 - July 2018
DOI: 10.19080/CTOIJ.2018.11.555813

Canc Therapy & Oncol Int J

A Plant-Based Diet Prevents and Treats Prostate Cancer

Stewart Rose and Amanda Strombom

Plant-Based Diets in Medicine, USA

Submission: June 20, 2018; **Published:** July 12. 2018

Correspondence Address: Stewart Rose, Vice President, Plant-Based Diets in Medicine, 12819 SE 38th St, #427, Bellevue, WA 98006.

Abstract

This review covers research done on the prevention and treatment of prostate cancer with a plant-based diet. Epidemiological studies have strongly implicated diet as a major modulator of prostate cancer risk. The risk of prostate cancer in vegetarians is less than half that of non-vegetarians. While plant-based foods have been shown to decrease the risk of prostate cancer, animal-derived foods increase the risk in a dose dependent manner. Intake of saturated fat and cholesterol found in animal-derived foods are independent risk factors for prostate cancer, contributing further to the higher risk that nonvegetarians have.

Other risk factors include a higher intake of carcinogenic persistent organic pollutants that bioconcentrate in animal adipose tissue, and known carcinogens such as heterocyclic amines and polycyclic aromatic hydrocarbons that result from consuming cooked, fried, or barbecued meats. Persistent organic pollutants have been shown to be etiologic factors.

Interventional studies have shown that a plant-based diet effectively halted or slowed the progression of most prostate cancer patients with a Gleason Score of less than seven. Results were maintained over a four-year period. Active tumor suppression for patients paced on a plant-based diet have been demonstrated.

While many patients are placed on a passive watchful waiting protocol adding a plant- based diet can transform the protocol to active treatment.

1. Introduction

Both patients and physicians are increasingly interested in the use of a healthy vegetarian diet composed fruits, vegetables, legumes, nuts and whole grains for the prevention and treatment of prostate cancer. This article discusses the research and the clinical application of vegetarian nutritional medicine to the prevention and treatment of prostate cancer.

Research has shed light on animal derived foods in the diet as a risk factor, and the value of plant foods in reducing the incidence of prostate cancer. The role of different constituents of animal derived foods in the pathogenesis of prostate cancer has also been studied, as have the chemoprotective properties of different plant foods.

Interventional studies using a plant-based diet in the treatment of early-stage low-grade prostate cancer have also been conducted. These studies document a dose response relationship between diet change and tumor suppression, strengthening the evidence for the efficacy of the treatment. Also studied are differences in gene expression between cancer patients treated with a plant- based diet and those in the control group, thus offering some biochemical basis for the treatment. Clinical compliance has been found to be enhanced when the patient's wife or partner's support and cooperation is incorporated in the treatment plan.

Treating a patient with a plant-based diet has essentially no adverse effects or contraindications, is cost effective, lowers the risk of, and can even help treat several common comorbidities such as metabolic syndrome, diabetes, coronary artery disease and hypertension.

2. Epidemiology, Pathogenesis and Etiology

Epidemiological studies of prostate cancer have strongly implicated diet as a major modulator of prostate cancer risk. Prostate cancer incidence and mortality varies among different geographic regions, with high prostate cancer risk in the United States and Europe, and low prostate cancer risk in Asia, especially in those following a low animal-food diet. When immigrants from low-risk regions move to high-risk regions, they typically adopt higher prostate cancer risks, particularly with cultural assimilation. (1, 2) This likely reflects dietary differences: either dietary habits in high risk regions promote prostate cancer, dietary habits in low risk regions prevent prostate cancer, or both. When examined in greater detail, the most consistent dietary association for prostate cancer appears to be intake of red meats and or animal fats. (3, 4)

As an overall dietary pattern, the risk of prostate cancer was 54% greater in the nonvegetarians (P=0.03) than vegetarians. (5) This dietary pattern includes a diet rich in fruits and vegetables, elimination of animal derived saturated fats, and elimination of cooked meats. In another study researchers found that inverse associations were observed with dietary intake of plant foods, suggesting decreased risk with a plant-based diet. (6) In summarizing, the research on diet for primary and secondary prostate prevention, many believe "heart healthy equals prostate healthy." (7)

2.1 Saturated Fat Consumption

The type of fatty acid consumed, rather than total amount, may play an important role in prostate cancer development and progression. (8) A study found plasma saturated fatty acids to be

How to cite this article: Rose S, Strombom A. A plant-based diet prevents and treats prostate cancer. Canc Therapy & Oncol Int J. 2018; 11(3): 555813.
DOI: 10.19080/CTOIJ.2018.11.555813.

positively associated with prostate cancer risk in a prospective cohort of 14,514 men of the Melbourne Collaborative Cohort Study. (9)

Another study prospectively followed 384 men diagnosed with prostate cancer in Canada. Proportional hazards models were used to estimate the relative risk of dying from prostate cancer associated with terciles of fat intake, expressed as percent of dietary energy, while controlling for prognostic factors and total energy. The median duration of follow up was 5.2 years. After controlling for grade, clinical stage, initial treatment, age and total energy intake, the study found that saturated fat consumption was significantly associated with disease specific survival ($p = 0.008$). Compared to men in the lower tercile of saturated fat, those in the upper tercile had three times the risk of dying from prostate cancer (hazards ratio 3.13, 95% confidence interval 1.28–7.67). (10)

Interestingly, another study found that eating more plant-based fat was associated with reduced prostate cancer risk. (11)

2.2 Cholesterol

Cholesterol is required for proliferation in all animal cells and is especially important for membrane formation. (12) Serum cholesterol has been identified as an independent risk factor for prostate cancer. For instance, in a study published in 2014, of 2,408 men scheduled for biopsy, serum cholesterol was independently associated with prediction of prostate cancer risk. (13)

Many pre-clinical studies have shown that the accumulation of cholesterol contributes to the progression of prostate cancer. (14, 15, 16) It has been suggested that high cholesterol in circulation may be a risk factor for solid tumors, primarily through the upregulation of cholesterol synthesis, inflammatory pathways (17) and intratumoral steroidogenesis. (18) In prostate cancer, cholesterol may also act as a substrate for intratumoral androgen biosynthesis, even after androgen deprivation therapy via the CPY17A1 enzyme. This is expressed by castration resistant prostate cancer cells that de-novo synthesize androgens. (19, 20)

Several lines of evidence link cholesterol metabolism and prostate cancer progression. Firstly, a positive association between serum cholesterol levels and high grade prostate cancer has been described. (21) Secondly, in vivo xenograft and in vitro cancer progression models have identified numerous aberrations in regulators of cholesterol metabolism. (22, 23, 24, 25) Thirdly, statin use as a cholesterol-lowering therapy has been associated with a lower risk of prostate cancer diagnosis, (26) advanced disease, (27) and mortality. (28)

Usage of statin cholesterol-lowering drugs, post radical prostatectomy (RP), was significantly associated with reduced risk of biochemical recurrence in 1,146 radical prostatectomy patients. (29) Another study also showed that statins may reduce prostate cancer risk by lowering progression. (30) Although the mechanism has not been established, more recent studies also showed that a low high-density lipoprotein (HDL) cholesterol level was associated with a higher risk for prostate cancer and, thus, a higher HDL was protective. (31, 32, 33)

However, a disturbing increase in the HGPCa (high grade prostate carcinoma) rate was observed in statin users who normalized their serum cholesterol. (13) These findings support the notion that a heart-healthy dietary intervention that lowers cholesterol may benefit prostate health, without any

How to cite this article: Rose S, Strombom A. A plant-based diet prevents and treats prostate cancer. Canc Therapy & Oncol Int J. 2018; 11(3): 555813.
DOI: 10.19080/CTOIJ.2018.11.555813.

other risks, whereas the statin approach, while reducing the general risk, may increase the risk of high grade lesions.

Vegetarians and vegans have lower total and LDL cholesterol levels on average. (34, 35) Vegans, or total vegetarians, have the lowest levels.

2.3 Persistent Organic Pollutants

Persistent organic pollutants (POPs) are synthetic organic chemicals that have an intrinsic resistance to natural degradation processes, and are therefore environmentally persistent and bioaccumulate through the food web. They include dioxins, furans, polychlorinated biphenyls (PCBs), and organochlorine pesticides, chemicals mainly created by industrial activities either intentionally or as by-products. (36) The introduction of POPs into the environment from anthropogenic activities resulted in their widespread dispersal and accumulation in soils and bodies of water, as well as in human and ecological food chains, where they are known to induce toxic effects.

There is evidence of long range transport of these substances to regions where they have never been used or produced, resulting in exposure of most human populations to POPs through consumption of fat-containing food such as fish, dairy products, and meat, (37, 38, 39) with the highest POP concentrations being commonly found in fatty fish. (36, 37, 38, 39, 40, 41, 42) Due to their ubiquity in the environment and lipophilic properties, there is mounting concern over the potential risks of human exposure to POPs. (37)

Total body concentrations of POPs showed positive associations with prostate cancer increasing cancer risk by 31%. (43) In a dose-response meta-analysis, 1 μg/g lipid of PCBs was found to be associated with a 49% increased risk of prostate cancer (OR 1.49, 95 % CI 1.07, 2.06). (43) Even one nanogram per gram lipid of trans-nonachlor still was found to be associated with approximately 2% increased risk of prostate cancer (OR = 1.02/1 ng/g lipid of trans-nonachlor, 95 % CI 1.00, 1.03). (43)

Some studies have found an even greater increased risk of prostate cancer with exposure to specific POPs. In one study, a greater than median concentration of one of the PCB congeners showed an increase 3.15 times and one chlordane type, trans-chlordane, showed a 3.49 times increased risk. In the group of case subjects with PSA levels greater than the median level of 16.5 ng/mL, the increased risk was even higher. (44) The available evidence suggests that body concentrations of POPs are positively associated with prostate cancer risk, which implies valuable evidence for prostate cancer prevention. (43)

2.4 Heterocyclic Amines and Polycyclic Aromatic Hydrocarbons

Cooking meat produces Heterocyclic Amines (HCAs) and Polycyclic Aromatic Hydrocarbons (PAHs). The fact that these are carcinogens is well established. Researchers found that high consumption of cooked, fried, or barbecued meats was associated with increased risk of prostate cancer. (45, 46) Additionally, the ability of these food-borne carcinogens to induce prostate cancer has been studied. (45, 46, 47, 48, 49)

2.5 Inflammatory Response

Most of the inflammation in the prostate is a consequence of damage to the prostate epithelium, which can be caused by dietary carcinogens, estrogens, and inflammatory oxidants. (50) Recently, molecular pathology insights have indicted chronic

How to cite this article: Rose S, Strombom A. A plant-based diet prevents and treats prostate cancer. Canc Therapy & Oncol Int J. 2018; 11(3): 555813.
DOI: 10.19080/CTOIJ.2018.11.555813.

or recurrent epithelial cell injury, accompanied by innate and adaptive inflammatory responses, in the early steps of prostate cancer development. (50)

As a consequence, dietary components capable of inducing such injury, such as the heterocyclic amines created by cooking meats, loom large as candidate prostate carcinogens, while dietary components able to limit cell and genome damage and/or attenuate prostate inflammation, may protect against prostate cancer development. (51) The best studied of these carcinogens for prostate cancer is 2-amino-1-methyl-6-phenylimidazopyridine (PhIP), the most abundant of the more than 20 heterocyclic amines that can appear in cooked meats. (51) Diets rich in inducers of phase 2 metabolic enzyme expression, which activate the Keap1-Nrf2 pathway, both reduce carcinogen damage generally in animal models, and lower prostate cancer risk in human epidemiology studies. (52, 53, 54)

2.6 Insulin-like Growth Factor-I

While research on IGF-I and prostate cancer has yielded somewhat inconsistent results, there are enough studies with positive results to warrant its inclusion here. One study found modestly lower IGF-I levels in vegan men. Mean serum IGF-I was 9% lower in 233 vegan men than in 226 meat eaters and 237 vegetarians (P= 0.002). Vegans had higher testosterone levels than vegetarians and meat-eaters, but this was offset by higher sex hormone binding globulin, and there were no differences between diet groups in free testosterone, androstanediol glucuronide or luteinizing hormone. (55) IGF-I may play an important role in the etiology of prostate cancer via its ability to interact with androgens to stimulate prostatic cell growth. (56) Chan et al. found that men who subsequently developed prostate cancer had 8% higher serum IGF-I concentrations than men who remained healthy, suggesting that the 9% difference we observed is large enough to significantly alter prostate cancer risk. (57) An increased risk from high IGF-1 and low binding protein (IGFBP-1) was confirmed just recently. (58)

2.7 Risk reduction with specific foods

The foods with the highest levels of phase 2 enzyme inducers, such as the isothiocyanate sulforaphane, are the cruciferous vegetables, such as broccoli, Brussels sprouts, cauliflower, and others. In a study of normal human volunteers, intake of cruciferous vegetables reduced PhIP adduction to DNA in response to a cooked meat meal. (59) The mechanism(s) by which dietary components, inherited susceptibility, and sex steroid hormones cause epithelial damage and/or drive inflammatory processes that lead to cancer as men age, if better understood, could provide new opportunities for prostate cancer prevention, improved prostate cancer screening strategies, and perhaps even better prostate cancer treatment outcomes. However, it is important to note that a vegetarian diet results in lower levels of C-reactive protein. (60, 61)

Several epidemiologic studies found inverse relationships between total fruit and vegetable intake, (62) including cruciferous vegetable intake, and PCa risk. (63, 64) In addition to the cruciferous vegetables discussed above, several other foods have been investigated, in particular green tea, tomato sauce and allium vegetables (onions, garlic, and scallions).

In a prospective randomized preprostatectomy trial, men consuming brewed green tea prior to surgery had increased levels of green tea polyphenols in their prostate tissue. (65) In a small proof of principle trial with 60 men, daily supplementation of 600 mg green tea catechin extract reduced PCa incidence by 90% (3% versus 30% in the placebo group). (66) Another small trial also showed that EGCG supplement resulted in a significant reduction in PSA, hepatocyte growth factor and vascular endothelial growth factor in men with prostate cancer. (67) These studies suggest green tea polyphenols may lower prostate incidence and reduce PCa progression.

Two short term preprostatectomy trials using tomato sauce or lycopene supplementation demonstrated lycopene uptake in prostate tissue and antioxidant and potential anticancer effects. (68, 69) While several clinical trials suggested an inverse relationship between lycopene supplementation, PSA levels and decreases in cancer related symptoms. (70, 71)

In a case study of several hundred subjects with incident histologically-confirmed prostate cancer and male control subjects, men in the highest of three intake categories of total allium vegetables (>10.0 g/day) had a statistically significantly lower risk (odds ratio [OR] = 0.51, 95% confidence interval [CI] = 0.34 to 0.76; P(trend)<.001) of prostate cancer than those in the lowest category (<2.2 g/day). Similar comparisons between categories showed reductions in risk for men in the highest intake categories for garlic (OR = 0.47, 95% CI = 0.31 to 0.71; P(trend)<.001) and scallions (OR = 0.30, 95% CI = 0.18 to 0.51; P(trend)<.001). The reduced risk of prostate cancer associated with allium vegetables was independent of body size, intake of other foods, and total calorie intake, and was more pronounced for men with localized than with advanced prostate cancer. (72)

3. Clinical Intervention

An important study examined whether comprehensive changes in diet to a plant-based diet (along with stress management) would affect the progression of prostate cancer, as measured by serial prostate specific antigen (PSA), treatment trends, and serum stimulated LNCaP cell growth, in men with early, biopsy-proven prostate cancer (Gleason score less than 7, PSA 4 to 10 ng/ml, stages T1 and T2). (73) Patient recruitment was limited to men who had chosen not to undergo any conventional treatment. The choice to perform watchful waiting was considered clinically reasonable in these men. The interventional diet consisted of fruits, vegetables, whole grains, legumes and soy products, with approximately 10% of calories from fat.

After one year, adherence to the intervention was 95% in the experimental group. There were no adverse events attributable to dietary intervention, and none of the patients in the experimental group required intervention with standard treatment, whereas 12% of the control group did. Serum from experimental group patients inhibited LNCaP cell growth by 70%, whereas serum from control group patients inhibited growth by only 9% (p<[1]0.001). Serum PSA decreased an average of 0.25 ng/ml or 4% of the baseline average in the experimental group, but it showed an average increase of 0.38 ng/ml or 6% of the baseline average in the control group (p < 0.016).

Patients with low grade prostate cancer were able to make and maintain comprehensive lifestyle changes for at least one year, resulting in significant decreases in serum PSA and a lower likelihood of needing standard treatment. In addition, substantially decreased growth of LNCaP prostate cancer cells was seen, when such cells were incubated in

How to cite this article: Rose S, Strombom A. A plant-based diet prevents and treats prostate cancer. Canc Therapy & Oncol Int J. 2018; 11(3): 555813.
DOI: 10.19080/CTOIJ.2018.11.555813.

the presence of serum from those who made lifestyle changes. These findings suggest that intensive changes in diet and lifestyle may beneficially affect the progression of early prostate cancer.

The observation that changes in PSA and in LNCaP cell growth were significantly related to the extent by which participants had changed their lifestyle, further supports the hypothesis that intensive changes in diet may affect the progression of prostate cancer.

A two-year follow up study revealed that only 5% of the experimental group required standard treatment, versus almost 25% in the control group, in addition to the 12% during the first year. (74) The authors conclude that patients with early stage prostate cancer choosing active surveillance might be able to avoid or delay conventional treatment for at least two years by making changes in their diet and lifestyle. (74)

A pilot study was conducted to examine changes in prostate gene expression in a unique population of men with low risk prostate cancer. These men had declined immediate surgery, hormonal therapy, or radiation, and participated in an intensive nutritional intervention (along with stress reduction activities) to a plant-based diet, while undergoing careful surveillance for tumor progression.

Gene expression profiles were obtained from 30 participants, pairing RNA samples from control prostate needle biopsy taken before intervention to RNA from the same patient's 3 month post intervention biopsy. Two class paired analysis of global gene expression using significance analysis of microarrays detected 48 up regulated and 453 down regulated transcripts after the intervention. Pathway analysis identified significant modulation of biological processes that have critical roles in tumorigenesis, including protein metabolism and modification, intracellular protein traffic, and protein phosphorylation (all $P < 0.05$). Intensive changes in nutrition may modulate gene expression in the prostate. (75) This study provides molecular hypotheses that may help explain some of the effects of comprehensive lifestyle changes.

4. Clinical Considerations

Evidence indicates that a healthy diet may improve overall clinical outcomes and quality of life in cancer survivors. (76, 77) In one study, greater exercise and better diet quality were associated with better physical quality of life outcomes (eg, better vitality and physical functioning; $P < .05$) in prostate cancer patients. (76)

Many men make positive dietary changes after PCa diagnosis, which are perceived by men and their partners to bring psychological and general health benefits, and could help future dietary intervention trials. Men and their partners desire more and better dietary information that may support PCa survivorship, particularly among those embarking on active surveillance/monitoring programs. There are opportunities for healthcare professionals to support PCa patients both clinically and psychologically, by the routine integration of healthy eating advice into survivorship care plans. (77)

One study found that prostate cancer patients' partners played a significant and multi-faceted role in their diets, often referring to dietary decisions being made jointly. While partners more often assumed responsibility for food purchasing and preparation, decisions about meal choices were mostly jointly made. Consequently, men typically described having considerable control or responsibility over their diet. Interest in dietary advice was

How to cite this article: Rose S, Strombom A. A plant-based diet prevents and treats prostate cancer. Canc Therapy & Oncol Int J. 2018; 11(3): 555813.
DOI: 10.19080/CTOIJ.2018.11.555813.

high among men both at elevated risk and men diagnosed with PCa, and their partners. (77) This study clearly indicates the value of soliciting the cooperation of the patient's partner when prescribing dietary changes in prostate cancer patients.

5. Discussion

It seems that there are several factors involved in the increased incidence of prostate cancer in men who consume animal derived foods. Lipophilic persistent organic pollutants bioconcentrate to significant levels in the adipose tissue of animals thus dosing their consumer with substantial amounts. These carcinogens play a role in raising the risk of prostate cancer. Polycyclic aromatic hydrocarbons and heterocyclic amines, formed when meat is cooked, cause a chronic inflammation of the prostate, thus playing a role in the development of malignant neoplasia. Consuming animal fat increases exposure to persistent organic pollutants, and is one way that they raise the risk of prostate cancer. Another way is that the saturated fats that animal fats contain raise serum cholesterol, which is now implicated in prostate cancer as well. On the other hand, several plant foods have been shown to lower the risk of prostate cancer. The mechanisms by which these factors induce a malignant transformation or exert a chemoprotective effect are being investigated, and have begun to yield some evidence by which they achieve of their effects.

In low-grade early-stage prostate cancer, a low-fat plant-based diet seems to have proven beneficial over a period of two years. Strengthening the findings was that the greater the level of patient adherence, the stronger the tumor suppressing effect, thus furthering strengthening the case for dietary intervention. Changes in gene expression were noted in other studies.

6. Conclusions

The plant-based diet, or vegan diet as it is also commonly known, is considered safe for all age groups by the American Academy of Nutrition and Dietetics, with recognized effects of lowering the risk of a number of diseases including ischemic heart disease and diabetes (78) which many prostate cancer patients, or those at risk for prostate cancer, either have or are at risk for, and even help treat those diseases. With no adverse effects noted and no contraindications, it would seem that dietary intervention would offer a cost effective way to reduce the risk of prostate cancer, and to treat those cases where watchful waiting is prescribed. It would likely enhance current standard treatments, while also lowering the risk of common comorbidities.

Future research is needed to further elucidate the mechanisms by which animal-derived foods induce prostate cancer and plant foods exert their chemoprotective effect. Further research is also needed to determine which plant foods, in addition to those already identified, have particular substantial chemoprotective effects. Research is needed to determine the efficacy of plant-based diets in high grade tumors, and advanced stages of prostate cancer with both high and low grade tumors. It also remains to be determined how important a risk factor the consumption of animal products is, compared to other risk factors such as age and family history.

References

1. Haenszel W, Kurihara M. (1968) Studies of Japanese migrants. I. Mortality from cancer and other diseases among Japanese in the United States. *J Natl Cancer Inst*. 40(1):43-68.
2. Shimizu H, Ross R, Bernstein L, Yatani R, Henderson B, et at. (1991) Cancers of the

How to cite this article: Rose S, Strombom A. A plant-based diet prevents and treats prostate cancer. Canc Therapy & Oncol Int J. 2018; 11(3): 555813.
DOI: 10.19080/CTOIJ.2018.11.555813.

prostate and breast among Japanese and white immigrants in Los Angeles County. *Br J Cancer*. 63(6):963-6.

3. Giovannucci E, Rimm E, Colditz G, Stampfer MJ, Ascherio A, et al. (1993) A prospective study of dietary fat and risk of prostate cancer. *J Natl Cancer Inst*. 85(19):1571-9.
4. Le Marchand L, Kolonel L, Wilkens L, Myers B, Hirohata T. (1994) Animal fat consumption and prostate cancer: a prospective study in Hawaii. *Epidemiology*. 5(3):276-82.
5. Fraser G. (1999) Associations between diet and cancer, ischemic heart disease, and all-cause mortality in non-Hispanic white California Seventh-day Adventists. *Am J Clin Nutr*. 70(3):532s-538s.
6. Stacewicz-Sapuntzakis M, Borthakur G, Burns J, Bowen P. (2008) Correlations of dietary patterns with prostate health. *Mol Nutr Food Res*. 52(1):114-130.
7. Lin P, Aronson W, Freedland S. (2015) Nutrition, dietary interventions and prostate cancer: the latest evidence. *BMC Medicine*. 13:3.
8. Ohwaki K, Endo F, Kachi Y, Hattori K, Muraishi O, et al. (2012) Relationship between dietary factors and prostate-specific antigen in healthy men. *Urol Int*. 89(3):270-4.
9. Bassett J, Severi G, Hodge A, MacInnis RJ, Gibson RA, et al. (2013) Plasma phospholipid fatty acids, dietary fatty acids and prostate cancer risk. *Int J Cancer*. 133(8):1882-91.
10. Fradet Y, Meyer F, Bairati I, Shadmani R, Moore L. (1999) Dietary fat and prostate cancer progression and survival. *Eur Urol*. 35(5-6):388-91.
11. Richman E, Kenfield S, Chavarro J, Stampfer MJ, Giovannucci EL, et al. (2013) Fat intake after diagnosis and risk of lethal prostate cancer and all-cause mortality. *JAMA Intern Med*. 173(14):1316-26.
12. Pelton K, Freeman M, Solomon K. (2012) Cholesterol and prostate cancer. *Curr Opin Pharmacol*. 12(6):751-759.
13. Morote J, Celma A, Planas J, Placer J, de Torres I, et al. (2014) Role of serum cholesterol and statin use in the risk of prostate cancer detection and tumor aggressiveness. *Int J Mol Sci*. 15(8):13615-23.
14. Yue S, Li J, Lee S, Lee HJ, Shao T, et al. (2014) Cholesteryl ester accumulation induced by PTEN loss and PI3K/AKT activation underlies human prostate cancer aggressiveness. *Cell Metab*. 19(3):393-406.
15. Sun Y, Sukumaran P, Varma A, Derry S, Sahmoun A, et al. (2014) Cholesterol-induced activation of TRPM7 regulates cell proliferation, migration, and viability of human prostate cells. *Biochem Biophys Acta*. 1843(9):1839-50.
16. Murai T. (2015) Cholesterol lowering: role in cancer prevention and treatment. *Biol Chem*. 396(1):1-11.
17. Zhuang L, Kim J, Adam R, Solomon K, Freeman M. (2005) Cholesterol targeting alters lipid raft composition and cell survival in prostate cancer cells and xenografts. *J Clin Invest*. 115(4):959-68.
18. Mostaghel E, Solomon K, Pelton K, Freeman M, Montgomery R. (2012) Impact of circulating cholesterol levels on growth and intratumoral androgen concentration of prostate tumors. *PLoS One*. 7(1):e30062.
19. Montgomery R, Mostaghel E, Vessella R, Hess DI, Kalhorn TF, et al. (2008) Maintenance of intratumoral androgens in metastatic prostate cancer: a mechanism for castration-resistant tumor growth. *Cancer Res*. 68(11):4447-54.
20. Stopsack K, Gerke T, Sinnott J, Penney KL, Tyekucheva S, et al. (2016) Cholesterol metabolism and prostate cancer lethality. *Cancer Res*. 76(16):4785-90.
21. Platz E, Clinton S, Giovannucci E. (2008) Association between plasma cholesterol and prostate cancer in the PSA. *Int J Cancer*. 123(7):1693-8.
22. Leon C, Locke J, Adomat H, Etinger SL, Twiddy AL, et al. (2010) Alterations in cholesterol

regulation contribute to the production of intratumoral androgens during progression to castration-resistant prostate cancer in a mouse xenograft model. *Prostate.* 70(4):390-400.

23. Lee B, Taylor M, Robinet P, Smith JD, Schweitzer J, et al. (2013) Dysregulation of cholesterol homeostasis in human prostate cancer through loss of ABCA1. *Cancer Res.* 73(3):1211-8.

24. Twiddy A, Cox M, Wasan K. (2012) Knockdown of scavenger receptor class B type I reduces prostate specific antigen secretion and viability of prostate cancer cells. *Prostate.* 72(9):955-65.

25. Murtola T, Syvälä H, Pennanen P, Bläuer M, Solakivi T. et al. (2012) The importance of LDL and cholesterol metabolism for prostate epithelial cell growth. *PLoS One.* 7(6):e39445.

26. Farwell W, D'Avolio L, Scranton R, Lawler E, Gaziano J. (2011) Statins and prostate cancer diagnosis and grade in a veterans population. *J Natl Cancer Inst.* 103(11):885-92.

27. Platz E, Leitzmann M, Visvanathan K, Rimm EB, Stampfer MJ, et al. (2006) Statin drugs and risk of advanced prostate cancer. *J Natl Cancer Inst.* 98(24):1819-25.

28. Yu O, Eberg M, Benayoun S, Aprikian S, Batist G, et al. (2014) Use of statins and the risk of death in patients with prostate cancer. *J Clin Oncol.* 32(1):5-11.

29. Allott E, Howard L, Cooperberg M, Kane CJ, Aronson WJ, et al. (2014) Postoperative statin use and risk of biochemical recurrence following radical prostatectomy: results from the Shared Equal Access Regional Cancer Hospital (SEARCH) database. *BJU Int.* 114(5):661-6.

30. Jespersen C, Nørgaard M, Friis S, Skriver C, Borre M. (2014) Statin use and risk of prostate cancer: A Danish population-based case–control study, 1997–2010. *Cancer Epidemiol.* 38(1):42-7.

31. Meyers C, Kashyap M. (2004) Pharmacologic elevation of high-density lipoproteins: recent insights on mechanism of action and atherosclerosis protection. *Curr Opin Cardiol.* 19(4):366-73.

32. Xia P, Vadas M, Rye K, Barter P, Gamble J. (1999) High density lipoproteins (HDL) interrupt the sphingosine kinase signaling pathway. A possible mechanism for protection against atherosclerosis by HDL. *J Biol Chem.* 274(46):33143-7.

33. Kotani K, Sekine Y, Ishikawa S, Ikpot I, Suzuki K, et al. (2013) High-density lipoprotein and prostate cancer: an overview. *J Epidemiol.* 23(5):313-9.

34. Thorogood M, Carter R, Benfield L, McPherson K, Mann JI. (1987) Plasma and lipoprotein cholesterol concentrations in people with different diets in Britain. *British Medical Journal (Clin Res Ed).* 295(6594):351–353.

35. Haddad EH, Berk LS, Kettering JD, Hubbard RW, Peters WR. (1999) Dietary intake and biochemical, hematologic, and immune status of vegans compared with nonvegetarians. *Am J Clin Nutr.* 70(3 Suppl):586S-593S.

36. Bergkvist C, Oberg M, Appelgren M, Becker W, Aune M, et al. (2008) Exposure to dioxin-like pollutants via different food commodities in Swedish children and young adults. *Food Chem Toxicol.* 46(11):3360-7.

37. Dougherty C, Henricks Holtz S, Reinert J, Panyacosit L, Axelrad D, et.al. (2000) Dietary exposures to food contaminants across the United States. *Environ Res.* 84(2):170-85.

38. Walker P, Rhubart-Berga P, McKenzie S, Kelling K, Lawrence R. (2005) Public health implications of meat production and consumption. *Public Health Nutrit.* 8(4):348-356.

39. Sasamoto T, Ushio F, Kikutani N, Saitoh Y, Yamaki Y, et al. (2006) Estimation of 1999-2004 dietary daily intake of PCDDs, PCDFs and dioxin-like PCBs by a total diet study in metropolitan Tokyo, Japan. *Chemosphere.* 64(4):634-41.

40. Bocio A, Domingo J. (2005) Daily intake of polychlorinated dibenzo-p-dioxins/polychlorinated dibenzofurans (PCDD/PCDFs) in

How to cite this article: Rose S, Strombom A. A plant-based diet prevents and treats prostate cancer. Canc Therapy & Oncol Int J. 2018; 11(3): 555813.
DOI: 10.19080/CTOIJ.2018.11.555813.

foodstuffs consumed in Tarragona, Spain: a review of recent studies (2001-2003) on human PCDD/PCDF exposure through the diet. *Environ Res*. 97(1):1-9.

41. Schecter A, Colacino J, Haffner D, Patel K, Opel M, et al. (2010) Perfluorinated compounds, polychlorinated biphenyls, and organochlorine pesticide contamination in composite food samples from Dallas, Texas, USA. *Environ Health Perspect*. 118(6):796-802.
42. Darnerud P, Atuma S, Aune M, Bierselius R, Glynn A, et.al. (2006) Dietary intake estimations of organohalogen contaminants (dioxins, PCB, PBDE and chlorinated pesticides, e.g. DDT) based on Swedish market basket data. *Food Chem Toxicol*. 44(9):1597-606.
43. Lim J, Park S, Jee S, Park H. (2015) Body concentrations of persistent organic pollutants and prostate cancer: a meta-analysis. *Environ Sci Pollut Res Int*. 22(15):11275-84.
44. Hardell L, Andersson S, Carlberg M, Bohr L, Van Bavel B, et al. (2006) Adipose tissue concentrations of persistent organic pollutants and the risk of prostate cancer. *J Occup Environ Med*. 48(7):700-7.
45. Cross A, Peters U, Kirsh V, Andriole GL, Reding D, et al. (2005) A prospective study of meat and meat mutagens and prostate cancer risk. *Cancer Res*. 65(24):11779-84.
46. Sinha R, Park Y, Graubard B, Leitzmann MF, Hollenbeck A, et al. (2009) Meat and meat-related compounds and risk of prostate cancer in a large prospective cohort study in the United States. *Am J Epidemiol*. 170(9):1165-77.
47. Powell J, Ghotbaddini M. (2014) Cancer-promoting and inhibiting effects of dietary compounds: role of the aryl hydrocarbon receptor (AhR). *Biochem Pharmacol (Los Angel)*. 3(1).
48. Sander A, Linseisen J, Rohrmann S. (2011) Intake of heterocyclic aromatic amines and the risk of prostate cancer in the EPIC-Heidelberg cohort. *Cancer Causes Control*. 22(1):109-14.
49. Zheng W, Lee S. (2009) Well-done meat intake, heterocyclic amine exposure, and cancer risk. *Nutr Cancer*. 61(4):437-46.
50. De Marzo A, Platz E, Sutcliffe S,Grönberg H, Drake CG, et al. (2007) Inflammation in prostate carcinogenesis. *Nat Rev Cancer*. 7(4):256-69.
51. Nelson W, Demarzo A, Yegnasubramanian S. (2014) The diet as a cause of human prostate cancer. *Cancer Treat Res*. 159:51-68.
52. Ahn YH, Hwang Y, Liu H, Wang XJ, Zhang Y, et al. (2010) Electrophilic tuning of the chemoprotective natural product sulforaphane. *Proc Natl Acad Sci USA*. 107(21):9590-9595.
53. Cohen J, Kristal A, Stanford J. (2000) Fruit and vegetable intakes and prostate cancer risk. *J Natl Cancer Inst*. 92(1):61-8.
54. Dinkova-Kostova A, Talalay P. (2008) Direct and indirect antioxidant properties of inducers of cytoprotective proteins. *Mol Nutr Food Res*. 52(Suppl 1):S128-38.
55. Allen N, Appleby P, Davey G, Key TJ. (2000) Hormones and diet: low insulin-like growth factor-I but normal bioavailable androgens in vegan men. *Br J Cancer*. 83(1):95-7.
56. Cohen P, Peehl D, Rosenfeld R. (1994) IGF axis in the prostate. *Horm Metab Res*. 26(2):81-4.
57. Chan J, Stampfer M, Giovannucci E, Gann PH, Ma J, et al. (1998) Plasma insulin-like growth factor-I and prostate cancer risk: a prospective study. *Science*. 279(5350):563-6.
58. Cao Y, Nimptsch K, Shui I, Platz EA, Wu K, et al. (2015) Prediagnostic plasma IGFBP-1, IGF-1 and risk of prostate cancer. *Int J Cancer*. 136(10):2418-26.
59. Walters D, Young P, Agus C, Knize MG, Boobis AR, et al. (2004) Cruciferous vegetable consumption alters the metabolism of the dietary carcinogen 2-amino-1-methyl-6-phenylimidazo[4,5-b]pyridine (PhIP) in humans. *Carcinogenesis*. 25(9):1659-69.

60. Krajcovicova-Kudlackova M, Blazicek P. (2005) C-reactive protein and nutrition. *Bratisl Lek Listy*. 106(11):345-7.

61. Chen C, Lin Y, Lin TK, Lin CT, Chan BC, et.al. (2008) Total cardiovascular risk profile of Taiwanese vegetarians. *Eur J Clin Nutr*. 62(1):138-44.

62. Askari F, Parizi M, Jessri M, Rashidkhani B. (2014) Fruit and vegetable intake in relation to prostate cancer in Iranian men: a case–control study. *Asian Pac J Cancer Prev*. 15(13):5223-7.

63. Liu B, Mao Q, Cao M, Xie L. (2012) Cruciferous vegetables intake and risk of prostate cancer: a meta-analysis. *Int J Urol*. 19(2):134-41.

64. Richman E, Carroll P, Chan J. (2012) Vegetable and fruit intake after diagnosis and risk of prostate cancer progression. *Int J Cancer*. 131(1):201-10.

65. Wang P, Aronson W, Huang M, Zhang Y, Lee RH. (2010) Green tea polyphenols and metabolites in prostatectomy tissue: implications for cancer prevention. *Cancer Prev Res (Phila)* 3(8):985-93.

66. Kurahashi N, Sasazuki S, Iwasaki M, Inoue M, Tsugane S, et al. (2008) Green tea consumption and prostate cancer risk in Japanese men: a prospective study. *Am J Epidemiol*. 167(1):71-7.

67. McLarty J, Bigelow R, Smith M, Elmajian D, Ankem M, et al. (2009) Tea polyphenols decrease serum levels of prostate-specific antigen, hepatocyte growth factor, and vascular endothelial growth factor in prostate cancer patients and inhibit production of hepatocyte growth factor and vascular endothelial growth factor in vitro. *Cancer Prev Res (Phila)*. 2(7):673-82.

68. Gann P, Ma J, Giovannucci E, Willett W, Sacks FM, et al. (1999) Lower prostate cancer risk in men with elevated plasma lycopene levels: results of a prospective analysis. *Cancer Res*. 59(6):1225-30.

69. Kucuk O, Sarkar F, Djuric Z, Sakr W, Pollak MN, et al. (2002) Effects of lycopene supplementation in patients with localized prostate cancer. *Exp Biol Med (Maywood)*. 227(10):881-5.

70. Chen L, Stacewicz-Sapuntzakis M, Duncan C, Sharifi R, Ghosh L, et al. (2001) Oxidative DNA damage in prostate cancer patients consuming tomato sauce-based entrees as a whole-food intervention. *J Natl Cancer Inst*. 93(24):1872-9.

71. van Breemen R, Sharifi R, Viana M, Pajkovic N,Zhu D, et al. (2011) Antioxidant effects of lycopene in African American men with prostate cancer or benign prostate hyperplasia: a randomized, controlled trial. *Cancer Prev Res (Phila)*. 4(5):711-8.

72. Hsing A, Chokkalingam A, Gao Y, Madigan MP, Deng J, et al. (2002) Allium vegetables and risk of prostate cancer: a population-based study. *J Natl Cancer Inst*. 94(21):1648-51.

73. Ornish D, Weidner G, Fair W, Marlin R, Pettengill EB, et al. (2005) Intensive lifestyle changes may affect the progression of prostate cancer. *J Urol*. 174(3):1065-9.

74. Frattaroli J, Weidner G, Dnistrian A, Kemp C, Daubenmier JJ, et al. (2008) Clinical events in prostate cancer lifestyle trial: results from two years of follow-up. *Urology*. 72(6):1319-23.

75. Ornish D, Magbanua M, Weidner G, Weinberg V, Kemp C, et al. (2008) Changes in prostate gene expression in men undergoing an intensive nutrition and lifestyle intervention. *Proc Natl Acad Sci USA*. 105(24):8369-74.

76. Mosher C, Sloane R, Morey M, Snyder DC, Cohen HJ, et al. (2009) Associations between lifestyle factors and quality of life among older long-term breast, prostate, and colorectal cancer survivors. *Cancer*. 115(17):4001-9.

77. Avery K, Donovan J, Horwood J, Neal DE, Hamdy FC, et al. (2014) The importance of dietary change for men diagnosed with and at risk of prostate cancer: a multi-centre interview study with men, their partners and health professionals. *BMC Fam Pract*. 15:81.

How to cite this article: Rose S, Strombom A. A plant-based diet prevents and treats prostate cancer. Canc Therapy & Oncol Int J. 2018; 11(3): 555813.
DOI: 10.19080/CTOIJ.2018.11.555813.

78. Melina V, Craig W, Levin S. (2016) Position of the academy of nutrition and dietetics: vegetarian diets. *J Acad Nutr Diet*. 116(12):1970-80.

Cancer Therapy & Oncology
International Journal
ISSN: 2473-554X

Juniper Publishers
key to the Researchers

Review Article
Volume 17 Issue 1 - October 2020
DOI: 10.19080/CTOIJ.2020.17.555955

Canc Therapy & Oncol Int J

Breast Cancer Prevention with a Plant-Based Diet

Stewart Rose and Amanda Strombom*

Plant-Based Diets in Medicine, USA

Submission: October 5, 2020; **Published:** October 22, 2020

***Correspondence Address:** Amanda Strombom, Plant-Based Diets in Medicine,
12819 SE 38th St, #427, Bellevue, WA 98006.

Abstract

Diet may be an independent risk factor for breast cancer, along with alcohol, physical activity, BMI and smoking. Several epidemiological studies show a decreased risk of breast cancer for vegetarians and vegans.

Studies show an increased risk in women exposed to heterocyclic amines (HCAs), polyaromatic hydrocarbons (PAHs) and persistent organic pollutants (POPs). POPs resist environmental degradation and accumulate in animal adipose tissue, while PAHs and HCAs are produced during cooking of meat. In addition to reducing their exposure to these carcinogenic compounds, those following a plant-based diet benefit from the increased consumption of phytochemicals and fiber found in plant foods. In particular, studies show that soy may reduce the risk of breast cancer and breast cancer recurrence, due to its isoflavone content. Dietary fiber also reduces the risk of breast cancer, most likely by affecting estrogen levels.

Most breast cancer patients tend to be older. The plant-based diet can reduce the risk of common comorbidities in post-menopausal women such as type II diabetes, coronary artery disease, arthritis, hypertension and thyroid disease. The plant-based diet is safe and has no adverse reactions or contraindications. It presents a valuable additional therapeutic measure to chemotherapy, radiation and surgery which will continue as standard of care.

Keywords

Breast cancer, carcinogens, dietary fiber, estrogen, heterocyclic amines, persistent organic pollutants, plant-based diet, polyaromatic hydrocarbons, phytochemicals, vegan

Abbreviations

BMI – Body mass index; ER+ – Estrogen receptor positive; HCAs – Heterocyclic amines; HER2 – Human epidermal growth factor receptor-2; PAHs – Polyaromatic hydrocarbons; PCBs – Polychlorinated biphenyls; POPs – Persistent organic pollutants; PR+ – Progesterone receptor positive.

Introduction

The World Cancer Research Fund (WCRF) and American Cancer Society (ACS) cancer prevention guidelines recommend maintaining a healthy weight, undertaking at least 150 minutes of moderate intensity exercise per week, limiting alcohol consumption, and eating a plant-based diet. (1) Recent expert reports estimate that successful lifestyle changes could prevent 25% to 30% of cases of breast cancer. (1)

In a study of post-menopausal women, the lowest quintile level of a combination of selected modifiable risk factors (diet, alcohol, physical activity, BMI, and smoking), compared to those in the highest quintile level had 30%, 37%, and 30% lower risk for overall, ER+/PR+, and HER2+ breast cancers respectively. (2) This study observed inverse associations between the modifiable factors and risk of breast cancer, irrespective of nodal status, tumor grade, and stage of the disease. Most individual lifestyle factors were independently associated with the risk of breast cancer.

It appears that diet may be an independent risk factor for breast cancer. In addition, studies show that those who follow a plant-based diet have lower rates of obesity, a risk factor for breast cancer independent of diet. For instance, in one study patients following a plant-based diet had an average BMI of only 23. (3) In light of the fact that a plant-based diet helps reduce the risk and recurrence of both prostate cancer (4) and colon cancer (5), it's not surprising that it is efficacious for breast cancer as well.

2. Epidemiology

Several studies show a decreased risk of breast cancer for vegetarians and vegans:

In a study of Taiwanese vegetarian women, long term vegetarians had a 58% reduced risk of breast cancer, compared to women following an omnivorous diet. Looking at specific foods, frequent consumption of meat and animal fat increased the risk of breast cancer 2.2 times, and processed meat increased the risk 49%, while soy isoflavones decreased the risk. (6)

In a study of women who follow a healthy lifestyle, those following a vegan diet showed a not-quite-significant 22% reduced risk of breast cancer. (7)

A study of lifelong South Asian vegetarians who migrated to Britain showed a not-quite-significant risk reduction of 23% for breast cancer. (8)

A metastudy study comparing the highest to the lowest category, red meat (unprocessed) consumption was associated with a 6% higher breast cancer risk and processed meat consumption was associated with a 9% higher breast cancer risk both before and after menopause, although results were not quite significant for premenopause. (9)

3. Carcinogenic compounds

Research has shown the carcinogenicity of persistent organic pollutants (POPs), heterocyclic amines (HCAs), and polyaromatic hydrocarbons (PAHs). Meat and other animal products are the main sources of these compounds in the human diet.

3.1 Persistent Organic Pollutants

Persistent organic pollutants (POPs) are a group of synthetic organic chemicals used for industrial, agricultural or domestic purposes, that persist in the environment and progressively bioaccumulate and concentrate in the food chain due to their

How to cite this article: Rose S, Strombom A. Breast cancer prevention with a plant-based diet. Canc Therapy & Oncol Int J. 2020; 17(1): 555955.
DOI: 10.19080/CTOIJ.2020.17.555955.

lipophilic properties. (10, 11) They include dioxins, furans, polychlorinated biphenyls (PCBs), and organochlorine pesticides, chemicals mainly created by industrial activities either intentionally or as by-products. (12) The introduction of POPs into the environment from anthropogenic activities has resulted in their widespread dispersal and accumulation in soils and bodies of water, ecological food chains, and in humans where they are known to induce toxic effects.

There is evidence of long range transport of these substances to regions where they have never been used or produced, resulting in exposure of most human populations to POPs through consumption of fat-containing food such as fish, dairy products, and meat, (13, 14, 15) with the highest POP concentrations being commonly found in fatty fish. (12, 13, 14, 15, 16, 17, 18) Due to their ubiquity in the environment and lipophilic properties, there is mounting concern over the potential risks of human exposure to POPs. (13)

A primary consideration in the evaluation of chemicals is the potential for substances to be absorbed and retained in an organism's tissues at concentrations sufficient to pose health concerns. Substances that exhibit properties that enable biomagnification in the food chain are of particular concern due to the elevated long-term exposures these substances pose to higher trophic organisms, including humans. (19)

POPs measured in breast adipose tissue are associated with higher breast cancer incidence. (20) Given the abundance of adipose tissue in the human breast, mammary epithelial cells' exposure to POPs sequestered in breast adipose tissue may promote carcinogenesis and progression of mammary cancers (21).

POPs measured in breast adipose tissue were associated with higher breast cancer incidence and were associated with worse breast cancer prognosis and mortality. (20)

3.2 Heterocyclic Amines

HCAs are mutagenic and carcinogenic compounds formed in meat and fish prepared by high temperature cooking methods, such as frying, grilling and barbecuing. The precursors are amino acids, reducing sugars and creatine, found specifically in muscle meat. (22)

Steck et al. found an association between higher lifetime consumption of grilled meats and fish and increased incidence of post-menopausal breast cancer. (23)

Laboratory studies of HCAs in systems using cultured breast cancer cells demonstrated that these chemicals can mimic estrogen, and they also can have direct effects on cell division processes in ways that might enhance the development of tumors. (24)

One of the HCAs, 2-amino-1-methyl-6-phenylimidazo[4,5-b]pyridine (PhIP), the most abundant HCA in the Western diet, has been found to be a mammary gland carcinogen in rats. (22) Studies demonstrate that PhIP is also a significant DNA-damaging agent in humans. (25)

Studies of both milk and cells from the ducts of women's breast revealed the presence of DNA adducts in association with HCAs (26, 27).

3.3 Polyaromatic Hydrocarbons

When meat and fish are cooked over an open flame or smoked, PAHs are formed. (28) If the grilled food is in direct contact with the flame, pyrolysis of the drippings from meat or fish generates PAHs that can be deposited on its surface. Even if not in direct contact, fat dripping onto the flame or hot coals generates these compounds that can then be carried back onto the surface of the food (29, 30).

PAHs are lipophilic and stored in fat tissue (31) and have been associated with breast cancer incidence. (23) The breasts are particularly susceptible to aromatic carcinogenesis, and the implementation of biomarkers has provided promising insights regarding PAH-DNA adducts in breast cancer. The use of biomarkers measuring these adducts assesses the exposure to eliminate bias inherent in self reporting measures, in case-control studies investigating the link between PAHs and cancer. (30)

PAH-DNA adducts are a biomarker of recent exposure and reflect DNA damage, a step in carcinogenesis. Detectable PAH-DNA adducts, or their proxy, have been consistently linked to breast cancer in previous studies (32, 33, 34) with one exception (35).

In 1996, Li et al. assessed aromatic adducts in human tissue from breast cancer patients undergoing mastectomy versus breast tissue from non-cancer patients undergoing reduction mammoplasty. Aromatic DNA adducts, although detected in all samples, were significantly higher in the breast cancer patients versus the healthy controls. These results indicate that PAHs may play a role in the development of breast cancer. (36) The association between PAH-DNA adducts and breast cancer incidence may be elevated even more among overweight/obese women. (31)

4. Chemoprotective effects of plant-foods

In addition to reducing the intake of harmful substances by not consuming animal products, those following a plant-based diet have the advantage of consuming large quantities of substances that help block the development of cancerous cells. These substances are called phytochemicals. Dietary fiber found in plant foods can also play a beneficial role.

Phytochemicals, often referred to as phytonutrients, are natural bioactive components rich in foods such as vegetables, fruits, whole grain products, nuts and seeds, and legumes. (37)

Cancerous tissue transformation, developing usually over years or even decades of life, is a highly complex process involving strong stressors damaging DNA, chronic inflammation, interaction between relevant molecular pathways, and cellular cross-talk within the neighboring tissues. (38)

The flavonoids, carotenoids, phenolic acids, and organosulfur compounds affect a number of cancer-related pathways. Phytochemicals may positively affect processes of cell signaling, cell cycle regulation, oxidative stress response, and inflammation. They can modulate non-coding RNAs, upregulate tumor suppressive miRNAs, and downregulate oncogenic miRNAs that synergically inhibits cancer cell growth and cancer stem cell self-renewal. (38)

4.1 Soy

The phytochemicals in soy have been the most studied. Questions were initially raised with regard to the isoflavone phytoestrogens found in soy, expressing concern that soy consumption could lead to the potential for an increased risk of breast cancer. However, these fears were unfounded. There is good evidence that soy foods not only do not raise the risk of breast cancer, but actually can lower it, especially when consumed early in life.

How to cite this article: Rose S, Strombom A. Breast cancer prevention with a plant-based diet. Canc Therapy & Oncol Int J. 2020; 17(1): 555955.
DOI: 10.19080/CTOIJ.2020.17.555955.

Soy may also lower the risk of recurrence of breast cancer in adults.

Phytoestrogens are naturally occurring polycyclic phenols found in certain plants, with high levels in soy. These are chemicals that may have very weak estrogenic effects when they are ingested and metabolized. One important group of phytoestrogens are isoflavones. (39) The absorption and metabolism of phytoestrogens demonstrate large interindividual variability, which may relate to differences in both human pharmacokinetics and metabolism by intestinal bacteria. (39)

Compared to physiologic estrogens such as 17β-estradiol, isoflavones have approximately 100 times weaker affinities. (40) A major difference between endogenous and dietary estrogens is that once made in the ovaries, the former reach responsive tissues in the unconjugated, i.e., biologically active, form whereas dietary estrogens are almost entirely conjugated, even in portal blood just after their absorption from the intestine. (41)

In an extensive and authoritative review, Messina finds that "clinical trials consistently show that isoflavone intake does not adversely affect markers of breast cancer risk, including mammographic density and cell proliferation. Furthermore, prospective epidemiologic studies involving over 11,000 women from the USA and China show that postdiagnosis soy intake statistically significantly reduces recurrence and improves survival." (42)

In one study, premenopausal women were fed soy isoflavones for approximately 100 days and urine samples were collected to quantify estrogen excretion levels (43). This study demonstrated that soy isoflavone consumption may exert cancer-preventive effects by decreasing estrogen synthesis, presumably by altering aromatase enzyme activity, based upon previously published reports. (43)

Research shows the consumption of soy does not increase the risk of breast cancer (44) and may significantly reduce the risk of recurrence. One study showed that generous amounts of soy lowered the risk of breast cancer. (45) Soy appears safe for breast cancer patients both premenopausal and post-menopausal.

Breast cancer is known to be less common in countries where soy consumption is common. (44) The difference in breast cancer incidence rates between Western and Eastern women are largely influenced by changes in lifestyle and diet rather than genetics (46). Several reports indicate that the occurrence of breast cancer is considerably lower in Asian women compared with other populations because they incorporate high levels of isoflavones as part of their regular diet (47, 48) The amount of dietary isoflavonoids consumed is geographically dependent. For instance, the mean daily isoflavone intake of 30 to 50mg among older individuals in Japan (49), whereas in the United States and Europe, per capita intake is less than 3mg. (50, 51)

As vegetarians and vegans are typically frequent soy consumers, serum isoflavone levels may increase dramatically in these groups (6). In one study it was found that the mean isoflavone level of vegetarians was 25.9mg. Therefore, in addition to finding that vegetarians had lower breast cancer risk, the results support a possible chemopreventive effect of isoflavones. (6)

Several reports demonstrate that high soy consumption during childhood may reduce one's risk of developing breast cancer later in life and that the risk may be further reduced by soy intake as an adult. (52, 53, 54, 55, 56)

In one study, substituting median intakes of dairy milk users with those of soy milk consumers was associated with 32% reduced risk of breast cancer. Similar-sized reductions of risk was found among pre- and post-menopausal cases. (57)

In another study, high dietary intake of soy isoflavones was associated with lower risk of recurrence among post-menopausal patients with breast cancer positive for estrogen and progesterone receptors, and for those who were receiving anastrozole as endocrine therapy. (58)

Soy does not appear to interfere with tamoxifen or anastrozole therapy (59) Among women with breast cancer, soy food consumption was significantly associated with decreased 34% risk of death and a 33% recurrence for the highest quartile of soy consumption. (60) The reduced risk was evident among women with either ER-positive or ER-negative breast cancer, and was present in both users and non-users of tamoxifen.

In one study, soy isoflavones consumed at levels comparable to those in Asian populations may reduce the risk of cancer recurrence in women receiving tamoxifen therapy and moreover, appears not to interfere with tamoxifen efficacy (61)

The positions of the American Cancer Society (62) and the American Institute for Cancer Research (63) are that soyfoods can be safely consumed by women with breast cancer. In addition, an evidence-based conclusion in response to a recent clinical inquiry published in the Journal of Family Practice, was that post-diagnosis soy intake improves the prognosis of breast cancer patients (64).

4.2 Dietary Fiber

Epidemiological studies have shown conflicting results for the relationship between intake of dietary fiber and breast cancer. (65) While there has been some inconsistency of results from studies of fiber and its association with breast cancer, a random-effects meta-analysis of prospective observational studies demonstrated that high total fiber consumption was associated with a reduced risk of breast cancer. This finding was consistent for soluble fiber as well as for women with premenopausal and postmenopausal breast cancer. (65)

Dietary fiber reduces the risk of breast cancer, most likely by decreasing the level of estrogen in the blood circulation. (66, 67, 68, 69, 70, 71, 72, 73) Results of the most recent meta-analysis published in 2012, which included 17 publications, supported this hypothesis (74). An increase in consumption of dietary fiber enhances its protective effect, indicating a possible dose response relationship. (75)

A study of vegetarian women found that they have an increased fecal output, which leads to increased fecal excretion of estrogen and a decreased plasma concentration of estrogen due to the much larger amount of fiber they consume. (66)

Components of dietary fiber not only absorb and retain moisture, but more importantly, combine with harmful and carcinogenic substances in the gut and promote their discharge and decomposition. (76)

It may be that fiber has a greater effect on breast cancer risk in the context of a vegetarian diet than in an omnivorous one. Further studies are needed.

5. Clinical considerations

Most breast cancer patients tend to be older. When treating these patients, comorbidities must

How to cite this article: Rose S, Strombom A. Breast cancer prevention with a plant-based diet. Canc Therapy & Oncol Int J. 2020; 17(1): 555955.
DOI: 10.19080/CTOIJ.2020.17.555955.

be taken into account. The prevalence of comorbidities among women treated for breast cancer aged older than 66 is 32.2%, a statistic comparable to those without cancer at 31.8% (77) The presence of comorbidities in patients with cancer has been negatively associated with patients' health outcomes. Poorer survival from cancer has been found overall in cancer survivors with comorbidities compared to those without. (78, 79)

In developed countries, 40% of breast cancer patients are older than 65 years of age at diagnosis, of whom 16% additionally suffer from diabetes. (80) Older women are more likely to die of diseases other than breast cancer, and cardiovascular disease (CVD) is the most frequent cause. (81, 82) In older, postmenopausal women, the risk of mortality attributable to CVD is higher in breast cancer survivors than in women without a history of breast cancer. This greater risk typically manifests itself 7 years after the diagnosis of breast cancer, which highlights the need to reduce the additional burden of CVD during this time frame with early recognition and treatment of CVD risk factors. (83)

One study of breast cancer patients showed that the prevalence of hypercholesterolemia at 22%, arthritis at 44% hypertension at 44% and thyroid disease at 30%. (84) A plant-based diet can help prevent and treat these diseases and can be very efficacious. (85, 86, 87, 88) For instance in one study a plant-based diet was found to be twice as efficacious in treating type 2 diabetes as Metformin. (89) A plant-based diet can also lower cholesterol as much as lovastatin. (90) Angina can also be treated with a plant-based diet, with one study showing 74% of patients put on a plant-based diet had no pain after 12 weeks and an additional 9% had pain reduction. (91) A plant based can lower the risk of both Grave's disease and Hashimoto's thyroiditis (88) and treat arthritis (86, 87). In treating their comorbidities, while also reducing the risk of breast cancer recurrence, the plant-based diet thus provides a double benefit for the patient.

Patient compliance on plant-based diets has been good in almost all studies. The degree of compliance has often been very high. For instance, one study obtained a 99% compliance. (92) In a 22-week study 94% of subjects on a vegan diet were compliant. (93) In a somewhat longer study, 84% of the participants in each group completed all 24 weeks. (94) In studies of patients placed on plant-based diets for coronary artery disease, high compliance has been noted even over several years. For instance, one study of patients placed on a plant-based diet showed 89% compliance for 3.7 years. (95)

Compliance may be enhanced when the rationale for the treatment, and that the treatment is backed by research, is explained to the patient. (96) The doctor should prescribe the treatment by writing it down on a prescription form or other stationery with the physician's name on it. This written prescription is not only valuable to the patient, but can also be valuable in enlisting the support of family, friends and social contacts.

It may take a few weeks for the treatment effects to become evident. Lab work and follow up visits should be scheduled accordingly.

6. Discussion

There are multiple risk factors for breast cancer. Some are not modifiable but other risk factors are modifiable, in particular those which are lifestyle related. A plant-based diet can help reduce the risk of breast cancer and its recurrence. While getting sufficient physical exercise, and reducing consumption of alcohol and cigarettes are well established, fewer patients are aware of the impact of their dietary choices. It is important for the physician to explain how their food choices impact their risk of breast cancer.

Some plant foods seem to be especially valuable. Soy, especially when its consumption starts before puberty, can reduce the risk of breast cancer. Soy may also have some efficacy in preventing recurrence of breast cancer especially when consumed in generous amounts. Soy is now widely considered safe.

The plant-based diet has no adverse reactions and no contraindications. It can safely be used as an adjunct to pharmacotherapy. It presents a valuable additional therapeutic measure to chemotherapy, radiation and surgery which will continue as standard of care. It also helps provide some sense of locus of control that many oncology patients desire.

Vegetarian and vegan diets are not so unusual as they once were. Patient awareness of these diets is much higher than they used to be, and thus prescribing a plant-based diet is likely to be met with higher patient acceptance than in the past.

References

1. Harvie M, Howell A, Evans DG. (2015) Can diet and lifestyle prevent breast cancer: what is the evidence? *Am Soc Clin Oncol Educ Book*. e66-e73.
2. Arthur R, Wassertheil-Smoller S, Manson JE, Luo J, Snetselaar L, et al. (2018) The Combined Association of Modifiable Risk Factors with Breast Cancer Risk in the Women's Health Initiative. *Cancer Prev Res*. 11(6):317–326.
3. Tonstad S, Butler T, Yan R, Fraser G. (2009) Type of Vegetarian Diet, Body Weight, and Prevalence of Type 2 Diabetes. *Diabetes Care*. 32(5):791–796.
4. Rose S, Strombom A. (2018) A plant-based diet prevents and treats prostate cancer. *Canc Therapy & Oncol Int J*. 11(3):555813.
5. Rose S, Strombom A. (2019) Colorectal Cancer Prevention with a Plant-Based Diet. *Canc Therapy & Oncol Int J*. 15(2):555906.
6. Chang YJ, Hou YC, Chen LJ, Wu JH, Wu CC, et al. (2017) Is vegetarian diet associated with a lower risk of breast cancer in Taiwanese women? *BMC Public Health*. 17(1):800.
7. Penniecook-Sawyers JA, Jaceldo-Siegl K, Fan J, Beeson L, Knutson S, et al. (2016) Vegetarian dietary patterns and the risk of breast cancer in a low-risk population. *Br J Nutr*. 115(10):1790-1797.
8. Silva IDS, Mangtani P, McCormack V, Bhakta D, Sevak L, et al. (2002) Lifelong vegetarianism and risk of breast cancer: a population-based case-control study among South Asian migrant women living in England. *Int J Cancer*. 99(2):238-44.
9. Farvid MS, Stern MC, Norat T, Sasazuki S, Vineis P, et al. (2018) Consumption of red and processed meat and breast cancer incidence: A systematic review and meta-analysis of prospective studies. *Int J Cancer*. 143(11):2787-2799.
10. Connell DW, Miller GJ, Mortimer MR, Shaw GR, Anderson SM. (1999) Persistent Lipophilic Contaminants and Other Chemical Residues in the Southern Hemisphere. *Crit Rev Environ Sci Technol*. 29:47–82.
11. Kelly BC, Ikonomou MG, Blair JD, Morin AE, Gobas FAPC. (2007) Food Web-Specific Biomagnification of Persistent Organic Pollutants. *Science*. 317:236–239.
12. Bergkvist C, Oberg M, Appelgren M, Becker W, Aune M, et al. (2008) Exposure to dioxin-like pollutants via different food commodities in Swedish children and young adults. *Food Chem Toxicol*. 11:3360-7.
13. Dougherty C, Henricks Holtz S, Reinert J, Panyacosit L, Axelrad D, et al. (2000) Dietary

How to cite this article: Rose S, Strombom A. Breast cancer prevention with a plant-based diet. Canc Therapy & Oncol Int J. 2020; 17(1): 555955.
DOI: 10.19080/CTOIJ.2020.17.555955.

exposures to food contaminants across the United States. *Environ Res*. 84(2):170-85.

14. Walker P, Rhubart-Berga P, McKenzie S, Kelling K, Lawrence R. (2005) Public health implications of meat production and consumption. *Public Health Nutrit*. 8(4):348-356.
15. Sasamoto T, Ushio F, Kikutani N, Saitoh Y, Yamaki Y, et al. (2006) Estimation of 1999-2004 dietary daily intake of PCDDs, PCDFs and dioxin-like PCBs by a total diet study in metropolitan Tokyo, Japan. *Chemosphere*. 64(4):634-41.
16. Bocio A, Domingo J. (2005) Daily intake of polychlorinated dibenzo-p-dioxins/polychlorinated dibenzofurans (PCDD/PCDFs) in foodstuffs consumed in Tarragona, Spain: a review of recent studies (2001-2003) on human PCDD/PCDF exposure through the diet. *Environ Res*. 97(1):1-9.
17. Schecter A, Colacino J, Haffner D, Patel K, Opel M, et al. (2010) Perfluorinated compounds, polychlorinated biphenyls, and organochlorine pesticide contamination in composite food samples from Dallas, Texas, USA. *Environ Health Perspect*. 118(6):796-802.
18. Darnerud P, Atuma S, Aune M, Bierselius R, Glynn A, et al. (2006) Dietary intake estimations of organohalogen contaminants (dioxins, PCB, PBDE and chlorinated pesticides, e.g. DDT) based on Swedish market basket data. *Food Chem Toxicol*. 44(9):1597-606.
19. Weisbrod AV, Woodburn KB, Koelmans AA, Parkerton TF, McElroy AE, et al. (2009) Evaluation of bioaccumulation using in vivo laboratory and field studies. *Integr Environ Assess Manag*. 5(4):598-623.
20. Ennour-Idrissi K, Ayotte P, Diorio C. (2019) Persistent Organic Pollutants and Breast Cancer: A Systematic Review and Critical Appraisal of the Literature. *Cancers (Basel)*. 11(8):1063.
21. Phillips KP, Foster WG. (2008) Key Developments in Endocrine Disrupter Research and Human Health. *J Toxicol Environ Health Part B*. 11:322–344.
22. Sinha R, Snyderwine E. (2001) Heterocyclic amines (HCAS) and risk of breast cancer. *Breast Cancer Res*. 3(Suppl 1):A60.
23. Steck SE, Gaudet MM, Eng SM, Britton JA, Teitelbaum SL, et al. (2007) Cooked meat and risk of breast cancer—lifetime versus recent dietary intake. *Epidemiology*. 18:373–382.
24. Gooderham NJ, Creton S, Lauber SN, Zhu H. (2006) Mechanisms of action of the carcinogenic heterocyclic amine PhIP. *Toxicol Lett*. 2006;168:269–277.
25. Bessette EE, Spivack SD, Goodenough AK, Wang T, Pinto S, et al. (2010) Identification of carcinogen DNA adducts in human saliva by linear quadrupole ion trap/multistage tandem mass spectrometry. *Chem Res Toxicol*. 23(7):1234-1244.
26. Thompson PA, DeMarini DM, Kadlubar FF, McClure GY, Brooks LR, et al. (2002) Evidence for the presence of mutagenic arylamines in human breast milk and DNA adducts in exfoliated breast ductal epithelial cells. *Environ Mol Mutagen*. 39:134–142.
27. Turesky J. (2007) Formation and biochemistry of carcinogenic heterocyclic aromatic amines in cooked meats. *Toxicol Lett*. 168:219–227.
28. Knize MG, Salmon CP, Pais P, Felton JS. (1999) Food heating and the formation of heterocyclic aromatic amine and polycyclic aromatic hydrocarbon mutagens/carcinogens. *Adv Exp Med Biol*. 459:179–193.
29. Lijinsky W, Shubik P. (1964) Benzo (a) pyrene and other polynuclear hydrocarbons in charcoal-broiled meat. *Science*. 145(3627):53-55.
30. Zelinkova Z, Wenzl T. (2015) The Occurrence of 16 EPA PAHs in Food – A Review. *Polycycl Aromat Compd*. 35(2-4):248-284.
31. Niehoff N, White AJ, McCullough LE, Steck SE, Beyea J, et al. (2017) Polycyclic aromatic hydrocarbons and postmenopausal breast cancer: An evaluation of effect measure

modification by body mass index and weight change. *Environ Res*. 152:17-25.

32. Gammon MD, Sagiv SK, Eng SM, Shantahumar S, Gaudet MM, et al. (2004) Polycyclic aromatic hydrocarbon-DNA adducts and breast cancer: a pooled analysis. *Arch Environ Health*. 59(12):640–649.
33. Li D, Zhang W, Sahin AA, Hittelman WN. (1999) DNA adducts in normal tissue adjacent to breast cancer: a review. *Cancer Detect Prev*. 23:454–462.
34. Rundle A, Tang D, Hibshoosh H, Estabrook A, Schnabel F, et al. (2000) The relationship between genetic damage from polycyclic aromatic hydrocarbons in breast tissue and breast cancer. *Carcinogenesis*. 21(7):1281–1289.
35. Saieva C, Peluso M, Masala G, Munnia A, Ceroti M, et al. (2011) Bulky DNA adducts and breast cancer risk in the prospective EPIC-Italy study. *Breast Cancer Res Treat.* 129:477–484.
36. Li D, Wang M, Dhingra K, Hittelman WN. (1996) Aromatic DNA adducts in adjacent tissues of breast cancer patients: clues to breast cancer etiology. *Cancer Res*. 56(2):287–293.
37. Xiao J, Bai W. (2019) Bioactive phytochemicals. *Critical Reviews in Food Science and Nutrition*. 59(6):827-829.
38. Kapinova A, Kubatka P, Golubnitschaja O, Kello M, Zubor P, et al. (2018) Dietary phytochemicals in breast cancer research: anticancer effects and potential utility for effective chemoprevention. *Environ Health Prev Med*. 23:36.
39. National Biomonitoring Program. (2017) Biomonitoring Summary. *Centers for Disease Control and Prevention*. Available at: https://www.cdc.gov/biomonitoring/Phytoestrogens_BiomonitoringSummary.html. Accessed Sept 30, 2020.
40. Kuiper G, Carlsson B, Grandien K, Enmark E, Häggblad J et al. (1997) Comparison of the ligand binding specificity and transcript tissue distribution of estrogen receptors alpha and beta. *Endocrinology*. 138(3):863–887.
41. Sfakianos J, Coward L, Kirk M, Barnes S. (1997) Intestinal uptake and biliary excretion of the isoflavone genistein in the rat. *J Nutr*. 127(7):1260–1268.
42. Messina M. (2016) Impact of soy foods on the development of breast cancer and the prognosis of breast cancer patients. *Forsch Komplementmed*. 23(2):75-80.
43. Xu X, Duncan AM, Merz BE, Kurzer MS. (1998) Effects of soy isoflavones on estrogen and phytoestrogen metabolism in premenopausal women. *Cancer Epidemiol Biomarkers Prev*. 7(12):1101–1108.
44. Pisani P, Parkin DM, Bray F, Ferlay J. (1999) Estimates of the worldwide mortality from 25 cancers in 1990. *Int J Cancer*. 83:18-29.
45. Wei Y, Lv J, Guo Y, Bian Z, Gao M, et al. (2020) Soy intake and breast cancer risk: a prospective study of 300,000 Chinese women and a dose–response meta-analysis. *Eur J Epidemiol*. 35:567–578.
46. Parkin DM, Khlat M. (1996) Studies of cancer in migrants: rationale and methodology. *Eur J Cancer*. 32A(5):761–771.
47. Mense SM, Hei TK, Ganju RK, Bhat HK. (2008) Phytoestrogens and breast cancer prevention: Possible mechanisms of action. *Environ Health Perspect*. 116(4):426–433.
48. Miller PE, Snyder DC. (2012) Phytochemicals and cancer risk: A review of the epidemiological evidence. *Nutr Clin Pract*. 27(5):599–612.
49. Messina M, Nagata C, Wu AH. (2006) Estimated asian adult soy protein and isoflavone intakes. *Nutr Cancer*. 55(1):1–12.
50. Bai W, Wang C, Ren C. (2014) Intakes of total and individual flavonoids by US adults. *Int J Food Sci Nutr*. 65(1):9–20.
51. Rizzo NS, Jaceldo-Siegl K, Sabate J, Fraser GE. (2013) Nutrient profiles of vegetarian and nonvegetarian dietary patterns. *J Acad Nutr Diet*. 113(12):1610–161.

How to cite this article: Rose S, Strombom A. Breast cancer prevention with a plant-based diet. Canc Therapy & Oncol Int J. 2020; 17(1): 555955.
DOI: 10.19080/CTOIJ.2020.17.555955.

52. Verheus M, van-Gils CH, Keinan-Boker L, Grace PB, Bingham SA. (2007) Plasma phytoestrogens and subsequent breast cancer risk. *J Clin Oncol*. 25(6):648–655.

53. Wu AH, Ziegler RG, Nomura AM, West DW, Kolonel LN, et al. (1998) Soy intake and risk of breast cancer in Asians and Asian Americans. *Am J Clin Nutr*. 68(6):1437S–1443S.

54. Shu XO, Jin F, Dai Q, Wen W, Potter JD, et al. (2001) Soyfood intake during adolescence and subsequent risk of breast cancer among Chinese women. *Cancer Epidemiol Biomark Prev*. 10(5):483–488.

55. Wu AH, Wan P, Hankin J, Tseng CC, Yu MC, et al. (2002) Adolescent and adult soy intake and risk of breast cancer in Asian-Americans. *Carcinogenesis*. 23(9):1491–1496.

56. Korde L, Wu A, Fears T, Nomura A, West D, et al. (2009) Childhood soy intake and breast cancer risk in Asian American women. *Cancer Epidemiol Biomark Prev*. 18(4):1050–1059.

57. Fraser GE, Jaceldo-Siegl K, Orlich M, Mashchak A, Sirirat R, et al. (2020) Dairy, soy, and risk of breast cancer: those confounded milks. *Int J Epidemiol*. dyaa007.

58. Kang X, Zhang Q, Wang S, Huang X, Jin S. (2010) Effect of soy isoflavones on breast cancer recurrence and death for patients receiving adjuvant endocrine therapy. *CMAJ*. 182(17):1857-1862.

59. Magee PJ, Rowland I. (2012) Soy products in the management of breast cancer. *Curr Opin Clin Nutr Metab Care*. 15(6):586-591.

60. Shu XO, Zheng Y, Cai H, Gu K, Chen Z, et al. (2009) Soy food intake and breast cancer survival. *JAMA*. 302(22):2437-2443.

61. Guha N, Kwan ML, Quesenberry-Jr CP, Weltzien EK, Castillo AL, et al. (2009) Soy isoflavones and risk of cancer recurrence in a cohort of breast cancer survivors: the Life After Cancer Epidemiology study. *Breast Cancer Res Treat.* 118(2):395-405.

62. Rock CL, Doyle C, Demark-Wahnefried W, Meyerhardt J, Courneya K, et al. (2012) Nutrition and physical activity guidelines for cancer survivors. *CA Cancer J Clin*. 62(4):242–274.

63. American Institute for Cancer Research. (2012) Study finds, soy foods and cruciferous vegetables may reduce side effects of breast cancer treatment. *American Institute for Cancer Research*. http://www.aicr.org/cancer-research-update/november_21_2012/cru-soy-safe.html. Accessed 2020.

64. Eakin A, Kelsberg G, Safranek S. (2015) Clinical inquiry: Does high dietary soy intake affect a woman's risk of primary or recurrent breast cancer? *J Fam Pract*. 64:660–662.

65. Farvid MS, Spence ND, Holmes MD, Barnett JB. (2020) Fiber consumption and breast cancer incidence: A systematic review and meta-analysis of prospective studies. *Cancer*. 126(13):3061-3075.

66. Goldin BR, Adlercreutz H, Gorbach SL, Warram JH, Dwyer JT, et al. (1982) Estrogen excretion patterns and plasma levels in vegetarian and omnivorous women. *N Engl J Med*. 307:1542–1547.

67. Rose D, Goldman M, Connolly J, Strong L. (1991) High-fiber diet reduces serum estrogen concentrations in premenopausal women. *Am J Clin Nutr*. 54(3):520-525.

68. Goldin B, Woods M, Spiegelman D, Longcope C, Morrill-LaBrode A, et al. (1994) The effect of dietary fat and fiber on serum estrogen concentrations in premenopausal women under controlled dietary conditions. *Cancer*. 74(3 Suppl):1125-1131.

69. Bagga D, Ashley J, Geffrey S, Wang H, Barnard R, et al. (1995) Effects of a very low fat, high fiber diet on serum hormones and menstrual function. Implications for breast cancer prevention. *Cancer*. 76(12):2491-2496.

70. Woods M, Barnett J, Spiegelman D, Trail N, Hertzmark E, et al. (1996) Hormone levels during dietary changes in premenopausal African-American women. *J Natl Cancer I*. 88(19):1369-1374.

How to cite this article: Rose S, Strombom A. Breast cancer prevention with a plant-based diet. Canc Therapy & Oncol Int J. 2020; 17(1): 555955.
DOI: 10.19080/CTOIJ.2020.17.555955.

71. Kaneda N, Nagata C, Kabuto M, Shimizu H. (1997) Fat and fiber intakes in relation to serum estrogen concentration in premenopausal Japanese women. *Nutr Cancer.* 27(3):279-83.

72. Gann P, Chatterton R, Gapstur S, Liu K, Garside D, et al. (2003) The effects of a low-fat/high-fiber diet on sex hormone levels and menstrual cycling in premenopausal women: a 12-month randomized trial (the diet and hormone study). *Cancer*. 98(9):1870-1879.

73. Aubertin-Leheudre M, Gorbach S, Woods M, Dwyer J, Goldin B, et al. (2008) Fat/Fiber intakes and sex hormones in healthy premenopausal women in USA. *J Steroid Biochem Mol Biol*. 112(1-3):32-39.

74. Aune D, Chan DSM, Greenwood DC, Vieira AR, Navarro Rosenblatt DA, et al. (2012) Dietary fibre and breast cancer risk: a systematic review and meta-analysis of prospective studies. *Ann Oncol*. 23(6):1394–1402.

75. Rock CL, Flatt SW, Thomson CA, Stefanick ML, Newman VA, et al. (2004) Effects of a high-fibre, low-fat diet intervention on serum concentrations of reproductive steroid hormones in women with a history of breast cancer. *J Clin Oncol*. 22(12):2379–2387.

76. Chen S, Chen Y, Ma S, Zheng R, Zhao P, et al. (2016) Dietary fibre intake and risk of breast cancer: A systematic review and meta-analysis of epidemiological studies. *Oncotarget*. 7(49):80980-80989.

77. Edwards BK, Noone A, Mariotto AB, Simard EP, Boscoe FP, et al. (2013) Annual Report to the Nation on the status of cancer, 1975–2010, featuring prevalence of comorbidity and impact on survival among persons with lung, colorectal, breast, or prostate cancer. *Cancer*. 120(9):1290-1314.

78. Braithwaite D, Moore DH, Satariano WA, Kwan ML, Hiatt RA, et al. (2012) Prognostic impact of comorbidity among long-term breast cancer survivors: Results from the lace study. *Cancer Epidemiol Biomar Prev*. 21(7):1115–1125.

79. Søgaard M, Thomsen RW, Bossen KS, Sørensen HT, Nørgaard M. (2013) The impact of comorbidity on cancer survival: A review. *J Clin Epidemiol*. 5(Suppl 1):3–29.

80. Kiderlen M, de-Glas NA, Bastiaannet E, Portielje JEA, van-de-Velde CJH, et al. (2013) Diabetes in relation to breast cancer relapse and all-cause mortality in elderly breast cancer patients: a FOCUS study analysis. *Annals of Oncology*. 24(12):P3011-P3016.

81. Chapman JAW, Meng D, Shepherd L, Parulekar W, Ingle J, et al. (2008) Competing causes of death from a randomized trial of extended adjuvant endocrine therapy for breast cancer. *J Natl Cancer Inst*. 100(4):252–260.

82. Hanrahan EO, Gonzalez-Angulo AM, Giordano SH, Rouzier R, Broglio KR, et al. (2007) Overall survival and cause-specific mortal-ity of patients with stage T1a,bN0M0 breast carcinoma. *J Clin Oncol*. 25(31):4952–4960.

83. Bradshaw PT, Stevens J, Khankari N, Teitelbaum SL, Neugut AI, et al. (2016) Cardiovascular disease mortality among breast cancer survivors. *Epidemiology*. 27(1):6–13.

84. Fu MR, Axelrod D, Guth AA, Cleland C, Ryan C, et al. (2015) Comorbidities and quality of life among breast cancer survivors: a prospective study. *J Pers Med*. 2015;5(3):229-242.

85. Rose S, Strombom A. (2018) A comprehensive review of the prevention and treatment of heart disease with a plant-based diet. *J Cardiol & Cardiovas Ther*. 12(5):555847.

86. Rose S, Strombom A. (2018) Rheumatoid Arthritis – Prevention and Treatment with a Plant-Based Diet. *Orth & Rheum Open Access J*. 13(1):555852.

87. Rose S, Strombom A. (2019) Osteoarthritis prevention and treatment with a plant-based diet. *Ortho & Rheum Open Access J*. 15(3):555914.

88. Rose S, Strombom A. (2020) Preventing thyroid diseases with a plant-based diet, while ensuring adequate iodine status. *Glob J Oto*. 21(4):556069.

How to cite this article: Rose S, Strombom A. Breast cancer prevention with a plant-based diet. Canc Therapy & Oncol Int J. 2020; 17(1): 555955.
DOI: 10.19080/CTOIJ.2020.17.555955.

89. Johansen K. (1999) Efficacy of metformin in the treatment of NIDDM. Meta-analysis. *Diabetes Care*. 22(1):33-37.

90. Jenkins D, Kendall C, Marchie A, Faulkner D, Wong J, et al. (2005) Direct comparison of a dietary portfolio of cholesterol-lowering foods with a statin in hypercholesterolemic participants. *Am J Clin Nutr*. 81(2):380-387.

91. Frattaroli J, Weidner G, Merritt-Worden T, Frenda S, Ornish D. (2008) Angina pectoris and atherosclerotic risk factors in the multisite cardiac lifestyle intervention program. *American Journal of Cardiology*. 101(7):911-8.

92. Bloomer R, Kabir M, Canale R, Trepanowski J, Marshall K, et al. (2010) Effect of a 21 day Daniel Fast on metabolic and cardiovascular disease risk factors in men and women. *Lipids Health Dis*. 9:94.

93. Barnard N, Cohen J, Jenkins D, Turner-McGrievy G, Gloede L, et al. (2006) A low-fat vegan diet improves glycemic control and cardiovascular risk factors in a randomized clinical trial in individuals with type 2 diabetes. *Diabetes Care*. 29(8):1777-83.

94. Kahleova H, Matoulek M, Bratova M, Malinska H, Kazdova L, et al. (2013) Vegetarian diet-induced increase in linoleic acid in serum phospholipids is associated with improved insulin sensitivity in subjects with type 2 diabetes. *Nutr Diabetes*. 3:e75.

95. Esselstyn CJ, Gendy G, Doyle J, Golubic M, Roizen M. (2014) A way to reverse CAD? *J Fam Pract*. 63(7):356-364b.

96. Drozek D, Diehl H, Nakazawa M, Kostohryz T, Morton D, et al. (2014) Short-term effectiveness of a lifestyle intervention program for reducing selected chronic disease risk factors in individuals living in rural appalachia: a pilot cohort study. *Advances in Preventive Medicine*. 2014:798184.

Cancer Therapy & Oncology
International Journal
ISSN: 2473-554X

Juniper PUBLISHERS
key to the Researchers

Review Article
Volume 15 Issue 2 - October 2019
DOI: 10.19080/CTOIJ.2019.15.555906

Canc Therapy & Oncol Int J

Colorectal Cancer Prevention with a Plant-Based Diet

Stewart Rose* **and Amanda Strombom**

Plant-Based Diets in Medicine, USA

Submission: October 13, 2019: **Published:** October 24, 2019

*Correspondence Author: Stewart Rose, Plant-based diets in Medicine, 12819 SE 38th St, #427, Bellevue, WA 98006, USA

Abstract

A plant-based diet is valuable in the primary and secondary prevention of colorectal cancer. Epidemiological studies show a 46%-88% reduced risk of colorectal cancer for those following a plant-based diet.

In light of evidence, the World Health Organization International Agency for Research on Cancer (IARC) has classified processed meat as a carcinogen and red meat as a probable carcinogen, and has since reaffirmed their decision in light of more recent studies.

The pathogenic mechanisms by which processed and red meat can cause colon cancer have been determined. Several exogenous carcinogens are contained in meat and others are formed as a byproduct of its preparation. Bacterial flora produce several carcinogens endogenously in response to processed and red meat intake.

Some of the ways plant foods and their phytonutrients protect against colon cancer are also now understood. The chemoprotective mechanisms of plant foods are through the direct actions of phytochemicals, through the action of fiber, and as a result of the anti-inflammatory environment produced by the colonic flora.

While colonoscopy and FIT-DNA tests remain very valuable for secondary prevention, a plant-based diet can provide both primary and secondary prevention of colorectal cancer. Making prevention of colon cancer with a plant-based diet all the more desirable is that it is also a safe and efficacious prophylaxis and treats common comorbidities such as coronary artery disease and type II diabetes.

Keywords:

Anti-Inflammatory; Bacterial Flora; Carcinogens; Colorectal Cancer; Diet; Fiber, Phytochemicals; Plant-Based Diet; Vegetarian, Vegan

1. Introduction

This review article takes a comprehensive look at the research currently available on the potential of diet to impact the primary and secondary prevention of colorectal cancer. It does not cover less common pathologies such as Familial Adenomatous Polyposis, Turcot Syndrome and Lynch Syndrome.

2. Prevention of Colorectal Cancer

2.1 General Epidemiology

Only 5-10% of all cancer cases can be attributed to genetic defects, whereas the remaining 90-95% have their roots in the environment and lifestyle. The lifestyle factors include cigarette smoking, diet – especially meat – alcohol, sun exposure, environmental pollutants, infections, stress, obesity, and physical inactivity. (1)

The link between diet and cancer is revealed by the large variation in rates of specific cancers in various countries, and by the observed changes in the incidence of cancer in migrating. For example, East Asians have been shown to have a 25 times lower rate of many forms of cancer, but these rates increase substantially in individuals who migrate to the West. (1) Since genetics don't change with migration, but diet usually does, the increase is most likely attributable to adopting the Standard American Diet.

While some lifestyle factors, such as cigarette smoking, are now well acknowledged as affecting cancer, the role of diet is less well known. However, diet may be linked to as many as 70% – 80% of cases of colorectal cancer. (2, 3, 4, 5, 6) What's more, we know which type of diet is the most beneficial. A Canadian study showed that a plant-based diet resulted in a 46% decreased risk of colon cancer and 73% decreased risk of rectal cancer. (7)

Literally hundreds of studies have been conducted addressing the relationship of some type of plant foods or plant food constituents and cancer risk. A clear majority of these studies demonstrate that fruits, vegetables, legumes, whole grains, tree nuts, spices, and seeds, as well as specific types of food within these categories including citrus fruit, tomatoes, cruciferous vegetables, soybeans, and wheat, for example, reduce the risk of one or more types of cancer. (8, 9, 10, 11)

On the other hand, a number of studies have examined relationships between processed and red meat intake and colorectal cancer, many of which have been summarized in at least one of four meta-analyses over the past decade. (8, 12, 13, 14) A systematic review and meta-analysis of epidemiological studies relating the amount of processed and red meat consumed to increased risk of colon cancer, showed that processed meat increased the risk of colon cancer by 58% per 100gm and red meat increased the risk of colorectal adenoma by 27% per 100gm. (15)

One particularly large, general food study, using data from the EPIC (European Prospective Investigation into Cancer) study, also showed an increased risk of colon cancer associated with processed and red meat consumption. Those consuming the most processed and red meat had a 35% increased risk of colorectal cancer (CRC) overall. This study also found a 55% increased risk per 100g of processed meat and a 25% increased risk of CRC per 100 g increase in red meat. No increased risk was found for poultry intake, and there was an inverse association with fish intake, but note that the risks were not being measured against a plant-based diet, only against varying levels of meat and fish consumption. (16)

How to cite this article: Rose S, Strombom A. Colorectal cancer prevention with a plant-based diet. Canc Therapy & Oncol Int J. 2019; 15(2): 555906.
DOI: 10.19080/CTOIJ.2019.15.555906

It has been well documented that most colorectal cancers arise from colorectal adenoma by a process referred to as the adenoma–carcinoma sequence. (17) Thus, identification of modifiable risk factors for colorectal adenoma is also helpful for modifying the correctable risk of colorectal adenoma and preventing colorectal cancer.

In a study comparing Buddhist priests, who are obligatory vegetarians, with matched controls, the risk of colon adenoma was 54% higher in non-vegetarians than in vegetarians. The risk for advanced adenoma was over 3 times higher in non-vegetarians than in vegetarians. (18) These results are especially notable because the meat intake of the non-vegetarians was relatively low.

Vegetarian and vegan diets increase beneficial plant foods and plant constituents, eliminate the intake of red and processed meat, and aid in achieving and maintaining a healthy weight. The direct and indirect evidence taken together suggests that vegetarian diets are a useful strategy for reducing the risk of colon cancer. (2)

This has been tested in a couple of significant studies. In a 6-year prospective study of people who otherwise have a healthy lifestyle, meat eaters had an 88% increased risk of colon cancer compared to long term vegetarians. In this study by Fraser et al, in contrast to other studies, white meat raised the risk of colon cancer at least as much as red meat. Those who ate legumes more than twice a week had a 47% decreased risk of colon cancer. Those with a high meat diet and low legume consumption, and who had an above normal BMI, had a threefold increased risk of colon cancer. (19)

In another study, Orlich et al. found that a plant-based diet offers a 49% decreased risk of colon cancer, compared with a typical American high meat diet. (20) According to the author, the meat-eaters in this study were consuming less than 2oz of meat a day, and so were already 27% less likely to get colon cancer. His results showed that those following the vegetarian diet had an additional 22% decreased risk of colon cancer compared to these meat eaters, so adding these factors together gave a 49% decreased risk. This study had some other significant limitations. Those following a plant-based diet had been doing so for less than half the amount of time the meat eaters were following their diet, and were also older, on average, than the meat eaters. This study did not compensate for these factors. Taking these limitations into account, it is possible that even better results could be obtained. (20)

2.2 Risk Factors for Colon Cancer

Age is a significant risk factor for colon cancer, but it is clearly unmodifiable. Alcohol consumption and cigarette smoking are also well-recognized, modifiable risk factors. Here we consider diet-related and other modifiable risk factors.

2.2.1 Dietary risk factors

In October 2015, processed meat was classified by the World Health Organization International Agency for Research on Cancer (IARC) as carcinogenic to humans (Group 1), based on strength of evidence in humans that the consumption of processed meat causes colorectal cancer. (21) Red meat was classified as probably carcinogenic to humans (Group 2A). (21) New epidemiological studies and reviews have been published since then, clearly supporting the IARC decision. (22)

2.2.2 Hyperinsulinemia

A number of epidemiological studies have consistently demonstrated that the risk for several types of cancer (including that of the breast, colorectum, liver, and pancreas) is higher in insulin-resistant patients. (23) Metabolic syndrome increases both insulin and insulin resistance, due to high body mass, high saturated fat intake, and high glycemic load, a synergism that implicates hyperinsulinemic exposure in colon carcinogenesis. (2, 19)

Vegetarians have a 70-80% reduced risk of hyperinsulinemia (24) and lower insulin levels. (25, 26) This likely is one of the factors causing their reduced risk of colon cancer.

2.2.3 Obesity

High body mass index (BMI) is a risk factor for colon cancer. (27)

Vegetarians and vegans have significantly lower BMI's on average. A study of American vegetarians and vegans found that that vegetarians had a mean BMI of 25.7 and vegans a mean BMI of 23.6. (28) A European study found the average BMI of vegetarians and vegans to be 23.3 and 22.4 respectively for men and 22.8 and 21.8 for women. (29) A study of German vegans found an average BMI of 22.3. (30) A study of vegetarian children found that they too had lower BMI's than their meat- eating counterparts with an average BMI of 17.3 in ages 6 to 11 and average of 20.0 ages 12-18. (31) One study found the risk of being overweight or obese is 65% less for vegans and 46% less for vegetarians. (32)

2.2.4 Crohn's Disease

There is an elevated risk of colon cancer in patients with Crohn's Disease. (33) However, a vegetarian diet reduces risk of Crohn's disease by 70% in girls, and 80% in boys. (34)

Therefore, a vegetarian diet reduces the risk of colon cancer by reducing the consumption of red and processed meat, and reducing the risk of hyperinsulinemia, obesity and Crohn's Disease.

Preventative Factors from Food

Epidemiologic studies have shown that the consumption of foods of plant origin is associated with lower risk of several cancers, including Colorectal Cancer (CRC). (8) The specific constituents in the dietary foods which are responsible for helping to prevent CRC and the possible mechanisms have also been investigated extensively. Various phytochemicals have been identified in fruits, vegetables, grains, nuts, and spices which exhibit chemo-preventive activity. (35) They have various cancer impeding activities, such as reducing DNA damage via antioxidant properties or interacting with inflammation pathways. (36) In this article we focus on just two phytochemicals as examples, sulforaphane and salicylate. However, there are many others that have chemo-protective effects.

2.3.1 Sulforaphane

Sulforaphane (SFN) is an isothiocyanate that is naturally present in cruciferous vegetables, with high concentration in broccoli. The results of the most recent studies indicate that multi-targeted sulforaphane actions may contribute to prevention and treatment of cancer. Protective properties of sulforaphane have been observed in every stage of carcinogenesis. (7) Due to their increased consumption of cruciferous vegetables, vegetarians will benefit from the protective properties of sulforaphane more than meat-eaters.

How to cite this article: Rose S, Strombom A. Colorectal cancer prevention with a plant-based diet. Canc Therapy & Oncol Int J. 2019; 15(2): 555906.
DOI: 10.19080/CTOIJ.2019.15.555906

2.3.2 Salicylates

The role of aspirin in cancer has been extensively investigated. (37, 38) Aspirin use is associated with decreased risk for colorectal, breast, esophageal, lung, stomach and ovarian cancer, and aspirin is both a chemo-preventive and chemo-therapeutic agent for breast and colon cancer. (39, 40, 41, 42, 43) A recent report on the chemo-preventive effects of aspirin showed that the incidence of colon cancer in Scotland was significantly decreased in the general population at the lowest daily dose of aspirin (75 mg), and that the decreased incidence was observed even after only 5 years of aspirin use. (42) Regular aspirin use after the diagnosis of colorectal cancer is associated with lower risk of colorectal cancer-specific and overall mortality, especially among individuals with colon cancer tumors that overexpress Cycloxogenase 2 (2 COX-2). (40)

After absorption, aspirin is very rapidly hydrolyzed to salicylic acid (2-hydroxybenzoic acid). (44) The reported high serum salicylate/aspirin ratios observed in human studies using aspirin suggest that salicylate may be an important contributor to the anticancer activity of aspirin, especially in colon cancer patients.

Salicylates are widely distributed throughout the plant kingdom, and they are therefore present in plant products of dietary relevance, such as fruit, vegetables, herbs and spices. Moreover, they appear to be readily absorbed from the food matrix. This has led some to suggest that the recognized effects of consuming fruit and vegetables on lowering the risk of several diseases, such as colon cancer, may be due, in part, to salicylates in plant-based foods. (45, 46)

2.3.3 Fiber

Inverse associations between dietary fiber intake and colorectal cancer risk have been reported in ecological and case-control studies. (47, 48) Inverse associations for fiber and colorectal adenoma (49) and colorectal cancer (50, 51, 52, 53) have also been reported in well-designed prospective studies. In the EPIC study, after an average 6.2 years of follow-up and 1,721 colorectal cancer cases, a 21% reduced risk amongst participants in the highest fiber intake quintile was observed when compared against the lowest intake group. (54, 55)

In a recent systematic review, in which a high concordance between study results was observed, the World Cancer Research Fund/American Institute for Cancer Research panel upgraded the association between fiber and colorectal cancer to "Convincing". (56)

Vegetarians and vegans, consuming a wide variety of plant-based foods, will naturally consume much more fiber than meat-eaters.

3. Pathophysiology

Research on the prevention of colon cancer with a vegetarian diet has gone beyond epidemiologic association. We now know of several mechanisms by which red and processed meat causes colon cancer and certain constituents of plant foods (phytonutrients) that help prevent it. For each of these mechanisms, vegetarians carry a distinct advantage. This helps explain why the risk of colon cancer is substantially lower in those who follow a plant-based diet.

Pathogenic factors explained below, include:

1. Carcinogens such as:
    1. heterocyclic amines (HCAs),

2. poly-aromatic hydrocarbons (PAHs)
3. nitrites, and
4. poly-chlorinated biphenyls (PCBs)

2. Insulin
3. Insulin-like Growth Factor (IGF)
4. Inflammation, as indicated by C-Reactive Protein (CRP)
5. Matrix metalloproteinases (MMPs)

Protective phytonutrients explained below include:

6. Salicylates
7. Sulforaphane
8. Phytic Acid and
9. Fiber

The microbiome also has a role in the pathogenesis of colon cancer. Heme iron promotes the bacterial production of Nitroso amines which are known carcinogens. While a meat-centered diet promotes the growth of bacteria which have an inflammatory action in the colon, a vegetarian diet results in a different composition of flora, favoring the growth of bacteria that produce anti-inflammatory metabolic byproducts such as butyrate.

3.1 Pathogenic Mechanisms

3.1.1 Carcinogens

Several individual compounds have been suggested to explain the underlying mechanisms by which red and processed meat may increase the risk of colorectal cancer, including heme iron, (57, 58) heterocyclic amines (HCAs), (57, 59) polycyclic aromatic hydrocarbons (PAHs), (60) nitrites and nitrates, (57, 61) and organochlorine compounds such as PCBs. (62) HCAs, PAHs, nitrites and nitrates may all be involved in colorectal cancer etiology. (63)

Heme iron is a pro carcinogen that becomes a carcinogen as a result of bacterial transformation to nitroso amines. Although there some preformed nitroso amine in the diet, the majority is produced by intestinal flora. Therefore, the role of heme iron in that pathogenesis of colon cancer will be discussed in the Microbiome section below.

Heterocyclic amines are mutagenic compounds formed when muscle meat is cooked using high-temperature methods, such as grilling, barbequing, and pan-frying. (64) They are formed when amino acids, sugars, and creatine react at high temperatures, especially those above 150 degrees Celsius. Cooking methods that result in the greatest amounts of HCAs include grilling and pan-frying. (65)

HCAs, measured using urine or leukocyte assays, have been associated with colon adenoma. (66, 67, 68) Many studies, examining interactions between meat intake and genetic polymorphisms that modulate metabolism of HCAs, also provide indirect yet compelling support for an association between these carcinogens and colorectal neoplasia. (69, 70, 71, 72, 73, 74, 75, 76, 77, 78) In one study, women with genotypes associated with rapid acetylation of meat-associated carcinogens, had a particularly high risk of colorectal cancer associated with red meat intake. (79) This strongly points to heterocyclic amines as carcinogenic for colon cancer.

Polycyclic aromatic hydrocarbons (PAHs) are well known to be carcinogenic. They are produced in many industrial situations, burning coal and wood, and by smoking cigarettes, but for a non-smoking person who hasn't been exposed to industrial processes, the prime source of PAHs comes through the diet. Some PAHs are deposited

How to cite this article: Rose S, Strombom A. Colorectal cancer prevention with a plant-based diet. Canc Therapy & Oncol Int J. 2019; 15(2): 555906.
DOI: 10.19080/CTOIJ.2019.15.555906

on plant foods through air pollution, which then bio-concentrate in animal adipose tissue through animals' consumption of plant foods over their lifespan, leading to much higher levels in animal tissue than in plant foods. However, the primary source of PAHs in the diet is as a result of thermal treatment of meat, especially barbecuing or grilling. (80, 81)

Meat that is cooked above an open flame, as with grilling and barbecuing, results in fat and juices dripping onto the fire, yielding flames that contain PAHs. These PAHs then adhere to the surface of the meat. (65) The smoking of meat, or other food preparation methods that expose meat to smoke or charring, also contributes to PAH formation.

As an important human exposure pathway of contaminants, dietary intake of PAHs is of increasing concern for assessing cancer risk in the human body. (82) Studies of PAH exposure indicate that the target organs for PAH compounds are the lung, oropharynx, breast and genitourinary and gastrointestinal tracts. (83) Dietary PAHs are of special concern to cancer of the gastrointestinal tract. In humans, there is specific evidence for the association of dietary PAH exposure with colon cancer. (84, 85)

The following significant positive associations were observed for meat-related PAH compounds: 2-amino-3,4,8-trimethylimidazo[4,5-f]quinoxaline (DiMeIQx) and colorectal, distal colon, and rectal tumors; 2-amino-3,8-dimethylimidazo[4,5-*f*]quinoxaline (MeIQx) and colorectal and colon cancer tumors; 2-amino-1-methyl-6-phenylimidazo[4,5-*b*]pyridine (PhIP) and rectal cancer; and benzo[a]pyrene and rectal cancer. (63)

One study determined a profile of 14 PAHs, frequently found in food: in cow's milk, human breast milk, and meat- and fish-based foods. The levels of PAHs were much higher than the permissible limits of 1 μg/kg in a large percentage of the foods sampled. (86)

Sodium nitrites and nitrates are added to meat for preservation and curing purposes. They are commonly found in processed meat products, such as ham, bacon, salami and hot dogs. These nitrites—and nitrates that are readily converted to nitrites by bacteria—react with amines or amides derived from protein, leading to the formation of N-nitroso compounds (NOCs), which are potent carcinogens. (87, 61) See the Microbiome section (Role of the Microbiome in the Pathogenesis of Colon Cancer) for more information on this process.

Organochlorine compounds, such as polychlorinated biphenyl (PCB) and organochlorine pesticides, have also been linked to increased risk of several cancers. Despite reductions in their use in the developed world, they remain one of the most important groups of persistent pollutants to which humans are exposed, primarily through dietary intake. They are deposited on plant foods through polluted water and air, but due to bioaccumulation in fatty tissue, meat and dairy products contain much greater levels of such compounds than plant products. (88, 89, 90) Some PCBs are not absorbed in the intestine and remain in the stool, potentially damaging the colon. A study found that an elevated risk of colorectal cancer was positively associated with the consumption of mono-ortho PCB congeners 28 and 118 in the diet. (62)

Another way that meat acts as carcinogen is in its activation of Toll Like Receptors (TLRs). A study showed that meat intake may activate TLRs

How to cite this article: Rose S, Strombom A. Colorectal cancer prevention with a plant-based diet. Canc Therapy & Oncol Int J. 2019; 15(2): 555906.
DOI: 10.19080/CTOIJ.2019.15.555906

at the epithelial surface. This can lead to colorectal cancer via nuclear factor-κB-initiated transcription of inflammatory genes. However, intake of fiber may protect against colorectal cancer via TLR4-mediated secretion of interleukin-10 and cyclooxygenase-2. (91)

3.1.2 Hyperinsulinemia

Insulin resistance is a pathological condition in which insulin action is impaired in peripheral target tissues including skeletal muscle, liver, and adipose tissue. Initially, in individuals destined to develop Type 2 Diabetes, the pancreatic beta cells increase insulin production to overcome insulin resistance and maintain euglycemia. (92)

Hyperinsulinemia promotes colon carcinogenesis, since insulin is an important growth factor of colonic epithelial cells and is a mitogen of tumor cell growth in vitro. (93) Insulin can exert its oncogenic potential via abnormal stimulation of multiple cellular signaling cascades, enhancing growth factor-dependent cell proliferation and/or by directly affecting cell metabolism. (92)

Insulin also increases the bioactivity of IGF-I by enhancing hepatic IGF-I synthesis and by reducing hepatic protein production of the insulin-like growth factor binding proteins 1 and 2 (IGFBP-1 and IGFBP-2). (94, 95) Therefore, although insulin can directly induce tumor growth, many of its mitogenic and antiapoptotic effects are operating through the IGF-I system, as reported in individuals with high levels of circulating IGF-I, in which an increased risk of developing certain types of tumors. (95, 96)

To date, two insulin receptor (IR) isoforms have been described. They differ in the presence of a short exon 11 that can be excised from (IR-A, short isoform) or included in (IR-B, long isoform) the IR coding sequence as a result of alternative splicing. (97, 98) While glucose uptake remains the main IR-mediated function, a growing body of evidence suggests that the two IR isoforms have different biological roles with IR-A mostly exerting mitogenic effects and IR-B modulating cell metabolism. (99)

Males with serum C-peptide concentration >3.3 ng/mL were 3.8 times more likely to have an adenoma relative to no polyp than those with C-peptide ≤1.8 ng/ml. (100) As therefore would be expected, serum insulin levels directly correlate with the presence of adenoma and hyperplastic polyps in the proximal colon, and also, but less strongly, correlate with the presence of distal adenoma. (101)

3.1.3 Insulin-Like Growth Factor

The insulin-like growth factor (IGF) system is a multifactorial signaling network that modulates energy metabolism, cell growth, and cancer. (97) IGFs are potent proliferation stimulators for numerous tumor cells and often function as autocrine growth factors. It has been shown that IGF-I and IGF-II enhance proliferation of colorectal carcinoma cells. The biological signal of both factors is transmitted through the IGF-I receptor (IGF-I-R). (102)

Breast, ovarian, prostate, lung, and colon cancer are the tumor tissues where the IGF system has been directly linked to tumor development and progression. (103, 104) As explained above, hyperinsulinemia makes IGF even more damaging.

The insulin/IGF biochemical system has also been associated with tumor formation and progression in breast, ovarian, prostate, lung, and colon cancer, especially the sporadic form of

How to cite this article: Rose S, Strombom A. Colorectal cancer prevention with a plant-based diet. Canc Therapy & Oncol Int J. 2019; 15(2): 555906.
DOI: 10.19080/CTOIJ.2019.15.555906

colorectal carcinoma that emerges through the adenoma–carcinoma pathway. (103, 104, 105)

Hyperinsulinemia has an effect on cell proliferation, not only through insulin receptor signaling, but also through the amplification of IGF-1 effect. (105, 106) iR-A receptors are overexpressed in tumors cells and both insulin and IGF-1 through its effect on HR/iR-A enhance cell proliferation. An overexpression of IGF receptors was found in human colon cancer cells, which was later on associated with formation of iRS-1 and iRS-2, and subsequently Akt activation and up regulation of the anti-apoptotic protein Bcl-xL, as well as activation of β catenin and its translocation into the nucleus, and subsequent promotion of cell proliferation gene transcription.

In a study comparing vegan women with meat-eating women, the mean serum IGF-I concentration was 13% lower in vegan women compared with meat-eaters. In line with these lower levels, the mean concentrations of both serum IGF-binding protein (IGFBP)-1 and IGFBP-2 were 20–40% higher in vegan women compared with meat-eaters. (107) Similar results have been obtained studying vegan men. (108)

3.1.4 C-Reactive Protein (CRP)

Cardio Reactive Protein (CRP), whose levels are of use in cardiology, also happens to be valuable as a prognostic factor in colon cancer. CRP is correlated with colon cancer prognosis and risk of death in colon cancer. One study showed a stage specific increase in poor prognosis and increased risk of death for high CRP levels: 7.37 for stage I and II, 3.29 for stage III, 2.24 for stage IV. (109)

A study of CRP and adenoma showed a positive association between plasma CRP concentration and the prevalence of colorectal adenoma. (110) Given that CRP is a preferable biomarker of systemic inflammation and a highly sensitive method that can evaluate low-grade inflammation, this finding of a positive association between higher CRP levels and an increased prevalence of adenoma supports the hypothesis that the development/growth of colorectal neoplasia likely involves a systemic, low-grade inflammatory state.

In another study, a dose response relationship with CRP level was observed for risk of multiple small tubular adenomas, increasing the risk 101% for the highest vs lowest tercile comparison, and increasing the risk of advanced adenomas by 81% for highest vs lowest tercile comparison. (111)

An elevated CRP is particularly associated with increased risk of colorectal cancer in patients with inflammatory bowel disease. A study showed an increased risk of colorectal cancer across quartiles of CRP elevation, with an increased risk of almost 200% for the highest versus the lowest quartile. (112)

The ability of a plant-based diet to lower CRP levels, and the fact that vegetarians have lower CRP levels (113), is very relevant to colorectal cancer risk. Lower levels of hs-CRP were found in those following a vegetarian diet for more than 2 years. (114) The fact that vegetarians have lower levels of CRP, decreases their chance of a poor prognosis for colon cancer.

3.1.5 Matrix Metalloproteinases

Matrix metalloproteinases (MMPs) consist of a multigene family of zinc dependent extracellular matrix (ECM) remodeling endopeptidases implicated in pathological processes, such as carcinogenesis. In this regard, their activity plays a pivotal

How to cite this article: Rose S, Strombom A. Colorectal cancer prevention with a plant-based diet. Canc Therapy & Oncol Int J. 2019; 15(2): 555906.
DOI: 10.19080/CTOIJ.2019.15.555906

role in tumor growth and the multistep processes of invasion and metastasis, including proteolytic degradation of ECM, alteration of the cell-cell and cell-ECM interactions, migration and angiogenesis. (115)

Considerable evidence has implicated the over expression of matrix metalloproteinases (MMPs) MMP-1, -2, -3. -7, -9, -13 in human colorectal cancers. The degree of over expression of some MMPs has been noted to correlate with stage of disease and prognosis. (116, 117)

One study examined circulating plasma concentrations of myeloperoxidase (MPO), matrix metalloproteinases MMP-9 and MMP-2, and tissue inhibitors of MMP TIMP-1 and TIMP-2, between healthy vegetarians and healthy omnivores. The study found significantly lower concentrations of MPO, MMP-9, MMP-2 and MMP-9/TIMP-1 ratio in vegetarians compared to omnivores. (116, 117)

3.2 Protective Mechanisms

Several phytonutrients found in plant foods have chemo-protective properties. While the number of different phytonutrients is considerable, in this section we consider some of the more important ones as examples, sulforaphane, salicylate, phytic acid (inositol hexaphophate), and fiber.

3.2.1 Sulforaphane

Various Brassica vegetables, especially broccoli, contain glucoraphanin (sulforophane or SFN). Following cutting or chewing, it is hydrolyzed into the corresponding isothiocyanate SFN either by the plant thioglucosidase myrosinase or by bacterial thioglucosidases in the colon. (118)

Because of its lipophilicity (119) and molecular size, SFN is likely to passively diffuse into the enterocytes. (120) After absorption, SFN is conjugated with glutathione (SF-GSH) by glutathione-S-transferase (GST) leading to maintenance of a concentration gradient and facilitating a fast passive absorption into the cell. (121) It is metabolized via the mercapturic acid pathway, producing predominantly cysteinylglycine (SF-CG), cysteine (SF-Cys), and N-acetyl-cysteine (SF-NAC) conjugates that are excreted in the urine. (122)

The mechanism of protection against the initiation of carcinogenesis by SFN includes modulation of phase I and II xenobiotic metabolizing enzymes, as well as direct blocking of specific binding sites of carcinogens with the DNA molecule. As a result, SFN inhibits DNA adduct formation, thus reducing the risk of mutations. Further SFN activity is targeted at cancer cells, and prevents their expansion due to regulation of proliferation and induction of differentiation and/or apoptosis. In vitro studies using various types of cancer cells have revealed the ability of SFN to arrest the cell cycle, particularly in G2/M, while SFN at higher concentration is shown to activate apoptotic pathways. The possible SFN anticancer effect in the progression stage of carcinogenesis has been proven by a few studies, which provide evidence for its anti-angiogenic and anti-metastatic influence. Additionally, SFN exhibits anti- inflammatory effects relevant to cancer prevention. (123)

The induction of cell cycle arrest and apoptosis is a key mechanism by which SFN exerts its colon cancer prevention effects on the growth and viability of Human Carcinoma Cells (HT29 cells) during their exponential growing phase. (124) It was observed that sulforaphane induced a cell cycle arrest in a dose dependent manner, followed by cell death. Moreover, the weak effect observed on

How to cite this article: Rose S, Strombom A. Colorectal cancer prevention with a plant-based diet. Canc Therapy & Oncol Int J. 2019; 15(2): 555906.
DOI: 10.19080/CTOIJ.2019.15.555906

differentiated Human Colon cells (CaCo2 cells) suggests a specific anticancer activity for this compound. (125)

3.2.2 Salicylates

The cancer preventive action of aspirin is due to its principal metabolite, salicylic acid. Sodium salicylate induces apoptosis in cancer cells. (126) Regular ingestion of aspirin can prevent cancer: observational studies, randomized polyp prevention studies, long-term cancer follow-up in cardiovascular aspirin trials and randomized trials with cancer as an endpoint confirm this relationship. (127) The first successful, double-blind randomized, controlled trial of aspirin chemoprevention (Cancer Prevention Programme–CAPP2) was carried out in 1009 carriers of Lynch syndrome (hereditary CRC). (127) Two aspirins taken daily for two years reduced CRC by more than 50% five years later. Obese participants were particularly protected. (128)

Aspirin's anti-neoplastic effects are generally attributed to salicylic acid inhibiting prostaglandin G/H-synthase 2 (PGHS2, commonly termed COX2) transcription, preventing PGHS2 from converting arachidonic acid to potentially tumor inducing prostaglandins. Aspirin down regulates Sp1, Sp3 and Sp4 transcription factors, reducing expression of proteins including VEGF (vascular epithelial growth factor), reducing tumor cell growth. (129) Additionally, aspirin may only be beneficial in CRCs characterized by a mutated, rather than wild type PIK3CA gene, explaining the effects of aspirin, independently of non steroidal anti inflammatory (NSAID) use. (130) Even 100 nmol/ml has an effect.

Assuming salicylic acid is the anti-neoplastic component in aspirin, inhibition of COX2 cannot be the only mechanism by which aspirin prevent cancers, because the anti-neoplastic effect of NSAID drugs does not vary in direct relation to COX2 inhibition. The inhibition and induction by salicylates include the following: (i) the interruption of nuclear factor kappa B (NF-κB), (ii) the interruption of extracellular signal-regulated kinases, (iii) the induction of caspase 8 and 9, and (iv) the inhibition of β-catenin signaling mechanism. These are therefore the mechanisms by which salicylates prevent cancer. (131)

Dietary salicylates can have the same effect. (132, 46) Median serum concentration in vegetarians not taking aspirin drugs is 107 nmol/ml; showing that diet can elevate serum salicylate levels enough to decrease COX2. In a study comparing vegetarians with meat-eaters taking 75mg of aspirin daily, some of the vegetarians achieved a serum salicylic acid level equal to those taking aspirin. (133) Lawrence et. al. show that urinary excretion of salicyluric acid (SU) and salicylic acid (SA) is significantly increased in vegetarians compared with non-vegetarians. (134) They previously reported that serum salicylic acid was also significantly increased in vegetarians compared with non-vegetarians. (133) Interestingly, urinary excretion of SA was similar in vegetarians and patients consuming 75 or 150 mg of aspirin/day, although SU excretion was substantially greater in the aspirin groups. It should also be noted that while studies of salicylate and colon cancer often use a time period of five to ten years, vegetarians, and even more so vegans, have often been consuming salicylate rich foods for much longer or even their whole lives.

3.2.3 Phytic Acid

Most of the research on the effects of phytic acid to prevent colon cancer has been in vitro on both human and animal cells and in vivo in rats,

How to cite this article: Rose S, Strombom A. Colorectal cancer prevention with a plant-based diet. Canc Therapy & Oncol Int J. 2019; 15(2): 555906.
DOI: 10.19080/CTOIJ.2019.15.555906

with just one in vivo study in humans. While they therefore must be interpreted with caution, there is a significant amount of research to indicate the likelihood that phytic acid has chemoprotective activity against colon cancer through several mechanisms.

Recently phytic acid (inositol hexaphosphate or IP_6) has received much attention for its role in cancer prevention and control of experimental tumor growth, progression, and metastasis. Exogenously administered IP_6 is rapidly taken up into the cells and dephosphorylated to lower inositol phosphates, which affect signal transduction pathways resulting in cell cycle arrest. A strong anticancer action of IP_6 was demonstrated in different experimental models. In addition to reducing cell proliferation, IP_6 also induces differentiation of malignant cells. Enhanced immunity and antioxidant properties also contribute to tumor cell destruction. (135)

IP_6 has been demonstrated to exert valuable anticancer effects in vivo when administered to cancer patients. An antitumor activity has been observed in advanced colon cancer patients, where inositol treatment is associated with appreciable reduction in tumor burden and improved quality of life. Moreover, if inositols were added along with conventional chemotherapy, colon cancer patients experienced significantly less side effects than controls, as reported in a pilot study. (136)

One mechanism by which IP_6 is chemoprotective is through modulating the gene expression. The results of a study show that IP_6 modulates MMP-2, TIMP-1 and TIMP-2 genes expression in human colon cancer cells at the transcriptional level in a way dependent on its concentration and time of interaction. (137) Vegetarians have lower levels of MMP-2 (116) and their greater intake of foods high in phytic acid may be one reason why.

Another mechanism is by phytic acid forming chelates with various metals and suppressing damaging iron-catalyzed redox reactions. Inasmuch as colonic bacteria have been shown to produce oxygen radicals in appreciable amounts, dietary phytic acid might suppress oxidant damage to intestinal epithelium and neighboring cells. (138)

One study sought to determine the potential of phytic acid extracted from rice bran in the suppression of colon carcinogenesis induced by azoxymethane in rats. Phytic acid significantly reduced the number of tumors in the distal, middle and proximal colon. (139)

In another study of azoxymethane induced colorectal cancer in rats, the administration of IP_6 markedly suppressed the incidence of tumors when compared to the control. Interestingly, the administration of IP_6 had also markedly decreased β-catenin and COX-2 in colon tumors. Thus, the downregulation of β-catenin and COX-2 could play a role in inhibiting the colorectal cancer development induced by IP_6 and thereby act as a potent anticancer agent. (140)

These are elements of rapidly accumulating data from animal models, indicating that dietary supplementation with phytic acid may provide substantial protection against experimentally induced colonic cancer. Should further investigations yield additional support for this hypothesis, purposeful amplification of dietary phytic acid content would represent a simple method for reducing the risk of colonic carcinogenesis. (138)

Preliminary studies in humans show that IP_6 and inositol, the precursor molecule of IP_6, appear to enhance the anticancer effect of conventional

How to cite this article: Rose S, Strombom A. Colorectal cancer prevention with a plant-based diet. Canc Therapy & Oncol Int J. 2019; 15(2): 555906.
DOI: 10.19080/CTOIJ.2019.15.555906

chemotherapy, control cancer metastases, and improve quality of life. Because it is efficiently absorbed from the gastrointestinal tract, and its safety is unquestioned, IP_6 and inositol, its parent compound, holds great promise in our strategies for cancer prevention and therapy. (135)

Since phytic acid can only be obtained from plant foods, vegetarians and especially vegans, naturally consume higher levels of phytic acid than meat eaters.

3.2.3 Fiber

The possible protective association between dietary fiber intake and colorectal cancer was first proposed by Burkitt in 1971. (141) In addition to the protective benefit of phytic acid, anti- carcinogenic mechanisms of dietary fiber within the bowel include:

1. the formation of short chain fatty acids from fermentation by colonic bacteria,
2. the reduction of secondary bile acid production,
3. the reduction in intestinal transit time, and increase of fecal bulk, and
4. a reduction in insulin resistance. (142, 143, 144)

The role of fiber is further discussed in the Microbiome section below.

3.3 The Role of the Gut Microbiome

Representing a vast ecosystem, the indigenous bacteria in the human gut have various physiological effects, and carry out multiple metabolic functions that can influence the health of the human host. Bacteria are thought to benefit the human host in many ways. These favorable effects include:

1. facilitating the metabolic conversion and uptake of beneficial dietary components;
2. producing beneficial fermentation end products that affect intestinal pH and interact with gut mucosa epithelial cells;
3. excluding pathogens by competing for attachment sites within the gut mucosa;
4. interacting with the intestinal immune system and contributing to the regulation of immune function;
5. transforming or eliminating toxic substances; and
6. generating fecal bulk that decreases transit time and dilutes toxic substances.(145)

Carcinogenesis has been associated with the microbiome through direct and indirect routes. Direct pathways include colonization of epithelia by pathogens, or direct interaction with the innate immune system via bacterial antigenic particles with pattern recognition receptors (PRR, e.g. toll-like receptor). Indirect pathways include bacterial production of carcinogens and the production of chemoprotective factors from exogenous sources, such as diet, or from endogenous sources, such as compounds resulting from human metabolism (e.g. bile acids). (146)

An expanding body of evidence supports a role for gut microbes in the etiology of colon cancer. Functional contributions of the gut microbiota that may influence colon cancer susceptibility include:

1. harvesting otherwise inaccessible nutrients and/or sources of energy from the diet (i.e., fermentation of dietary fibers and resistant starch),

2. metabolism of xenobiotics, both potentially beneficial or detrimental (i.e., dietary constituents, drugs, carcinogens, etc.),
3. renewal of gut epithelial cells and maintenance of mucosal integrity, and
4. affecting immune system development and activity.

Diet and energy balance influence colorectal cancer (CRC) by multiple mechanisms via the gut microbiome. They modulate the composition and function of gut microbiota, which have a prodigious metabolic capacity and can produce oncometabolites or tumor suppressive metabolites depending, in part, on which dietary factors and digestive components are present in the GI tract. Gut microbiota also have a profound effect on immune cells in the lamina propria, which influences inflammation and subsequently CRC.

Nutrient availability, which is an outcome of diet and energy balance, determines the abundance of certain energy metabolites that are essential cofactors for epigenetic enzymes, and therefore impinges upon epigenetic regulation of gene expression. Aberrant epigenetic marks accumulate during CRC, and epimutations that are selected for drive tumorigenesis by causing transcriptome profiles to diverge from the cell of origin. In some instances, the above mechanisms are intertwined, as exemplified by dietary fiber being metabolized by colonic bacteria into butyrate, which is both a short chain fatty acid and a histone deacetylase inhibitor that epigenetically upregulates tumor suppressor genes in CRC cells and anti-inflammatory genes in immune cells. (147)

Understanding the complex and dynamic interplay between the gut microbiome, human host immune system, and dietary exposures may help elucidate mechanisms for carcinogenesis and guide future cancer prevention and treatment strategies. (146)

3.3.1 The Role of the Microbiome in the Pathogenesis of Colon Cancer

The colon flora in meat eaters produce more carcinogens, such as N-Nitroso Compounds (NOC), Hydrogen Sulphide (H_2S) and Deoxycholic Acid (DCA), than the flora in vegetarians. Bacteria produce carcinogens by their actions on both exogenous material, such as the production of Nitroso amines from Heme iron, and by their actions on endogenously produced substances, such as bile acids, to produce Deoxycholic acid.

3.3.1.1 N-Nitroso compounds (NOC)

Numerous constituents in red and processed meats may contribute to the increased risk of colon cancer associated with red and processed meat consumption. (58) These include protein and other nitrogenous residues which allow for increased gut bacterial production of N-nitroso compounds (NOC). (148) Nitrate can be reduced endogenously to nitrite via nitrate reductase produced by the gut bacteria, and nitrite can interact with organic compounds to form NOC. Many classes of NOC have been identified in feces, including nitrosamines, nitrosamides, and nitrosoguanidine. (149) NOC can form DNA adducts which induce mutations. For example, it has been shown that some NOC are alkylating agents that induce GC to AT transitions at the second base of codon 12 or 13 of the K-ras gene—this is a common mutation found in colorectal tumors with K-ras mutations. (149)

Diet can influence NOC concentrations. Meat consumption increases the amount of nitrogenous residues in the colon, (150) and in a controlled

How to cite this article: Rose S, Strombom A. Colorectal cancer prevention with a plant-based diet. Canc Therapy & Oncol Int J. 2019; 15(2): 555906.
DOI: 10.19080/CTOIJ.2019.15.555906

feeding study in eight men, there was a dose-response between intake of meat and fecal concentrations of NOC. (151) Fecal water genotoxicity correlated with colonic gene expression changes in pro-carcinogenic pathways, including DNA damage repair, cell cycle, and apoptosis pathways in a 7-day dietary intervention with red meat. (152) Additional controlled feeding studies in men showed that, while heme iron increased fecal NOC, protein sources low in heme (protein from vegetable sources) did not increase fecal NOC. (153, 154) The independent effect of heme on NOC suggested that chemical catalysis, in addition to bacterial N-nitrosation, may be responsible for the dose-dependent effect of red meat on increasing endogenous intestinal N-nitrosation. (154) The addition of soy to the diet statistically significantly suppressed fecal NOC. (155)

3.3.1.2 Hydrogen sulfide (H_2S)

Hydrogen sulfide (H_2S) is produced by sulfate-reducing bacteria (SRB) and has been shown to have both cytotoxic and genotoxic effects in cell culture studies. (156, 157, 158) For example, using a modified comet assay, Attene-Ramos et al. (156) showed that H_2S resulted in genomic DNA damage. H_2S has also been shown to prevent the oxidation of butyrate by colonic epithelial cells, thereby reducing ATP formation and energy harvest. (159) This lowers the absorption of ions, mucus formation, and cellular detoxification. Roediger et al. (160, 161) reported decreased fatty acid oxidation in colonocytes exposed to H_2S, and there is evidence that sulfide alters cellular redox potential which, in turn, alters cell proliferation. (157)

The role of SRB in inflammatory bowel disease and colorectal cancer has been evaluated in several epidemiologic and clinical studies. (146) Genomic instability associated with sporadic colon cancer and ulcerative colitis, a risk factor for colon cancer, is thought to result in part from H_2S exposure. (162) In a population-based study, the prevalence of SRB was associated with the diets of groups having higher rates of colon cancer. (163)

SRB are often members of the normal gut microbiota, and diet can influence their distribution and activity. Dietary protein, especially sulfur-containing amino acids, and inorganic sulfur sources (SO_4 in water) contribute to H_2S production. (164) In a controlled feeding study, Magee et al. (165) showed that H_2S was significantly related to the amount of meat protein consumed.

3.3.1.3 Dietary fat

Cani et al. (166) found that a high fat diet resulted in a significant change in the composition of the dominant bacterial populations within the gut microflora, including a decrease in the number of Bifidobacteria, Eubacterium, rectal Clostridium coccoides group, and Bacteroides, thus favoring an increase in the gram-negative to gram-positive ratio. This change in gut microflora composition was associated with a significant increase in plasma lipopolysaccharide (LPS) levels, fat mass, body weight gain, liver hepatic triglyceride accumulation, insulin resistance, and diabetes. (166, 167) In addition, de Wit et al. (168) observed that a high saturated fatty acid diet enhanced an overflow of dietary fat to the distal intestine, which affected the gut microbiota composition.

Lipopolysaccharide (LPS, also known as endotoxin) is a bacterial cell wall component in gram-negative bacteria that is associated with low grade, chronic inflammation in obesity (166, 169, 170) and colorectal cancer. (171) LPS acts through toll-like receptor-4 (TLR-4), a PRR associated with

How to cite this article: Rose S, Strombom A. Colorectal cancer prevention with a plant-based diet. Canc Therapy & Oncol Int J. 2019; 15(2): 555906.
DOI: 10.19080/CTOIJ.2019.15.555906

innate immunity, which triggers TGF-β-mediated pathways. (172, 173) This leads to the expression of various genes that promote neoplasia, including those of growth factors and inflammatory mediators. Serum LPS binding protein (LBP), a protein that binds LPS upon activation of TLR-4, is correlated with circulating concentrations of LPS, (174, 175) and a recent prospective study showed that polymorphisms in the LBP gene were associated with increased colorectal cancer risk. (176)

3.3.1.4 Deoxycholic acid (DCA)

The secondary bile acid, deoxycholic acid (DCA), a colonic bacterial transformation product, has been implicated in gallstone formation and colorectal carcinogenesis. (177, 178)

Serum DCA levels, which may reflect the bile acid pool more accurately, also have been shown to be higher in patients with colon cancer than in healthy individuals. (179, 180) Vegetarian diets result in significantly lower levels of DCA than the standard American diet. (181, 182) A proposed mechanism for associations between DCA and colon cancer is that DCA may change the balance between apoptosis, proliferation, and differentiation in the intestinal epithelium, (183) acting through interference of tumor suppression and enhancing stimulation of growth via cell signaling pathways. In addition, the higher fiber intake of the vegetarian diet results in increased fecal bulk, thus lessening the concentration of DCA in the colon. The more rapid transit time that results from a high fiber diet further reduces exposure to DCA. (184, 185)

3.3.2 How the microbiome can prevent colon cancer

Among the dietary factors, several plant-derived compounds have been found to afford colon cancer protection. These compounds influence many aspects of colonic cellular regulation and develop complex interrelationships with the colonic microbiome. Increasing understanding of the role of microorganisms in determining the colonic environment has led to awareness of this important interrelationship among dietary factors and the microbial population.

3.3.2.1 Butyrate

The gut microbiota can ferment complex dietary residues that are resistant to digestion by enteric enzymes. This process provides energy for the microbiota, and culminates in the release of short chain fatty acids including butyrate, propionate and acetate. Propionate and acetate are beneficial in lowering the pH of the stool, whereas butyrate is utilized for the metabolic needs of the colon and the body.

Butyrate has a remarkable array of colonic health promoting and antineoplastic properties: it is the preferred energy source for colonocytes, it maintains mucosal integrity, and it suppresses inflammation and carcinogenesis through effects on immunity, gene expression and epigenetic modulation. (186)

3.3.2.2 Polyphenols

Plant-derived polyphenols are active mediators of cellular events, targeting key carcinogenic pathways, and modulating colonic microbial populations. In turn, the colonic microorganisms metabolize dietary compounds and mediate

How to cite this article: Rose S, Strombom A. Colorectal cancer prevention with a plant-based diet. Canc Therapy & Oncol Int J. 2019; 15(2): 555906.
DOI: 10.19080/CTOIJ.2019.15.555906

cellular events. Hence, dietary bioactive compounds and the intestinal microbiota create a complex milieu that directly affects the carcinogenic events of the colon. (187)

Consumption of cruciferous or Brassica vegetables has been shown to be inversely associated with risk of some cancers. (188) Glucosinolates are converted into isothiocyanates (ITCs) by bacterially produced thioglucosidases. Previous studies have shown that certain species of bacteria, such as Escherichia coli, Bacteroides thetaiotaomicron, Enterococcus faecalis, E. faecium, Peptostreptococcus sp., and Bifidobacterium sp., isolated from the human gut or feces, can convert glucosinolates into ITC and other derivatives. (189, 190, 191)

Isothiocyanates (ITCs) have been shown to have anti carcinogenic properties both in vitro and in vivo. (192) The biologic effects of ITCs are diverse, including interaction with multiple signaling pathways important to carcinogenesis as well as cross talk between pathways. As explained in the section on Sulforaphane (an example of ITC), the inhibitory activity of ITCs against tumorigenesis is inferred by its ability to modulate Phase 1 and 2 biotransformation enzyme activities, thereby affecting several processes related to chemical carcinogenesis, such as the metabolism and DNA binding of carcinogens. In vivo studies have also indicated that ITCs induce apoptosis. (193)

3.3.2.3 Fiber

Dietary fiber appears critical in influencing the composition and metabolic activity of the microbiome, determining levels of short chain fatty acids important for intestinal health. Western style diets, high in fat and sugar, and low in fiber decrease beneficial Firmicutes that metabolize dietary-fiber-derived polysaccharides to short chain fatty acids. (194) However, in healthy individuals, fiber intake improves the gut microbiota. (195)

Dietary fiber of edible plants comprises insoluble and soluble carbohydrates including cellulose, lignin, and nonstarch polysaccharides such as hemicelluloses, pectins and arabinoxylan oligosaccharides. (196, 194) Other dietary fiber components include nondigestible oligosaccharides such as inulin and oligofructose, as well as resistant starch. (196, 194, 197) They demonstrate resistance to digestion in the human small intestine, allowing passage largely intact into the colon where they increase viscosity and bulking of the fecal matter. (198) Importantly, it is here that dietary fiber undergoes fermentation by the resident colonic microbiota to short chain fatty acids (primarily butyrate, acetate and propionate) that act as the primary carbon energy source for colonocytes. (199, 200, 201) In particular, butyrate has been reported to be protective against development of colitis (202) and colorectal cancer. (203, 204)

3.3.3 The Vegan Advantage

When vegan diets are directly compared to vegetarian and omnivorous diets, a pattern of protective health benefits emerges. The relatively recent inclusion of vegan diets in studies of gut microbiota and health allows us the opportunity to assess whether the vegan gut microbiota is distinct, and whether the many health advantages characteristic of a vegan diet may be partially explained by the associated microbiota profile. The relationship between diet and the intestinal microbial profile appears to follow a continuum, with vegans displaying a gut microbiota most distinct from that of omnivores. (205)

How to cite this article: Rose S, Strombom A. Colorectal cancer prevention with a plant-based diet. Canc Therapy & Oncol Int J. 2019; 15(2): 555906.
DOI: 10.19080/CTOIJ.2019.15.555906

The vegan gut profile appears to be unique in several characteristics, including a reduced abundance of pathobionts and a greater abundance of protective species. Reduced levels of inflammation may be the key feature linking the vegan gut microbiota with protective health effects. (205)

Vegans have a higher ratio than meat eaters of Faecalibacterium prausnitzii, an anti inflammatory bacterium and abundant butyrate producer in the class Clostridia (phylum Firmicutes), purported to play a protective role for colonocytes. (205)

A recent, large-scale study by Zimmer et al. (206) set out to distinguish the fecal microbiota profile of vegans from that of vegetarians, and from an equal number of controls consuming an omnivorous diet. Vegan and vegetarian subjects had adhered to their proclaimed diet for at least 4 weeks prior to the study. Vegan samples had significantly lower microbial counts than their omnivore counterparts for four bacterial taxa: Bacteroides, Bifidobacterium, E. coli and Enterobacteriaceae. Interestingly, the vegetarian sample also showed significantly reduced Bacteroides and Bifidobacteria, a result found 37 years earlier by Reddy. (181)

In a small Indian study, the dominant phylum from healthy vegetarians was found to be Firmicutes (34%), followed by Bacteroidetes (15%). The balance was reversed in non vegetarian (Bacteroidetes 84%, Firmicutes 4%). The colon cancer and IBD patients had higher percentages of Bacteroidetes (55% in both) than Firmicutes (26% and 12%, respectively) than the healthy non vegetarian. (207) This difference may help account for the lower risk vegetarians have of colon cancer.

4. Secondary Prevention

While there are currently no studies on the effect of an overall vegetarian diet on those who already have colon cancer, recurrence studies have shown a substantially raised risk of recurrence of colon cancer for those consuming processed meat. However, those consuming plant foods such as legumes and tree nuts had the risk of recurrence lowered. The studies on recurrence that are available are detailed below. This field warrants further study.

Disease-free survival among colorectal cancer patients was significantly worsened among patients with a high processed meat dietary pattern raising the risk of recurrence by 85%. (208)

However, certain plant foods, in particular beans, cereals and nuts, have been shown to be especially efficacious in preventing colon cancer recurrence. Those colon cancer patients who are in the highest quartile of bean consumption reduced the risk of advanced adenomas recurrence by 65%. Those in the highest quartile of peas and green beans consumption reduced the risk of advanced adenoma recurrence by 49%. (209)

In a recent prospective study involving 1575 patients with Stage I to III colorectal cancer, high fiber intake especially from cereals was associated with a low colorectal-cancer-specific mortality and overall mortality. (210)

In the past few years, an inverse correlation between nut consumption and major chronic diseases such as cardiovascular diseases, metabolic syndrome, and type 2 diabetes has been established. (211, 212, 213, 214, 215) In addition, studies have suggested that nut consumption could also have a chemopreventive effect, especially on colorectal and prostate cancer. (216, 217) Recent epidemiological studies have confirmed an inverse association between frequent nut consumption and cancer mortality. (218, 219, 220)

How to cite this article: Rose S, Strombom A. Colorectal cancer prevention with a plant-based diet. Canc Therapy & Oncol Int J. 2019; 15(2): 555906.
DOI: 10.19080/CTOIJ.2019.15.555906

An observational study of 826 patients with stage III colon cancer showed that those who consumed two ounces or more of tree nuts per week had a 42% lower chance of cancer recurrence and 57% lower chance of death than those who did not eat nuts. (221)

Nuts contain many bioactive compounds that have been found to affect several cellular processes involved in tumor development and progression, including cell survival, cell proliferation, cell invasion, and angiogenesis (222, 223) and therefore can account for the anticancer properties of nuts.

5. Clinical Considerations

The benefits of a plant-based diet in reducing the risk of colon cancer, and in preventing recurrence, should be explained to every patient, and they can be presented with the option to change their diet.

A quality of life study found that colorectal patients following a "Western" meat centered diet had a 45% lower chance to improve in physical functioning, 30% lower chance to improve constipation and a 44% lower chance to improve diarrhea over time compared to patients following a fruit and vegetable diet who also reported a better quality of life. (224) These are symptoms that no patient would wish to prolong.

The plant-based diet has the distinct advantage of having no contraindications or adverse reactions. Since age is a major risk factor for colon cancer, many colon cancer patients are also at higher risk of coronary artery disease and Type 2 Diabetes. The plant-based diet is both safe and efficacious for these comorbidities as well. (225, 226)

When treating patients with a plant-based diet, physicians should also monitor those patients with such comorbidities, and be careful not to underestimate the efficacy of a plant-based to treat these common comorbidities. For instance, the plant-based diet can lower glycosylated Hb significantly more than the frontline drug, Metformin (227, 228) and is as efficacious for the treatment of treatment of hypercholesterolemia as the reductase inhibitor, Lovostatin. (229) Therefore, medications should be titrated as the treatment effects for comorbidities become evident.

6. Discussion

The WHO and the ACIR have classified processed meats as a group 1 carcinogen based on the strength of evidence. This is the same category as tobacco. While tobacco probably has an even greater deleterious effect on overall public health, the potential negative impact of consuming processed meats should be explained to all patients. They should also be informed that red meat is in group 2A as a probable carcinogen.

The plant-based diet very significantly treats several risk factors for colon cancer while reducing the risk of colon cancer itself. We now know of several mechanisms by which this occurs. This should increase the confidence of physicians when prescribing a plant-based diet for the primary prevention of colon cancer.

Currently, the prevention of colon cancer is carried out by the widespread use of fecal testing, colonoscopies and tomography followed by polypectomy. But colonoscopy, with excision of a pedunculated or sessile polyps, is really secondary prevention and it comes at quite a price tag for the country. According to a New York Times article, the price tag for colonoscopies averages $1,185 and is often much, much more — as much as $4,090 in the Twin Cities, according to Healthcare Blue Book data. That's less than New York City's $8,517, but much more than Baltimore's $1,908. Data from the Centers for Disease Control and Prevention suggests that more than 10 million people have a colonoscopy each year, adding up to more than $10 billion in annual costs. Also, let's not forget that the procedure is not risk free and is unpleasant for the patient at best. About one in three adults aged 50 to 75 years have not been tested for colorectal cancer as recommended by the United States Preventive Services Task Force. This may be due in part to the expense and the discomfort anticipated by the patients about the procedure.

With all these disadvantages, the question that naturally comes to mind is what can the patient be offered for primary prevention? Evidence shows that a plant-based diet is both safe and efficacious for the primary prevention of colon cancer. The advantage of at least a 50% reduction in colon cancer risk is too significant to be overlooked, especially for one of the more common malignant pathologies. Diet is also a significant factor in reducing colon cancer recurrence.

References

1. Anand P, Kunnumakara A, Sundaram C, Harikumar K, Tharakan S, et al. (2008) Cancer is a Preventable Disease that Requires Major Lifestyle Changes. *Pharm Res.* 25(9):2097-2116.
2. Singh P, Fraser G. (1998) Dietary risk factors for colon cancer in a low-risk population. *Am J Epidemiol.* 148(8):761-74.
3. Bingham S. (2000) Diet and colorectal cancer prevention. *Biochem Soc Trans.* 28(2):12-6.
4. Willett W. (1995) Diet, nutrition, and avoidable cancer. *Environ Health Perspect.* 103(Suppl 8):165-70.
5. Boutron M, Wilpart M, Faivre J. (1991) Diet and colorectal cancer. *Eur J Cancer Prev.* 1(Suppl 2):13-20.
6. Potter J. (1996) Nutrition and Colorectal Cancer. *Cancer Causes Control.* 7(1):127-46.
7. Chen Z, Wang P, Woodrow J, Zhu Y, Roebothan B et al. (2015) Dietary patterns and colorectal cancer: results from a Canadian population-based study. *Nutr J.* 14:8.
8. World Cancer Research Fund / American Institute for Cancer Research. (2007) *Food, Nutrition, Physical Activity, and the Prevention of Cancer: a Global Perspective.* Washington DC: AICR.
9. Lanou A, Svenson B. (2011) Reduced cancer risk in vegetarians: an analysis of recent reports. *Cancer Manag Res.* 3:1-8.
10. Tabung F, Brown L, Fung T. (2018) Dietary patterns and colorectal cancer risk: a review of 17 years of evidence (2000–2016). *Curr Colorectal Cancer Rep.* 13(6):440-454.
11. Schwingshackl L, Schwedhelm C, Hoffmann G, Knüppel S, Laure Preterre A, et al. (2018) Food groups and risk of colorectal cancer. *Int J Cancer.* 142(9):1748-1758.
12. Sandhu M, White I, McPherson K. (2001) Systematic review of the prospective cohort studies on meat consumption and colorectal cancer risk: a meta-analytical approach. *Cancer Epidemiol Biomarkers Prev.* 10(5):439-46.
13. Larsson S, Wolk A. (2006) Meat consumption and risk of colorectal cancer: a meta-analysis of prospective studies. *Int J Cancer.* 119(11):2657-64.
14. Norat T, Lukanova A, Ferrari P, Riboli E. (2002) Meat consumption and colorectal cancer risk: dose-response meta-analysis of epidemiological studies. *Int J Cancer.* 98(2):241-56.
15. Aune D, Chan D, Vieira A, Navarro Rosenblatt DA, Vieira R et al. (2013) Red and processed meat intake and risk of colorectal adenomas: a systematic review and meta-analysis of epidemiological studies. *Cancer Causes Control.* 24(4):611-27.

How to cite this article: Rose S, Strombom A. Colorectal cancer prevention with a plant-based diet. Canc Therapy & Oncol Int J. 2019; 15(2): 555906.
DOI: 10.19080/CTOIJ.2019.15.555906

16. Norat T, Bingham S, Ferrari P, Slimani N, Jenab M et al. (2005) Meat, fish, and colorectal cancer risk: the European prospective investigation into cancer and nutrition. *J Natl Cancer Inst*. 97(12):906-16.

17. Muto T, Bussey H, Morson B. (1975) The evolution of cancer of the colon and rectum. *Cancer*. 36(6):2251-70.

18. Lee C, Hahn S, Song M, Lee JK, Kim JH, et al. (2014) Vegetarianism as a Protective Factor for Colorectal Adenoma and Advanced Adenoma in Asians. *Dig Dis Sci*. May 2014;59(5):1025-35.

19. Fraser G. (1999) Associations between diet and cancer, ischemic heart disease, and all-cause mortality in non-Hispanic white California Seventh-day Adventists. *Am J Clin Nutr.* 70(3):532s-538s.

20. Orlich M, Singh P, Sabate Jea. (2015) Vegetarian dietary patterns and the risk of colorectal cancers. *JAMA Intern Med*. 175(5):767-76.

21. Bouvard V, Loomis D, Guyton K, Grosse Y, Ghissassi F, et al. (2015) Carcinogenicity of consumption of red and processed meat. *Lancet. Oncol*. 16(16):1599-600.

22. Domingo J, Nadal M. (2017) Carcinogenicity of consumption of red meat and processed meat: A review of scientific news since the IARC decision. *Food Chem Toxicol*. 105:256-261.

23. Kaaks R, Lukanova A. (2001) Energy balance and cancer: the role of insulin and insulin-like growth factor-I. *Proc Nutr Soc*. 60(1):91-106.

24. Rizzo N, Sabaté J, Jaceldo-Siegl K, Fraser G. (2011) Vegetarian dietary patterns are associated with a lower risk of metabolic syndrome: the adventist health study 2. *Diabetes Care*. 34(5):1225-7.

25. Valachovicová M, Krajcovicová-Kudlácková M, Blazícek P, Babinská K. (2006) No evidence of insulin resistance in normal weight vegetarians: A case control study. *Eur J Nutr*. 45(1):52-4.

26. Kuo C, Lai N, Ho L, Lin C. (2004) Insulin sensitivity in Chinese ovo-lactovegetarians compared with omnivores. *Eur J Clin Nutr*. 58(2):312-6.

27. Ma Y, Yang Y, Wang F, Zhang P, Shi C, et al. (2013) Obesity and Risk of Colorectal Cancer: A Systematic Review of Prospective Studies. *PLoS One*. 8(1):e53916.

28. Tonstad S, Butler T, Yan R, Fraser G. (2009) Type of Vegetarian Diet, Body Weight, and Prevalence of Type 2 Diabetes. *Diabetes Care*. 32(5):791–796.

29. Bradbury K, Crowe F, Appleby P, Schmidt J, Travis R, et al. (2014) Serum concentrations of cholesterol, apolipoprotein A-I, and apolipoprotein B in a total of 1694 meat-eaters, fish-eaters, vegetarians, and vegans. *Eur J Clin Nutr.* 68(2):178-183.

30. Waldmann A, Koschizke J, Leitzmann C, Hahn A. (2005)German vegan study: diet, life-style factors, and cardiovascular risk profile. *Ann Nutr Metab*. 49(6):366-72.

31. Haddad E, Tanzman J. (2003) What do vegetarians in the United States eat? *Am J Clin Nutr*. 78(3):626S-632S.

32. Newby P, Tucker K, Wolk A. (2005) Risk of overweight and obesity among semivegetarian, lactovegetarian, and vegan women. *Am J Clin Nutr*. 81(6):1267-74.

33. Freeman H. (2008) Colorectal cancer risk in Crohn's disease. *World J Gastroenterol*. 14(12):1810-1811.

34. D'Souza S, Levy E, Mack D, Israel D, Lambrette P, et al. (2008) Dietary patterns and risk for Crohn's disease in children. *Inflamm Bowel Dis*. 14(3):367-73.

35. Li Y, Niu Y, Sun Y, Zhang F, Liu C, et al. (2015) Role of phytochemicals in colorectal cancer prevention. *World J Gastroenterol*. 21(31):9262-72.

36. Spencer JP, Crozier A, eds. (2012) *Flavonoids and related compounds.* Boca Raton: CRC Press, Taylor & Francis Group.

How to cite this article: Rose S, Strombom A. Colorectal cancer prevention with a plant-based diet. Canc Therapy & Oncol Int J. 2019; 15(2): 555906.
DOI: 10.19080/CTOIJ.2019.15.555906

37. Baron J. (2003) Epidemiology of non-steroidal anti-inflammatory drugs and cancer. *Prog Exp Tumor Res*. 37:1-24.

38. Elwood P, Gallagher A, Duthie G, Mur LA, Morgan G. (2009) Aspirin, salicylates, and cancer. *Lancet*. 373(9671):1301-9.

39. Sandler R, Halabi S, Baron J, Budinger S, Paskett E, et al. (2003) A randomized trial of aspirin to prevent colorectal adenomas in patients with previous colorectal cancer. *N Engl J Med*. 348(10):883-90.

40. Chan A, Ogino S, Fuchs C. (2009) Aspirin use and survival after diagnosis of colorectal cancer. *JAMA*. 302(6):649-58.

41. Jacobs E, Thun M, Bain E, Rodriguez C, Henley SJ, et al. (2007) A large cohort study of long-term daily use of adult-strength aspirin and cancer incidence. *J Natl Cancer Inst*. 99(8):608-15.

42. Din F, Theodoratou E, Farrington S, Tenesa A, Barnetson RA, et al. (2010) Effect of aspirin and NSAIDs on risk and survival from colorectal cancer. *Gut*. 59(12):1670-9.

43. Holmes M, Chen W, Li L, Hertzmark E, Spiegelman D, et al. (2010) Aspirin intake and survival after breast cancer. *J Clin Oncol*. 28(9):1467-72.

44. Juárez Olguín H, Flores Pérez J, Lares Asseff I, Loredo Abdala A, Carbajal Rodriguez L et al. (2004) Comparative pharmacokinetics of acetyl salicylic acid and its metabolites in children suffering from autoimmune diseases. *Biopharm Drug Dispos*. 25(1):1-7.

45. Duthie G, Wood A. (2011) Natural salicylates: Foods, functions and disease prevention. *Food Funct*. 2(9):515-20.

46. Paterson J, Baxter GLJ, Duthie G. (2006) Is there a role for dietary salicylates in health? *Proc Nutr Soc*. 65(1):93-96.

47. Jansen M, Bueno-de-Mesquita H, Buzina R, Fidanza F, Menotti A, et al. (1999) Dietary fiber and plant foods in relation to colorectal cancer mortality: The Seven Countries Study. *Int J Cancer*. 81(2):174-9.

48. Howe G, Benito E, Castelleto R, Cornée J, Estève J, et al. (1992) Dietary Intake of Fiber and Decreased Risk of Cancers of the Colon and Rectum: Evidence From the Combined Analysis of 13 Case-Control Studies. *J Natl Cancer Ins*. 84(24):1887-96.

49. Peters U, Sinha R, Chatterjee N, Subar A, Ziegler R, et al. (2003) Dietary fibre and colorectal adenoma in a colorectal cancer early detection programme. *Lancet*. 361(9368):1491-5.

50. Nomura A, Hankin J, Henderson B, Wilkens L, Murphy S, et al. (2007) Dietary fiber and colorectal cancer risk: the multiethnic cohort study. *Cancer Causes Control*. 18(7):753-64.

51. Wakai K, Date C, Fukui M, Tamakoshi K, Watanabe Y, et al. (2007) Dietary Fiber and Risk of Colorectal Cancer in the Japan Collaborative Cohort Study. *Cancer Epidemiol Biomarkers Prev*. 16(4):668-75.

52. Dahm C, Keogh R, Spencer E, Greenwood D, Key T, et al. (2010) Dietary Fiber and Colorectal Cancer Risk: A Nested Case-Control Study Using Food Diaries. *J Natl Cancer Inst*. 102(9):614-26.

53. McCarl M, Harnack L, Limburg P, Anderson K, Folsom A. (2006) Incidence of colorectal cancer in relation to glycemic index and load in a cohort of women. *Cancer Epidemiol Biomarkers Prev*. 15(5):892-6.

54. Bingham S, Norat T, Moskal A, Ferrari P, Slimani N, et al. (2005) Is the Association with Fiber from Foods in Colorectal Cancer Confounded by Folate Intake? *Cancer Epidemiol Biomarkers Prev*. 14(6):1552-6.

55. Murphy N, Norat T, Ferrari P, Jenab M, Bueno-de-Mesquita B, et al. (2012) Dietary Fibre Intake and Risks of Cancers of the Colon and Rectum in the European Prospective Investigation into Cancer and Nutrition (EPIC). *PLoS One*. 7(6):e39361.

56. World Cancer Research Fund / American Institute for Cancer Research. (2011) *Continuous Update Project Report Summary.*

How to cite this article: Rose S, Strombom A. Colorectal cancer prevention with a plant-based diet. Canc Therapy & Oncol Int J. 2019; 15(2): 555906.
DOI: 10.19080/CTOIJ.2019.15.555906

Food, Nutrition, Physical Activity, and the Prevention of Colorectal Cancer. Washington DC: AICR.

57. Cross A, Ferrucci L, Risch A, Graubard B, Ward M, et al. (2010) A large prospective study of meat consumption and colorectal cancer risk: an investigation of potential mechanisms underlying this association. *Cancer Res*. 70(6):2406-14.
58. Bastide N, Pierre F, Corpet D. (2011) Heme iron from meat and risk of colorectal cancer: a meta-analysis and a review of the mechanisms involved. *Cancer Prev Res (Phila)*. 4(2):177-84.
59. Zheng W, Lee S. (2009) Well-done meat intake, heterocyclic amine exposure, and cancer risk. *Nutr Cancer*. 61(4):437-46.
60. Sinha R, Peters U, Cross A, Kulldorff M, Weissfeld J, et al. (2005) Meat, meat cooking methods and preservation, and risk for colorectal adenoma. *Cancer Res*. 65(17):8034-41.
61. Ward M, Cross A, Divan H, Kulldorff M, Nowell-Kadlubar S, et al. (2007) Processed meat intake, CYP2A6 activity and risk of colorectal adenoma. *Carcinogenesis*. 28(6):1210-6.
62. Howsam M, Grimalt J, Guinó E, Navarro M, Martí-Ragué J, et al. (2004) Organochlorine Exposure and Colorectal Cancer Risk. *Environ Health Perspect*. 112(15):1460-6.
63. Miller P, Lazarus P, Lesko S, Cross AJ, Sinha R, et al. (2013) Meat-Related Compounds and Colorectal Cancer Risk by Anatomical Subsite. *Nutr Cancer*. 65(2):202-26.
64. Turteltaub K, Dingley K, Curtis K, Malfatti M, Turesky R, et al. (1999) Macromolecular adduct formation and metabolism of heterocyclic amines in humans and rodents at low doses. *Cancer Lett*. 143(2):149-55.
65. Cross A, Sinha R. (2004) Meat-related mutagens/carcinogens in the etiology of colorectal cancer. *Environ Mol Mutagen*. 44(1):44-55.
66. Gunter M, Divi R, Kulldorff M, Vermeulen R, Haverkos K, et al. (2007) Leukocyte polycyclic aromatic hydrocarbon-DNA adduct formation and colorectal adenoma. *Carcinogenesis*. 28(7):1426-9.
67. Peters U, DeMarini D, Sinha R, Brooks L, Warren S, et al. (2003) Urinary mutagenicity and colorectal adenoma risk. *Cancer epidemiol biomarkers prev*. 12(11 Pt 1):1253-6.
68. Shin A, Shrubsole M, Rice J, Cai Q, Doll M, et al. (2008) Meat intake, heterocyclic amine exposure, and metabolizing enzyme polymorphisms in relation to colorectal polyp risk. *Cancer Epidemiol Biomarkers Prev*. 17(2):320-9.
69. Kampman E, Slattery M, Bigler J, Leppert M, Samowitz W, et al. (1999) Meat consumption, genetic susceptibility, and colon cancer risk: a United States multicenter case-control study. *Cancer Epidemiol Biomarkers Prev*. 8(1):15-24.
70. Le Marchand L, Hankin J, Pierce L, Sinha R, Nerurkar P, et al. (2002) Well-done red meat, metabolic phenotypes and colorectal cancer in Hawaii. *Mutat Res*. 506-507:205-214.
71. Nowell S, Coles B, Sinha R, MacLeod S, Luke Ratnasinghe D, et al. (2002) Analysis of total meat intake and exposure to individual heterocyclic amines in a case-control study of colorectal cancer: contribution of metabolic variation to risk. *Mutat Res*. 506-507:175-85.
72. Butler L, Millikan R, Sinha R, Keku T, Winkel S, et al. (2008) Modification by N-acetyltransferase 1 genotype on the association between dietary heterocyclic amines and colon cancer in a multiethnic study. *Mutat Res*. 638(1-2):162-74.
73. Chen J, Stampfer M, Hough H, Garcia-Closas M, Willett W, et al. (1998) A prospective study of N-acetyltransferase genotype, red meat intake, and risk of colorectal cancer. *Cancer Res*. 58(15):3307-11.
74. Joshi A, Corral R, Siegmund K, Haile R, Le Marchand L, et al. (2009) Red meat and poultry intake, polymorphisms in the nucleotide excision repair and mismatch repair pathways and colorectal cancer risk. *Carcinogenesis*. 30(3):472-9.

75. Lang N, Butler M, Massengill J, Lawson M, Stotts R, et al. (1994) Rapid metabolic phenotypes for acetyltransferase and cytochrome P4501A2 and putative exposure to food-borne heterocyclic amines increase the risk for colorectal cancer or polyps. *Cancer Epidemiol Biomarkers Prev*. 3(8):675-82.
76. Le Marchand L, Hankin J, Wilkens L, Pierce L, Franke A, et al. (2001) Combined effects of well-done red meat, smoking, and rapid N-acetyltransferase 2 and CYP1A2 phenotypes in increasing colorectal cancer risk. *Cancer Epidemiol Biomarkers Prev*. 10(12):1259-66.
77. Probst-Hensch N, Haile R, Ingles S, Longnecker M, Han C, et al. (1995) Acetylation polymorphism and prevalence of colorectal adenomas. *Cancer Res*. 55(10):2017-20.
78. Roberts-Thomson I, Ryan P, Khoo K, Hart W, McMichael A, et al. (1996) Diet, acetylator phenotype, and risk of colorectal neoplasia. *Lancet*. 347(9012):1372-4.
79. Chan A, Tranah G, Giovannucci E, Willett W, Hunter D, et al. (2005) Prospective study of N-acetyltransferase-2 genotypes, meat intake, smoking and risk of colorectal cancer. *Intl J Cancer*. 115(4):648-52.
80. Phillips D. (1999) Polycyclic aromatic hydrocarbons in the diet. *Mutat Res*. 443(1-2):139-47.
81. Buckley T, Lioy P. (1992) An examination of the time course from human dietary exposure to polycyclic aromatic hydrocarbons to urinary elimination of 1-hydroxypyrene. *Br J Ind Med*. 49(2):113-24.
82. Hamidi E, Hajeb P, Selamat J, Abdull Razis A. (2016) Polycyclic Aromatic Hydrocarbons (PAHs) and their Bioaccessibility in Meat: a Tool for Assessing Human Cancer. *Asian Pac J Cancer Prev*. 17(1):15-23.
83. Goldman R, Shields P. (2003) Food Mutagens. *J Nutr*. 133(3):965S-973S.
84. Probst-Hensch N, Sinha R, Longnecker M, Witte J, Ingles S, et al. (1997) Meat preparation and colorectal adenomas in a large sigmoidoscopy-based case-control study in California (United States). *Cancer Causes Control*. 8(2):175-83.
85. Giovannucci E, Rimm E, Stampfer M, Colditz G, Ascherio A, et al. (1994) Intake of fat, meat, and fiber in relation to risk of colon cancer in men. *Cancer Res*. 54(9):2390-7.
86. Santonicola S, Albrizio S, Murru N, Ferrante M, Mercogliano R. (2017) Study on the occurrence of polycyclic aromatic hydrocarbons in milk and meat/fish-based baby food available in Italy. *Chemosphere*. 184:467-472.
87. Tricker A, Preussmann R. (1991) Carcinogenic N-nitrosamines in the diet: occurrence, formation, mechanisms and carcinogenic potential. *Mutat Res*. 259(3-4):277-89.
88. Fisher B. (1999) Most Unwanted. *Environ Health Perspect*. 107(1):A18-23.
89. Dougherty C, Henricks Holtz S, Reinert J, Panyacosit L, Axelrad D, et al. (2000) Dietary exposures to food contaminants across the United States. *Environ Res*. 84(2):170-85.
90. Kiviranta H, Tuomisto J, Tuomisto J, Tukiainen E, Vartiainen T. (2005) Polychlorinated dibenzo-p-dioxins, dibenzofurans, and biphenyls in the general population in Finland. *Chemosphere*. 60(7):854-69.
91. Kopp T, Vogel U, Tjonneland A, Andersen V. (2018) Meat and fiber intake and interaction with pattern recognition receptors (TLR1, TLR2, TLR4, and TLR10) in relation to colorectal cancer in a Danish prospective, case-cohort study. *Am J Clin Nutr*. 107(3):465-479.
92. Arcidiacono B, Iiritano S, Nocera A, Possidente K, Nevolo M, et al. (2012) Insulin Resistance and Cancer Risk: An Overview of the Pathogenetic Mechanisms. *Exp Diabetes Res*. 2012:789174.
93. Giovannucci E. (1995) Insulin and Colon Cancer. *Cancer Causes Control*. 6(2):164-79.
94. 94. Pollak M. (2008) Insulin and insulin-like growth factor signaling in neoplasia. *Nature Reviews. Cancer*. 8(12):915-28.

How to cite this article: Rose S, Strombom A. Colorectal cancer prevention with a plant-based diet. Canc Therapy & Oncol Int J. 2019; 15(2): 555906.
DOI: 10.19080/CTOIJ.2019.15.555906

95. Frasca F, Pandini G, Scalia P, Sciacca L, Mineo R, et al. (1999) Insulin receptor isoform A, a newly recognized, high-affinity insulin- like growth factor II receptor in fetal and cancer cells. *Mol Cell Biol*. 19(5):3278-3288.

96. Vigneri P, Frasca F, Sciacca L, Pandini G, Vigneri R. (2009) Diabetes and cancer. *Endocr Relat Cancer*. 16(4):1103-23.

97. Nakae J, Kido Y, Accili D. (2001) Distinct and overlapping functions of insulin and IGF-I receptors. *Endocr Rev*. 22(6):818-35.

98. Siddle K. (2011) Signalling by insulin and IGF receptors: supporting acts and new players. J *Mol Endocrinol*. 47(1):R1-10.

99. Mosthaf L, Grako K, Dull T, Coussens L, Ullrich A, et al. (1990) Functionally distinct insulin receptors generated by tissue-specific alternative splicing. *EMBO J*. 9(8):2409-13.

100. Comstock S, Xu D, Hortos K, Kovan B, McCaskey S, et al. (2014) Association of insulin-related serum factors with colorectal polyp number and type in adult males. *Cancer Epidemiol Biomarkers Prev*. 23(9):1843-51.

101. Yoshida I, Suzuki A, Vallée M, Matano Y, Masunaga T, et al. (2006) Serum insulin levels and the prevalence of adenomatous and hyperplastic polyps in the proximal colon. *Clin Gastroenterol Hepatol*. 4(10):1225-31.

102. Lahm H, Amstad P, Wyniger J, Yilmaz A, Fischer J, et al. (1994) Blockade of the insulin-like growth-factor-I receptor inhibits growth of human colorectal cancer cells: evidence of a functional IGF-II-mediated autocrine loop. *Intl J Cancer*. 58(3):452-9.

103. Bowers L, Rossi E, O'Flanagan C, deGraffenried L, Hursting S. (2015) The role of the insulin/IGF system in cancer: lessons learned from clinical trials and the energy balance-cancer link. *Front Endocrinol (Lausanne)*. 6:77.

104. Frasca F, Pandini G, Sciacca L, Pezzino V, Squatrito S, et al. (2008) The role of insulin receptors and IGF-I receptors in cancer and other diseases. *Arch Physiol Biochem*. 114(1):23-37.

105. Stojsavljević S, Virović Jukić L, Kralj D, Duvnjak M. (2016) The relationship between insulin resistance and colon cancer. *Endocr Oncol Metab*. 24-33.

106. Giovannucci E. (2001) Insulin, insulin-like growth factors and colon cancer: a review of the evidence. *J Nutr*. 131(11 Suppl):3109S-20S.

107. Allen N, Appleby P, Davey G, Kaaks R, Rinaldi S, et al. (2002) The associations of diet with serum insulin-like growth factor I and its main binding proteins in 292 women meat-eaters, vegetarians, and vegans. *Cancer Epidemiol Biomarkers Prev*. 11(11):1441-8.

108. Allen N, Appleby P, Davey G, Key T. (2000) Hormones and diet: low insulin-like growth factor-I but normal bioavailable androgens in vegan men. *Br J Cancer*. 83(1):95-7.

109. Kersten C, Louhimo J, Ålgars A, Lahdesmaki A, Cvancerova M, et al. (2013) Increased C-reactive protein implies a poorer stage-specific prognosis in colon cancer. *Acta Oncologica (Stockholm, Sweden)*. 52(8):1691-8.

110. Kigawa N, Budhathoki S, Yamaji, T, Iwasaki M, Inoue M, et al. (2017) Association of plasma C-reactive protein level with the prevalence of colorectal adenoma: the Colorectal Adenoma Study in Tokyo. *Sci Rep*. 7(1):4456.

111. Davenport J, Cai Q, Ness R, Milne G, Zhao Z, et al. (2016) Evaluation of Pro-inflammatory Markers Plasma C-reactive Protein and Urinary Prostaglandin-E2 Metabolite in Colorectal Adenoma Risk. *Mol Carcinogenesis*. 55(8):1251-61.

112. Ananthakrishnan A, Cheng S, Cai T, Cagan A, Gainer V, et al. (2014) Serum Inflammatory Markers and Risk of Colorectal Cancer in Patients with Inflammatory Bowel Diseases. *Clin Gastroenterol Hepatol*. 12(8):1342-8.

113. Szeto Y, Kwok T, Benzie I. (2004) Effects of long-term vegetarian diet on biomarkers of antioxidant status and cardiovascular disease risk. *Nutr*. 20(10):863-6.

114. Haghighatdoost F, Bellissimo N, Totosy de Zepetnek J, Rouhani M. (2017) Association of

vegetarian diet with inflammatory biomarkers: a systematic review and meta-analysis of observational studies. *Public Health Nutr*. 1-9.

115. Gialeli C, Theocharis A, Karamanos N. (2011) Roles of matrix metalloproteinases in cancer progression and their pharmacological targeting. *FEBS J*. 278(1):16-27.

116. Navarro J, de Gouveia L, Rocha-Penha L, Cinegaglia N, Belo V, et al. (2016) Reduced levels of potential circulating biomarkers of cardiovascular diseases in apparently healthy vegetarian men. *Clinica Chimica Acta*. 461:110-113.

117. Zucker S, Vacirca J. (2004) Role of matrix metalloproteinases (MMPs) in colorectal cancer. *Cancer Metastisis Rev*. 23(1-2):101-17.

118. Matusheski N, Juvik J, Jeffery E. (2004) Heating decreases epithiospecifier protein activity and increases sulforaphane formation in broccoli. *Phytochemistry*. 65(9):1273-81.

119. Cooper D, Webb D, JC P. (1997) Evaluation of the potential for olestra to affect the availability of dietary phytochemicals. *J Nutr*. 127((8 Suppl)):1699S-1709S.

120. Winiwarter S, Bonham N, Ax F, Hallberg A, Lennernäs H, et al. (1998) Correlation of human jejunal permeability (in vivo) of drugs with experimentally and theoretically derived parameters. A multivariate data analysis approach. *J Med Chem*. 41(25):4939-49.

121. Zhang Y, Callaway E. (2002) High cellular accumulation of sulphoraphane, a dietary anticarcinogen, is followed by rapid transporter-mediated export as a glutathione conjugate. *Biochem J*. 364(Pt 1):301-7.

122. Kassahun K, Davis M, Hu P, Martin B, Baillie T. (1997) Biotransformation of the naturally occurring isothiocyanate sulforaphane in the rat: identification of phase I metabolites and glutathione conjugates. *Chem res toxicol*. 10(11):1228-33.

123. Tomczyk J, Olejnik A. (2010) Sulforaphane–a possible agent in prevention and therapy of cancer. *Postepy Hig Med Dosw (online)*. 64:590-603.

124. Zeng H, Trujillo O, Moyer M, Botnen J. (2011) Prolonged sulforaphane treatment activates survival signaling in nontumorigenic NCM460 colon cells but apoptotic signaling in tumorigenic HCT116 colon cells. *Nutr Cancer*. 63(2):248-55.

125. Gamet-Payrastre L, Li P, Lumeau S, Cassar G, Dupont M, et al. (2000) Sulforaphane, a naturally occurring isothiocyanate, induces cell cycle arrest and apoptosis in HT29 human colon cancer cells. *Cancer Res*. 60(5):1426-33.

126. Burn J, Chapman P, Bishop D, Mathers J. (1998) Diet and cancer prevention: the concerted action polyp prevention (CAPP) studies. *Proc Nutr Soc*. 57(2):183-6.

127. Burn J, Gerdes A, Macrae F, Mecklin J, Moeslein G, et al. (2011) Long-term effect of aspirin on cancer risk in carriers of hereditary colorectal cancer: an analysis from the CAPP2 randomised controlled trial. *Lancet*. 378(9809):2081-7.

128. Movahedi M, Bishop D, Macrae F, Mecklin J, Moeslein G, et al. (2015) Obesity, aspirin, and risk of colorectal cancer in carriers of hereditary colorectal cancer: a prospective investigation in the CAPP2 study. *J Clin Oncol*. 33(31):3591-7.

129. Chung Y, Bae Y, Lee S. (2003) Molecular ordering of ROS production, mitochondrial changes, and caspase activation during sodium salicylate-induced apoptosis. *Free Radic Biol Med*. 34(4):434-42.

130. Liao X, Lochhead P, Nishihara R, Morikawa T, Kuchiba A, et al. (2012) Aspirin use, tumor PIK3CA mutation, and colorectal-cancer survival. *N Engl J Med*. 367(17):1596-606.

131. Dhanoya T, Burn J. (2016) Colon cancer and Salicylates. *Evol Med Public Health*. 2016(1):146-7.

132. Paterson J, Lawrence J. (2001) Salicylic acid: a link between aspirin, diet and the prevention of colorectal cancer. *QJM*. 94(8):445-8.

How to cite this article: Rose S, Strombom A. Colorectal cancer prevention with a plant-based diet. Canc Therapy & Oncol Int J. 2019; 15(2): 555906.
DOI: 10.19080/CTOIJ.2019.15.555906

133. Blacklock C, Lawrence J, Wiles D, Malcolm E, Gibson I, et al. (2001) Salicylic acid in the serum of subjects not taking aspirin. Comparison of salicylic acid. *J Clin Pathol.* 54(7):553-5.

134. Lawrence J, Peter R, Baxter G, Robson J, Graham A, et al. (2003) Urinary excretion of salicyluric and salicylic acids by non-vegetarians, vegetarians and patients taking low-dose aspirin. *J Clin Pathol.* 56(9):651-3.

135. Vucenik I, Shamsuddin A. (2006) Protection against cancer by dietary IP6 and inositol. *Nutr Cancer.* 55(2):109-25.

136. Druzijanic N, Juricic J, Perko Z, Kraljevic D. (2004) IP6 + Inositol as adjuvant to chemotherapy of colon cancer: our clinical experience. *Anticancer Res.* 24(5):3474-75.

137. Kapral M, Wawszczyk J, Jurzak M, Dymitruk D, Weglarz L. (2010) Evaluation of the expression of metalloproteinases 2 and 9 and their tissue inhibitors in colon cancer cells treated with phytic acid. *Acta Poloniae Pharmaceutica.* 67(6):625-9.

138. Graf E, Eaton J. (1993) Suppression of colonic cancer by dietary phytic acid. *Nutr Cancer.* 19(1):11-19.

139. Norazalina S, Norhaizan M, Hairuszah I, Norashareena M. (2010) Anticarcinogenic efficacy of phytic acid extracted from rice bran on azoxymethane-induced colon carcinogenesis in rats. *Exp Toxicol Pathol.* 62(3):259-68.

140. Shafie N, Mohd Esa N, Ithnin H, Md Akim A, Saad N, et al. (2013) Preventive inositol hexaphosphate extracted from rice bran inhibits colorectal cancer through involvement of Wnt/β-catenin and COX-2 pathways. *Biomed Res Intl.* 2013:681027.

141. Burkitt D. (1971) Epidemiology of cancer of the colon and rectum. *Cancer.* 28(1):3-13.

142. Bingham S. (1990) Mechanisms and experimental and epidemiological evidence relating dietary fibre (non-starch polysaccharides) and starch to protection against large bowel cancer. *Proc Nutr Soc.* 49(2):153-71.

143. Young G, Hu Y, Le Leu R, Nyskohus L. (2005) Dietary fibre and colorectal cancer: A model for environment-gene interactions. *Mol Nutr Food Res.* 49(6):571-84.

144. Slavin J. (2000) Mechanisms for the Impact of Whole Grain Foods on Cancer Risk. *J Am Coll Nutr.* 19(3 Suppl):300S-307S.

145. Rowland I. (1999) Toxicological implications of the normal microflora. In: Tannock GW, ed. *Med Imp Normal Microflora.* Dordrecht: Kluwer Academic Publishers.

146. Hullar M, Burnett-Hartman A, Lampe J. (2014) Gut microbes, diet, and cancer. *Cancer Treat Res.* 159:377-99.

147. Bultman S. (2017) Interplay between diet, gut microbiota, epigenetic events, and colorectal cancer. *Mol Nutr Food Res.* 61(1).

148. Bingham S, Hughes R, Cross A. (2002) Effect of white versus red meat on endogenous N-nitrosation in the human colon and further evidence of a dose response. *J Nutr.* 132(11 Suppl):3522S-3525S.

149. Bos J. (1989) ras oncogenes in human cancer: a review. *Cancer Res.* 49(17):4682-9.

150. Silvester K, Cummings J. (1995) Does digestibility of meat protein help explain large bowel cancer risk? *Nutr Cancer.* 24(3):279-88.

151. Hughes R, Cross A, Pollock J, Bingham S. (2001) Dose-dependent effect of dietary meat on endogenous colonic N-nitrosation. *Carcinogenesis.* 22(1):199-202.

152. Hebels D, Sveje K, de Kok M, van Herwijnen MH, Kuhnle GG, et al. (2012) Red meat intake-induced increases in fecal water genotoxicity correlate with pro-carcinogenic gene expression changes in the human colon. *Food Chem Toxicol.* 50(2):95-103.

153. Blaser M. (2008) Understanding microbe-induced cancers. *Cancer Prev Res (Philadel).* 1(1):15-20.

154. Cross A, Pollock J, Bingham S. (2003) Haem, not protein or inorganic iron, is responsible for

endogenous intestinal N-nitrosation arising from red meat. *Cancer Res*. 63(10):2358-60.

155. Hughes R, Pollock J, Bingham S. (2002) Effect of vegetables, tea, and soy on endogenous N-nitrosation, fecal ammonia, and fecal water genotoxicity during a high red meat diet in humans. *Nutr Cancer*. 42(1):70-77.
156. Attene-Ramos M, Wagner E, Plewa M, Gaskins H. (2006) Evidence that hydrogen sulfide is a genotoxic agent. *Mol Cancer Res*. 4(1):9-14.
157. Deplancke B, Gaskins H. (2003) Hydrogen sulfide induces serum-independent cell cycle entry in nontransformed rat intestinal epithelial cells. *FASEB J*. 17(10):1310-2.
158. Huycke M, Gaskins H. (2004) Commensal bacteria, redox stress, and colorectal cancer: mechanisms and models. *Exp Biol Med (Maywood)*. 229(7):586-97.
159. Christl S, Eisner H, Dusel G. (1996) Antagonistic effects of sulfide and butyrate on proliferation of colonic mucosa: a potential role for these agents in the pathogenesis of ulcerative colitis. *Dig Dis Sci*. 41(12):2477-81.
160. Roediger W. (1998) Decreased sulphur amino acid intake in ulcerative colitis. *Lancet*. 351(9115):1555.
161. Roediger W, Moore J, Babidge W. (1997) Colonic sulfide in pathogenesis and treatment of ulcerative colitis. *Dig Dis Sci*. 42(8):1571-9.
162. Attene-Ramos M, Wagner E, Gaskins H, Plewa M. (2007) Hydrogen sulfide induces direct radical-associated DNA damage. *Mol Cancer Res*. 5(5):455-9.
163. O'Keefe S, Carrim Y, van der Merwe C, Hylemon P, Hertzler S. (2004) Differences in Diet and Colonic Bacterial Metabolism That Might Account for the Low Risk of Colon Cancer in Native Africans Compared with Americans. *J Nutr*. 134:3521S–3547S.
164. Deplancke B, Finster K, Graham W. (2003) Gastrointestinal and microbial responses to sulfate-supplemented drinking water in mice. *Exp Biol Med (Maywood)*. 228(4):424-33.
165. Magee E, Curno R, Edmond L, Cummings J. (2004) Contribution of dietary protein and inorganic sulfur to urinary sulfate: toward a biomarker of inorganic sulfur intake. *Am J Clin Nutr*. 80(1):137-42.
166. Cani P, Neyrinck A, Fava F, Knauf C, Burcelin R, et al. (2007) Selective increases of bifidobacteria in gut microflora improve high-fat-diet-induced diabetes in mice through a mechanism associated with endotoxaemia. *Diabetologia*. 50(11):2374-83.
167. Delzenne N, Cani P. (2011) Interaction between obesity and the gut microbiota: relevance in nutrition. *Ann Rev Nutr*. 31:15-31.
168. de Wit N, Derrien M, Bosch-Vermeulen H, Oosterink E, Keshtkar S, et al. (2012) Saturated fat stimulates obesity and hepatic steatosis and affects gut microbiota composition by an enhanced overflow of dietary fat to the distal intestine. *Am J Physiol Gastrointest Liver Physiol*. 303(5):589-99.
169. Cani P, Amar J, Iglesias M, Poggi M, Knauf C, et al. (2007) Metabolic endotoxemia initiates obesity and insulin resistance. *Diabetes*. 56(7):1761-72.
170. Creely S, McTernan P, Kusminski C, Fisher fM, Da Silva N, et al. (2007) Lipopolysaccharide activates an innate immune system response in human adipose tissue in obesity and type 2 diabetes. *Am J Physiol Endocrinol Metab*. 292(3):E740-7.
171. Cammarota R, Bertolini V, Pennesi G, Bucci EO, Gottardi O, et al. (2010) The tumor microenvironment of colorectal cancer: stromal TLR-4 expression as a potential prognostic marker. *J Transl Med*. 8:112.
172. Fukata M, Abreu M. (2007) TLR4 signaling in the intestine in health and disease. *Biochem Soc Transac*. 35(Pt 6):1473-8.
173. Abreu M. (2010) Toll-like receptor signaling in the intestinal epithelium: how bacterial recognition shapes intestinal function. *Nat Rev Immunol*. 10(2):131-44.

How to cite this article: Rose S, Strombom A. Colorectal cancer prevention with a plant-based diet. Canc Therapy & Oncol Int J. 2019; 15(2): 555906.
DOI: 10.19080/CTOIJ.2019.15.555906

174. Manco M, Putignani L, Bottazzo G. (2010) Gut microbiota, lipopolysaccharides, and innate immunity in the pathogenesis of obesity and cardiovascular risk. *Endocr Rev*. 31(6):817-44.

175. Pastor Rojo O, López San Román A, Albéniz Arbizu E. (2007) Serum lipopolysaccharide-binding protein in endotoxemic patients with inflammatory bowel disease. *Inflamm Bowel Dis*. 13(3):269-77.

176. Chen R, Luo F, Wang Y, Tang J, Liu Y. (2011) LBP and CD14 polymorphisms correlate with increased colorectal carcinoma risk in Han Chinese. *World J Gastroenterol*. 17(18):2326-31.

177. Bernstein C, Holubec H, Bhattacharyya A, Nguyen H, Payne C, et al. (2011) Carcinogenicity of deoxycholate, a secondary bile acid. *Arch Toxicol*. 85(8):863-71.

178. Mower H, Ray R, Shoff R, Stemmermann G, Nomura A, et al. (1979) Fecal bile acids in two Japanese populations with different colon cancer risks. *Cancer Res*. 39(2 Pt 1):328-31.

179. Bayerdörffer E, Mannes G, Richter W. (1993) Increased serum deoxycholic acid levels in men with colorectal adenomas. *Gastroenterol*. 104(1):145-51.

180. Bayerdörffer E, Mannes G, Ochsenkühn T, Dirschedl P, Paumgartner G. (1994) Variation of serum bile acids in patients with colorectal adenomas during a one-year follow-up. *Digestion*. 55(2):121-9.

181. Reddy B, Weisburger J, Wynder E. (1975) Effect of high-risk and low-risk diets for colon carcinogenesis on focal microflora and steroids in man. *J Nutr*. 105(7):878-84.

182. Reddy B. (1981) Diet and excretion of bile acids. *Cancer Res*. 41(9 Pt 2):3766-8.

183. Hague A, Elder D, Hicks D, Paraskeva C. (1995) Apoptosis in colorectal tumour cells: induction by the short chain fatty acids butyrate, propionate and acetate and by the bile salt deoxycholate. *Intl J Cancer*. 60(3):400-6.

184. Reddy B, Hedges A, Laakso K, Wynder E. (1978) Metabolic epidemiology of large bowel cancer: fecal bulk and constituents of high-risk North American and low-risk Finnish population. *Cancer*. 42(6):2832-8.

185. Reddy B, Watanabe K, Sheinfil A. (1980) Effect of dietary wheat bran, alfalfa, pectin and carrageenan on plasma cholesterol and fecal bile acid and neutral sterol excretion in rats. *J Nutr*. 110(6):1247-54.

186. O'Keefe S. (2016) Diet, microorganisms and their metabolites, and colon cancer. *Nat Rev Gastroenterol Hepatol*. 13: 691–706.

187. Macdonald R, Wagner K. (2012) Influence of dietary phytochemicals and microbiota on colon cancer risk. *J Agric Food Chem*. 60(27):6728-35.

188. Kristal A, Lampe J. (2002) Brassica vegetables and prostate cancer risk: a review of the epidemiological evidence. *Nutr Cancer*. 42(1):1-9.

189. Brabban A, Edwards C. (1994) Isolation of glucosinolate degrading microorganisms and their potential for reducing the glucosinolate content of rapemeal. *FEMS Microbiol Lett*. 119(1-2):83-8.

190. Elfoul L, Rabot S, Khelifa N, Quinsac A, Duguay A, et al. (2001) Formation of allyl isothiocyanate from sinigrin in the digestive tract of rats monoassociated with a human colonic strain of Bacteroides thetaiotaomicron. *FEMS Microbiol Lett*. 197(1):99-103.

191. Holst B, Williamson G. (2004) A critical review of the bioavailability of glucosinolates and related compounds. *Nat Prod Rep*. 21(3):425-47.

192. Navarro S, Li F, Lampe J. (2011) Mechanisms of action of isothiocyanates in cancer chemoprevention: an update. *Food Func*. 2(10):579-87.

193. Myzak M, Tong P, Dashwood W, Dashwood R, Ho E. (2007) Sulforaphane inhibits HDAC activity in prostate cancer cells, retards growth of PC3 xenografts, and inhibits HDAC activity in human subjects. *Exp Biol Med(Maywood, NJ)*. 232(2):227-34.

How to cite this article: Rose S, Strombom A. Colorectal cancer prevention with a plant-based diet. Canc Therapy & Oncol Int J. 2019; 15(2): 555906.
DOI: 10.19080/CTOIJ.2019.15.555906

194. Simpson H, Campbell B. (2015) Review article: dietary fibre-microbiota interactions. *Aliment Pharmacol Therap*. 42(2):158-79.

195. Lin D, Peters B, Friedlander C, Freiman H, Goedert J, et al. (2018) Association of dietary fibre intake and gut microbiota in adults. *Br J Nutr*. 120(9):1014-1022.

196. Fry S. (2004) Primary cell wall metabolism: tracking the careers of wall polymers in living plant cells. *New Phytologist*. 161(3):641-675.

197. Chassard C, Lacroix C. (2013) Carbohydrates and the human gut microbiota. *Cur Opin Clin Nutr Metab Care*. 16(4):453-60.

198. Lattimer J, Haub M. (2010) Effects of dietary fiber and its components on metabolic health. *Nutr*. 2(12):1266-89.

199. Macfarlane G, Gibson G. (1997) Carbohydrate fermentation, energy transduction and gas metabolism in the human large intestine. In: Mackie R, White B, eds. *Gastrointest Microbiol*. Vol 1 Gastrointestinal Ecosystems and Fermentations. New York: Chapman & Hall.

200. Flint H, Bayer E, Rincon M, Lamed R, White B. (2008) Polysaccharide utilization by gut bacteria: potential for new insights from genomic analysis. *Nat Rev Microbiol*. 6(2):121-31.

201. Hamer H, Jonkers D, Venema K, Vanhoutvin S, Troost F, et al. (2008) Review article: the role of butyrate on colonic function. *Ailment Pharmacol Ther*. 27(2):104-19.

202. Vinolo M, Rodrigues H, Nachbar R, Curi R. (2011) Regulation of inflammation by short chain fatty acids. *Nutrients*. 3(10):858-76.

203. Sengupta S, Muir J, Gibson P. (2006) Does butyrate protect from colorectal cancer? *J Gastroenterol Hepatol*. 21(1 Pt 2):209-18.

204. Donohoe D, Holley D, Collins L. (2014) A gnotobiotic mouse model demonstrates that dietary fiber protects against colorectal tumorigenesis in a microbiota- and butyrate-dependent manner. *Cancer Discov*. 4(12):1387-97.

205. Glick-Bauer M, Yeh MC. (2014) The Health Advantage of a Vegan Diet: Exploring the Gut Microbiota Connection. *Nutrients*. 6(11):4822-38.

206. Zimmer J, Lange B, Frick J, Sauer H, Zimmermann K, et al. (2012) A vegan or vegetarian diet substantially alters the human colonic faecal microbiota. *Eur J Clin Nutr*. 66(1):53-60.

207. Bamola V, Ghosh A, Kapardar R, Lal B, Cheema S, et al. (2017) Gut microbial diversity in health and disease: experience of healthy Indian subjects, and colon carcinoma and inflammatory bowel disease patients. *Microb ecol health dis*. 28(1):1322447.

208. Zhu Y, Wu H, Wang P, Savas S, Woodrow J, et al. (2013) Dietary patterns and colorectal cancer recurrence and survival: a cohort study. *BMJ Open*. 3(e002270).

209. Lanza E, Hartman T, Albert P, Shields R, Slattery M, et al. (2006) High Dry Bean Intake and Reduced Risk of Advanced Colorectal Adenoma Recurrence among Participants in the Polyp Prevention Trial. *J Nutr*. 136(7):1896-903.

210. Song M, Wu K, Meyerhardt J, Ogino S, Wang M, et al. (2018) Fiber intake and survival after colorectal cancer diagnosis. *JAMA Oncol*. 4(1):71-79.

211. Jiang R, Manson J, Stampfer M, Liu S, Willett W, et al. (2002) Nut and peanut butter consumption and risk of type 2 diabetes in women. *JAMA*. 288(20):2554-60.

212. Salas-Salvadó J, Fernández-Ballart J, Ros E, Martínez-González M, Fitó M, et al. (2008) Effect of a Mediterranean diet supplemented with nuts on metabolic syndrome status: one-year results of the PREDIMED randomized trial. *Arch Inter Med*. 168(22):2449-58.

213. Casas-Agustench P, Bulló M, Ros E, Basora J, Salas-Salvadó J. (2011) Cross-sectional association of nut intake with adiposity in a Mediterranean population. *Nutr Metab Cardiovasc Dis*. 21(7):518-25.

How to cite this article: Rose S, Strombom A. Colorectal cancer prevention with a plant-based diet. Canc Therapy & Oncol Int J. 2019; 15(2): 555906.
DOI: 10.19080/CTOIJ.2019.15.555906

214. Kelly JJ, Sabaté J. (2006) Nuts and coronary heart disease: an epidemiological perspective. *Br J Nutr*. 96(Suppl 2):S61-7.

215. Ibarrola-Jurado N, Bulló M, Guasch-Ferré M, Ros E, Martínez-González M, et al. (2013) Cross-sectional assessment of nut consumption and obesity, metabolic syndrome and other cardiometabolic risk factors: the PREDIMED study. *PLoS One*. 8(2):e57367.

216. González C, Salas-Salvadó J. (2006) The potential of nuts in the prevention of cancer. *Br J Nutr*. 96(Suppl 2):S87-94.

217. Falasca M, Casari I, Maffucci T. (2014) Cancer Chemoprevention with nuts. *J Natl Cancer Inst*. 106(9):dju238.

218. Falasca M, Casari I. (2012) Cancer chemoprevention by nuts: evidence and promises. *Front Biosci*. 4:109-20.

219. Bao Y, Han J, Hu F, Giovannucci E, Stampfer M, et al. (2013) Association of nut consumption with total and cause-specific mortality. *New Engl J Med*. 369(21):2001-11.

220. Guasch-Ferré M, Bulló M, Martínez-González M, Ros E, Corella D, et al. (2013) Frequency of nut consumption and mortality risk in the PREDIMED nutrition intervention trial. *BMC Med*. 11:164.

221. Fadelu T, Niedzwiecki D, Zhang S, Ye X, Saltz L, et al. (2017) Nut consumption and survival in stage III colon cancer patients: Results from CALGB 89803 (Alliance). *J Clin Oncol*. 35(suppl abstr 3517).

222. Bao Y, Hu F, Giovannucci E, Wolpin B, Stampfer M, et al. (2013) Nut consumption and risk of pancreatic cancer in women. *Br J Cancer*. 109(11):2911-6.

223. Gupta S, Kim J, Prasad S, Aggarwal B. (2010) Regulation of survival, proliferation, invasion, angiogenesis, and metastasis of tumor cells through modulation of inflammatory pathways by nutraceuticals. *Cancer Metastasis Rev*. 29(3):405-34.

224. Gigic B, Boeing H, Toth R, Böhm J, Habermann N, et al. (2018) Associations between dietary patterns and longitudinal quality of life changes in colorectal cancer patients: The ColoCare Study. *Nutr Cancer*. 70(1):51-60.

225. Rose S, Strombom A. (2018) A comprehensive review of the prevention and treatment of heart disease with a plant-based diet. *J Cardiol Cardiovas Ther*. 12(5):555847.

226. Strombom A, Rose S. (2017) The prevention and treatment of Type II Diabetes Mellitus with a plant-based diet. *Endocrin Metab Int J*.5(5):00138.

227. Barnard N, Cohen J, Jenkins D, Turner-McGrievy G, Gloede L, et al. (2006) A low-fat vegan diet improves glycemic control and cardiovascular risk factors in a randomized clinical trial in individuals with type 2 diabetes. *Diabetes Care*. 29(8):1777-83.

228. Lancet. (1998) Effect of intensive blood-glucose control with metformin on complications in overweight patients with type 2 diabetes (UKPDS 34). UK Prospective Diabetes Study (UKPDS) Group. *Lancet*. 352(9131):854-865.

229. Jenkins D, Kendall C, Marchie A, Faulkner D, Wong J, et al. (2005) Direct comparison of a dietary portfolio of cholesterol-lowering foods with a statin in hypercholesterolemic participants. *Am J Clin Nutr*. 81(2):380-7.

Advanced Research in Gastroenterology & Hepatology
ISSN: 2472-6400

Juniper Publishers
key to the Researchers

Mini Review
Volume 9 Issue 1 - February 2018
DOI: 10.19080/CTOIJ.2019.15.555906

Adv Res Gastroenterol Hepatol

Crohn's Disease Prevention and Treatment with a Plant-Based Diet

Stewart D Rose and Amanda J Strombom*

Plant-Based Diets in Medicine, USA

Submission: February 08, 2018; **Published:** February 16, 2018

***Corresponding Author:** Amanda J Strombom, Plant-Based Diets in Medicine, 12819 SE 38th St, #427, Bellevue, WA 98006, USA

Abstract

Epidemiologic studies show that IBD is prevalent in wealthy nations where dietary westernization usually occurs. Dietary westernization is characterized by increased consumption of animal protein, animal fat, and sugar. An epidemiological study found that the risk of Crohn's disease reduced by 70% in females and 80% in males following a vegetarian diet.

Treatment with medications, though efficacious to a degree, all have significant adverse reactions. Many of these medications will also be contraindicated in a significant number of patients.

Treatment is aimed at inducing remission. A semi-vegetarian diet has been shown to achieve a 100% remission rate at 1 year and 92% at 2 years. Plant-based diets are rich in phytochemicals that help reduce inflammation by modifying several inflammatory mechanisms.

A study of treatment with infliximab and a plant-based diet showed a remission rate of 96%, substantial reduction in CRP and CDAI and improvements in mucosa healing. This study shows that combining infliximab with a plant-based diet results in a strong clinical response.

Plant-based diets promote a more favorable gut microbial profile that is anti-inflammatory. Naturally occurring substances in plant foods, having anti-inflammatory bowel actions include phytochemicals, antioxidants, dietary fibers, and lipids. Many of these natural products exert their beneficial action by altering cytokine production.

The plant-based diet has no adverse reactions or contra-indications and is affordable, so physicians can initiate therapy with a plant-based diet immediately, and prescribe it as a prophylaxis for all patients at risk of Crohn's disease.

Keywords:
Crohn's Disease; Plant-based diet; Vegetarian; Vegan; Biologics; Microbiota; Cytokines; Inflammatory bowel disease; Phytochemicals

1. Introduction

Crohn's disease is difficult to treat and can be frustrating for both the patient and their physician. Safer and more efficacious treatments are needed for this disease.

The current standard treatment for Crohn's disease involves medication to manage symptoms and induce remission, and when necessary, bowel resection. Medications used in the treatment of Crohn's disease include the following:

- 5-Aminosalicylic acid derivative agents (eg. mesalamine rectal, mesalamine, balsalazide)
- Corticosteroids (eg. prednisone, methylprednisolone, budesonide)
- Immunosuppressive agents (eg. mercaptopurine, methotrexate, tacrolimus)
- Biologics (eg. infliximab, adalimumab, certolizumab pegol, natalizumab, vedolizumab)
- Antibiotics (eg. metronidazole, ciprofloxacin)
- Antidiarrheal agents (eg. loperamide, diphenoxylate-atropine)
- Bile acid sequestrants (eg. cholestyramine, colestipol)
- Anticholinergic agents (eg. dicyclomine, hyoscyamine, propantheline)

These medications, though efficacious to a degree, all have significant adverse reactions. Many of these medications will also be contraindicated in a significant number of patients.

Most patients with Crohn's disease require surgical intervention during their lifetime, as it plays an integral role in controlling the symptoms and treating the complications of Crohn's disease, but operative resection is not curative. Because of the high rate of disease recurrence after segmental bowel resection, the guiding principle of surgical management of Crohn's disease is preservation of intestinal length and function. (1)

Mean annual costs for Crohn's disease are about $8265. 31% of costs were attributable to hospitalization, 33% to outpatient care, and 35% to pharmaceutical claims. The annual dollar cost for Crohn's disease in the United States is $3.6 billion. (2) It can reasonably be concluded that Crohn's is both difficult and expensive to treat.

Symptoms of Crohn's disease may subside with total parenteral nutrition or total enteral nutrition, but it is well known to flare up after the resumption of meals. Therefore, the food in patient's meals are thought to be an etiologic factor in gut inflammation. (3)

While parenteral nutrition is possible, nutrition taken orally is to be preferred if it won't cause a flare up, or even better, if it can prevent flare ups and induce remission. This is what a vegetarian diet seems to accomplish.

2. Prevention

The etiology of Crohn's disease is unknown. Genetic, microbial, immunologic, environmental, dietary, vascular, and psychosocial factors have been implicated, as have smoking and the use of

How to cite this article: Rose S, Strombom A. Crohn's disease prevention and treatment with a plant-based diet. Adv Res Gastroentero Hepatol 2018; 9(1): 555753.
DOI: 10.19080/ARGH.2018.09.555753.

oral contraceptives and nonsteroidal anti-inflammatory agents (NSAIDs).

Epidemiology shows that IBD is prevalent in wealthy nations (4, 5, 6) where dietary westernization inevitably occurs (7, 8). Dietary westernization is characterized by increased consumption of animal protein, animal fat, and sugar. Diets rich in animal protein and animal fat cause a decrease in beneficial bacteria in the intestine (9, 10).

However, the risk of Crohn's disease was found to be reduced by 70% in female and 80% in male young people following a nearly vegetarian diet. (11)

3. Treatment

Treatment is aimed at inducing remission. An important and well-designed study published in 2010, using a semi-vegetarian diet, achieved a 100% remission rate at 1 year and 92% at 2 years. (12)

A more advanced study published in 2017 examined whether a substantial improvement of the relapse-free rate in Crohn's Disease could be obtained by incorporating three recently developed concepts in medicine: biologics, a plant-based diet and window of opportunity. This was followed by maintenance of remission with a plant-based diet, rather than further use of biologics with or without immunosuppressants. (13)

Patients were treated with infliximab and a plant-based diet. The primary end point was clinical remission at week 6. Secondary end points were normalization of C-reactive protein (CRP) concentration at week 6 and mucosal healing. Crohn Disease Activity Index (CDAI) score was also evaluated. (13)

All patients in this study who completed the protocol achieved remission at week 6. Remission rates by intention-to-treat and per protocol analysis were 96% and 100%, respectively. The rates of CRP normalization at week 6 were 92% among adults with a new diagnosis, 82% among children with a new diagnosis and 67% among relapsing adults. The mean CDAI score was significantly decreased from 314 before treatment to 163 after the first week. The scores were further decreased chronologically: 115, 98, 82, 74, and 63 at weeks 2, 3, 4, 5, and 6, respectively. Mucosal healing was achieved in 46% patients. This study has shown that a plant-based diet can improve the efficacy of biologics such as infliximab. (13)

Plant-based dietary patterns may promote a more favorable gut microbial profile. Such diets are high in dietary fiber and fermentable substrate (i.e. non digestible or undigested carbohydrates), which are sources of metabolic fuel for gut microbial fermentation and, in turn, result in end products that may be used by the host (i.e. short chain fatty acids such as butyrate). These end products may have direct or indirect effects on modulating the health of their host. (14)

The naturally occurring substances in plant foods having anti-inflammatory bowel actions include phytochemicals, antioxidants, microorganisms, dietary fibers, and lipids. The literature indicates that many of these natural products exert their beneficial action by altering cytokine production. Specifically, phytochemicals such as polyphenols or flavonoids are the most abundant, naturally occurring anti-inflammatory substances. The effects of lipids are primarily related to the n-3 polyunsaturated fatty acids. The effects of phytochemicals are associated with modulating the levels of tumor necrosis factor α (TNF-α), interleukin

How to cite this article: Rose S, Strombom A. Crohn's disease prevention and treatment with a plant-based diet. Adv Res Gastroentero Hepatol 2018; 9(1): 555753.
DOI: 10.19080/ARGH.2018.09.555753.

(IL)-1, IL-6, inducible nitric oxide synthase, and myeloperoxide. The anti-IBD effects of dietary fiber are mainly mediated via peroxisome proliferator-activated receptor-γ, TNF-α, nitric oxide, and IL-2, whereas the effects of lactic acid bacteria are reported to influence interferon-γ, IL-6, IL-12, TNF-α, and nuclear factor-κ light-chain enhancer of activated B cells. These results suggest that the anti-IBD effects exhibited by natural products are mainly caused by their ability to modulate cytokine production. (15)

Studies, conducted using in vivo and in vitro models, provide evidence that pure polyphenolic compounds and natural polyphenolic plant extracts can modulate intestinal inflammation. (16) Polyphenols may thus be considered able to prevent or delay the progression of Crohn's disease, especially because they reach higher concentrations in the gut than in other tissues. (17)

While not perfect, of all the laboratory markers, C-Reactive Protein (CRP) is the most studied and has been shown to have the best overall performance. CRP is an objective marker of inflammation and correlates well with disease activity in Crohn's disease. (18) It is produced as an acute phase reactant predominantly in the liver, in response to stimulation by interleukin (IL)-6, TNF-α and IL-1β, which are produced at the site of inflammation. (19)

Adipocytes in hypertrophied mesenteric adipose tissue produce and secrete significant amounts of adiponectin, which may be involved in the regulation of intestinal inflammation associated with Crohn's disease. Furthermore, adiponectin concentrations in hypertrophied mesenteric adipose tissues of Crohn's disease patients correlated inversely with serum CRP levels ($r=-0.51$, $p=0.015$) (20) There is a good correlation between CRP and other measures of inflammation such as the Crohn's Disease Activity Index, radioactive labelled fecal granulocyte excretion and fecal calprotectin. (21, 22, 23)

Plant-based diets have been shown to increase adiponectin in diabetics, and reduce CRP in both diabetics and patients with coronary artery disease, and may well be doing the same in Crohn's disease patients. (24, 25, 26) This improved profile of cytokines may be part of the therapeutic efficacy of plant-based diets in Crohn's disease.

4. Discussion

To put the efficacy of a vegetarian diet into perspective one must compare it to standard treatments. Overall, despite the use of oral mesalamine treatment in the past, new evidence suggests that this approach is minimally effective as compared with a placebo, and less effective than budesonide or conventional corticosteroids. Induction of remission was noted in 52% of Crohn's disease patients.

Maintenance of remission was reported in 71% of Crohn's disease patients on azathioprine over a 6-month to 2-year period. Induction and maintenance of remission was noted in 70% of Crohn's disease patients on methotrexate over a 40-week period. Induction of remission was reported in 32%, 26%, and 20% of Crohn's Disease patients on infliximab, adalimumab or certolizumab, respectively. Approximately one-fifth of Crohn's disease patients treated with biologicals require intestinal resection after 2–5 years in referral-center studies. (27) The adverse reactions of the above medications are well-known, as are the risks and complications of surgery.

How to cite this article: Rose S, Strombom A. Crohn's disease prevention and treatment with a plant-based diet. Adv Res Gastroentero Hepatol 2018; 9(1): 555753.
DOI: 10.19080/ARGH.2018.09.555753.

The safety and efficacy of a plant-based diet to treat Crohn's disease would seem quite advantageous. It has no contraindications and no adverse reactions. Therefore, it may be safely combined with standard treatments.

Treatment with a plant-based diet also reduces the risk of common diseases that the Crohn's patient will face in common with all patients, such as coronary artery disease and type II diabetes mellitus.

Given the substantial advantages more study is warranted. However, given its safety the physician can institute therapy with a plant-based diet immediately.

Finally, every physician should practice prevention. The decreased risk of Crohn's disease obtained with a plant-based diet is considerable. It is a safe prophylaxis, and should especially be prescribed for patients at risk because of family history or because of cigarette smoking.

References

1. Kornbluth A, Sachar D, Salomon P. (1998) Crohn's disease. In: Feldman M, Scharschmidt B, Friedman L, Sleisenger M, eds. *Sleisenger & Fordtran's Gastrointestinal and Liver Disease: Pathophysiology/Diagnosis/ Management 6th Edition*. Vol 2. 6th ed. Philadelphia: WB Saunders Co.Pages 1708–1734
2. Kappelman M, Rifas-Shiman S, Porter C, Ollendorf DA, Sandler RS, et al. (2008) Direct Health Care Costs of Crohn's Disease and Ulcerative Colitis in US Children and Adults. *Gastroenterology*. 135(6):1907-1913.
3. Chiba M, Ohno H, Ishii H, Komatsu M. (2014) Plant-Based Diets in Crohn's Disease. *Perm J*. 18(4):94.
4. Bernstein C, Shanahan F. (2008) Disorders of a modern lifestyle: reconciling the epidemiology of inflammatory bowel diseases. *Gut*. 57(9):1185-1191.
5. Whelan G. (1995) Inflammatory bowel disease: epidemiology. In: Haubrich W, Schaffner F, Berk J, eds. *Bockus Gastroenterology*. Vol 2. 5th ed. Philadelphia: WB Saunders. Pages 1318–1325
6. Shivananda S, Lennard-Jones J, Logan R, Fear N, Price A, et al. (1996) Incidence of inflammatory bowel disease across Europe: is there a difference between north and south? Results of the European Collaborative Study on Inflammatory Bowel Disease (EC-IBD). *Gut*. 39(5):690-697.
7. US Dept of Health and Human Services. (1981) Report of the Working Group on Arteriosclerosis of the National Heart, Lung and Blood Institute. *Arteriosclerosis*. Vol 2. Philadelphia: WB Saunders
8. Popkin B. (1994) The nutrition transition in low-income countries: an emerging crisis. *Nutr Rev*. 52(9):285-298.
9. Hentges D, Maier B, Burton G, Flynn M, Tsutakawa R. (1977) Effect of a high-beef diet on the fecal bacterial flora of humans. *Cancer Research*. 37(2):568-571.
10. Benno Y, Suzuki K, Suzuki K, Narisawa K, Bruce W, Mitsuoka T. (1986) Comparison of the fecal microflora in rural Japanese and urban Canadians. *Microbiol Immunol*. 30(6):521-32.
11. D'Souza S, Levy E, Mack D, Israel D, Lambrette P, et al. (2008) Dietary patterns and risk for Crohn's disease in children. *Inflamm Bowel Dis*. 14(3):367-73.
12. Chiba M, Abe T, Tsuda H, Sugawara T, Tsuda S, et al. (2010) Lifestyle-related disease in Crohn's disease: Relapse prevention by a semi-vegetarian diet. *World J Gastroenterol*. 16(20):2484–2495.
13. Chiba M, Tsuji T, Nakane K, Tsuda S, Ishii H, et al. (2017) Induction with Infliximab and a plant-based diet as first-line (IPF) therapy for Crohn disease: a single-group trial. *Perm J*.21:17-009.

How to cite this article: Rose S, Strombom A. Crohn's disease prevention and treatment with a plant-based diet. Adv Res Gastroentero Hepatol 2018; 9(1): 555753.
DOI: 10.19080/ARGH.2018.09.555753.

14. Wong J. (2014) Gut microbiota and cardiometabolic outcomes: influence of dietary patterns and their associated components. *Am J Clin Nutr*. 100(Suppl 1):369S-77S.
15. Hur SJ, Kang SH, Jung HS, Kim SC, Jeon HS, et al. (2012) Review of natural products actions on cytokines in inflammatory bowel disease. *Nutr Res*. 32(11):801-16.
16. Romier B, Schneider Y, Larondelle Y, During A. (2009) Dietary polyphenols can modulate the intestinal inflammatory response. *Nutr Rev*. 67(7):363-78.
17. Biasi F, Astegiano M, Maina M, Leonarduzzi G, Poli G. (2011) Polyphenol supplementation as a complementary medicinal approach to treating inflammatory bowel disease. *Curr Med Chem*. 18(31):4851-65.
18. Vermeire S, Van Assche G, Rutgeerts P. (2006) Laboratory markers in IBD: useful, magic, or unnecessary toys? *Gut*. 55(3):426-431.
19. Vermeire S, Van Assche G, Rutgeerts P. (2004) C-reactive protein as a marker for inflammatory bowel disease. *Inflamm Bowel Dis*. 10(5):661-5.
20. Yamamoto K, Kiyohara T, Murayama Y, Kihara S, Okamoto T, et al. (2005) Production of adiponectin, an anti-inflammatory protein, in mesenteric adipose tissue in Crohn's disease. *Gut*. 54(6):789-96.
21. Fagan EA, Dyck RF, Maton PN, Hodgson HJ, Chadwick VS, et al. (1982) Serum levels of C-reactive protein in Crohn's disease and ulcerative colitis. *Eur J Clin Invest*. 12(4):351-9.
22. Saverymuttu S, Hodgson H, Chadwick V, Pepys M. (1986) Differing acute phase responses in Crohn's disease and ulcerative colitis. *Gut*. 27(7):809–813.
23. Hammer H, Kvien T, Glennås A, Melby K. (1995) A longitudinal study of calprotectin as an inflammatory marker in patients with reactive arthritis. *Clin Exp Rheumatol*. 13(1):59-64.
24. Kahleova H, Matoulek M, Malinska H, Oliyarnik O, Kazdova L, et al. (2011) Vegetarian diet improves insulin resistance and oxidative stress markers more than conventional diet in subjects with Type 2 diabetes. *Diabet Med*. 28(5):549-59.
25. Krajcovicova-Kudlackova M, Blazicek P. (2005) C-reactive protein and nutrition. *Bratisl Lek Listy*. 106(11):345-7.
26. Chen C, Lin Y, Lin T, Lin C, Chen B, Lin C. (2008) Total cardiovascular risk profile of Taiwanese vegetarians. *Eur J Clin Nutr*. 62(1):138-44.
27. Peyrin-Biroulet L, Lémann M. (2011) Review article: remission rates achievable by current therapies for inflammatory bowel disease. *Aliment Pharmacol Ther*. 33(8):870-9.

How to cite this article: Rose S, Strombom A. Crohn's disease prevention and treatment with a plant-based diet. Adv Res Gastroentero Hepatol 2018; 9(1): 555753.
DOI: 10.19080/ARGH.2018.09.555753.

Advanced Research in Gastroenterology & Hepatology
ISSN: 2472-6400

Juniper Publishers
key to the Researchers

Review Article
Volume 15 Issue 2 – June 2020
DOI: 10.19080/ARGH.2020.15.555908

Adv Res Gastroenterol Hepatol

Ulcerative Colitis - Prevention and Treatment with a Plant-Based Diet

Stewart D Rose and Amanda J Strombom*

Plant-Based Diets in Medicine, USA

Submission: May 21, 2020: **Published:** June 05, 2020

***Corresponding Author:** Amanda Strombom, Plant-Based Diets in Medicine, 12819 SE 38th St, #427, Bellevue, WA 98006, USA

Abstract

Treating ulcerative colitis (UC) can be frustrating for doctor and patient alike. Therefore, practicing prevention with this disease is particularly desirable. Significant changes in dietary intake during the past decades have been associated with the increase in incidence of UC. A meta-analysis of seven epidemiological studies found meat intake to raise the risk of ulcerative colitis by 47%. Consumption of fruits and vegetables have been found to significantly decrease the risk.

A plant-based diet can significantly reduce the risk or relapse in ulcerative colitis patients, almost as effectively as the leading drug, Mesalamine. Changes in the gut microbiome can be a potential prognostic feature. Improved biodiversity when consuming prebiotic plant foods, resulted in a significant increase in fecal butyrate levels. Fish oil and essential fatty acid supplements have not been found to be effective in the treatment and or maintenance of remission in ulcerative colitis.

Treating the ulcerative colitis patient with a plant-based diet has no contraindications or adverse reactions, is affordable and can prevent and treat common comorbidities such as type 2 diabetes and coronary artery disease. Vitamin D deficiency is common in people with ulcerative colitis and may be a contributing factor in the development of the disease, and should be part of every workup.

Keywords:

Butyrate; Inflammatory bowel disease; Meat intake; Microbiome; Plant-based diet; Prebiotics; Ulcerative colitis; Vegan; Vegetarian

Abbreviations:

UC: Ulcerative Colitis; IBD: Inflammatory Bowel Disease; MCHC: Mean Corpuscular Hemoglobin Concentration; MCV: Mean Corpuscular Volume; IL: Interleukin; TNF-α: Tumor Necrosis Factor α

1. Introduction

Samuel Wilks first described ulcerative colitis (UC) in 1859. (1) Ulcerative colitis is a type of inflammatory bowel disease (IBD). It is characterized by continuous and diffuse inflammation that is limited to the colonic mucosa and extends proximally from the rectum. The disease develops most often in the second or third decade of life. The classic symptoms are bloody diarrhea, abdominal pain, and tenesmus. (2) Because the natural history of the disease is periods of remission and flares, medications are used in most cases to induce and maintain a long-term corticosteroid-free remission. Despite available medical treatments, approximately 15% of patients will require surgery for their disease. (3, 4)

2. Epidemiology

Genetic factors are attributed to the risk of developing the disease, accompanied by epithelial barrier defects and environmental factors. Currently, a number of genetic and environmental factors that increase the risk of developing UC have been identified. (5) A westernized lifestyle and diet including cessation of tobacco use, consumption of animal products, stress, medication use and high socioeconomic status are all associated with the development of IBD. (6) Among many such factors, tobacco smoking and appendectomy are linked to milder disease, fewer hospitalizations, and decreased incidence of UC, but the reverse is true for Crohn's disease. (7, 8)

Significant changes in dietary intake during the past decades have been associated with the increase in incidence of UC. The relationship between diet and UC development has been indicated in several epidemiological studies. (9)

One study found a significant association between meat intake, red meat in particular, and UC risk. This meta-analysis of seven epidemiological studies found meat intake to raise the risk of ulcerative colitis by 47%. (10) Another study found that a high fat intake was associated with an increased risk for UC; this was particularly marked for animal fat which quadrupled the risk of ulcerative colitis. (11) A meta-analysis of fruit and vegetable consumption found that fruits and vegetables are associated with a significantly decreased risk of ulcerative colitis. (12)

3. Interventional studies

A year-long prospective cohort study was performed with UC patients in remission who were followed for a year to determine the effect of habitual diet on relapse. High sulfur or sulfate intake increased the risk of relapse 2.7 times. (13)

In a study of patients with mild UC or UC in remission who did not need immediate treatment, a residential program including a plant-based diet and dietary guidance was provided during a two-week period. The majority (77%) of patients experienced improvements in symptoms and laboratory data during treatment. These same patients were then followed for 5 years and at 1, 2, 3, 4, and 5 years, the relapse rates were 2%, 4%, 7%, 19%, and 19%, respectively. (14) These relapse rates are far better than those previously reported. For instance,

How to cite this article: Rose S, Strombom A. Ulcerative Colitis – prevention and treatment with a plant-based diet. Adv Res Gastroentero Hepatol, 2020;15(2): 555908.
DOI: 10.19080/ARGH.2020.15.555908

a study of patients treated with aminosalicylates showed a relapse rate of 16% after only one year. (15) Other studies, without treatment with a plant-based diet, also showed higher rates of relapse. (16, 17, 18, 19, 20, 21, 22)

A study characterizing the gut microbiome in a large cohort of pediatric patients with severe UC was the first to describe changes in the gut microbiome as a potential prognostic feature. (23) Richness, evenness, and biodiversity of the gut microbiome were remarkably reduced in children with UC compared with healthy controls. Children who did not respond to steroids harbored a microbiome that was even less rich than steroid responders.

Prebiotics are defined as non-digestible food ingredients that beneficially affect the host by selectively stimulating the growth or activity of bacterial species already present in the gut. Prebiotics, such as psyllium, are found in plant foods. (24) Because colonic fermentation of Plantago ovata seeds (psyllium) supports the bacteria that produce butyrate, it may have efficacy in treating ulcerative colitis. In a one-year study, consumption of 10mg BID Plantago ovata seeds was almost as effective as Mesalamine in maintaining remission. A significant increase in fecal butyrate levels was observed after Plantago ovata seed administration, thus reducing inflammation. (25)

Fish oil and essential fatty acid supplements have not been found to be effective in the treatment and or maintenance of remission in ulcerative colitis. (26) Five placebo-controlled double-blind studies found no overall convincing clinical benefit of dietary fish oil supplementation for 4–12 months in the treatment of patients with active UC. (27, 28, 29, 30, 31)

4. Pathophysiology

The multifactorial pathophysiology of UC includes genetic predisposition, epithelial barrier defects, dysregulated immune responses, microbial dysbiosis, and environmental factors. (32, 33)

Dietary factors can be related to UC pathogenesis or disease course through direct effects on the host, or through indirect effects through modulations of composition or function of gut microbiota. Diet plays a major role in shaping gut microbial composition (34, 35) Although the exact pathophysiological mechanisms in which diet plays a role in ulcerative colitis development remain unknown, several plausible explanations have been proposed, including its effects on the composition of gut microbiota, production of microbial metabolites, alterations in mucosal immunity, and mucosal barrier function (36)

A plant-based diet produces a greater quantity of butyrate and other short chain fatty acids, as well as supplying phytochemicals with anti inflammatory properties. Plant-based dietary patterns may promote a more favorable gut microbial profile. Such diets are high in dietary fiber and fermentable substrate (i.e. non digestible or undigested carbohydrates), which are sources of metabolic fuel for gut microbial fermentation and, in turn, result in end products that may be used by the host (i.e. short chain fatty acids such as butyrate). These end products may have direct or indirect effects on modulating the health of their host. (37)

The naturally occurring substances in plant foods having anti-inflammatory bowel actions include phytochemicals, antioxidants, dietary fibers, and lipids. The literature indicates that many of these compounds of plant foods exert their beneficial action by altering cytokine production.

How to cite this article: Rose S, Strombom A. Ulcerative Colitis – prevention and treatment with a plant-based diet. Adv Res Gastroentero Hepatol, 2020;15(2): 555908.
DOI: 10.19080/ARGH.2020.15.555908

Specifically, phytochemicals such as polyphenols or flavonoids are the most abundant, naturally occurring anti-inflammatory substances. The effects of phytochemicals are associated with modulating the levels of tumor necrosis factor α (TNF-α), interleukin (IL)-1, IL-6, inducible nitric oxide synthase, and myeloperoxide. The anti-ulcerative effects of dietary fiber are mainly mediated via peroxisome proliferator-activated receptor-γ, TNF-α, nitric oxide, and IL-2, whereas the effects of lactic acid bacteria are reported to influence interferon-γ, IL-6, IL-12, TNF-α, and nuclear factor-κ light-chain enhancer of activated B cells. These results suggest that the anti-IBD effects exhibited by natural products are mainly caused by their ability to modulate cytokine production. (38)

Studies, conducted using in vivo and in vitro models, provide evidence that polyphenolic compounds and natural polyphenolic plant extracts can modulate intestinal inflammation. (39) Polyphenols may thus be considered able to prevent or delay the progression of ulcerative colitis, especially because they reach higher concentrations in the gut than in other tissues. (40)

It is thought that sulfide toxicity may be important in the pathogenesis of UC. (41, 42) The initial evidence in this regard was a demonstration that experimental exposure of colonic tissue to sulfide causes inhibition of butyrate use, a defect similar to that observed in mucosal biopsies obtained from UC patients. (43) UC patients have significantly higher luminal concentrations of hydrogen sulfide than controls, and disease activity correlates with sulfide production rates. (44) Hydrogen sulfide induces hyperproliferation of colonic mucosa and this effect is antagonized by butyrate. (45) Treatment with 5-aminosalicylates and bismuth subsalicylates has been shown to reduce hydrogen sulfide production in the colonic lumen. (46)

Exogenous sources, such as red meat, cheese, milk, fish and eggs, contribute to the colonic pool of sulfur, (26, 47, 48) whereas endogenous sources do not seem to make a significant contribution to the colonic pool of sulfur. (44) The major exogenous sources of sulfur are the sulfur amino acids found in high protein foods and inorganic sulfate (in brassica vegetables and as preservatives in processed foods, particularly commercial breads, beers, sausages, and dried fruit.) (49) Sulfur amino acids and inorganic sulfate reach the colon where they are converted to sulfides by fermentation with colonic bacteria or by sulfate-reducing bacteria. (50, 51) Fecal hydrogen sulfide concentration increases when either the sulfur amino acid content (as meat) (52) or sulfate content (as additives) of the diet increase. (53) Generation of hydrogen sulfide by sulfate- reducing bacteria is modest compared with total fecal sulfide concentration, (47, 54) suggesting that fermentation of sulfur amino acids may be the more important of the two mechanisms of generation of hydrogen sulfide.

Fecal sulfide levels increase after consumption of increasing amounts of meat, (26, 47) providing evidence that meat is an important substrate for sulfide generation by bacteria in the human large intestine. In a pilot study in which the intake of sulfur amino acids was limited, clinical improvement, in terms of stool frequency, was demonstrated in patients with UC. (42)

The toxic effects of sulfur-reducing compounds, particularly hydrogen sulfide, at concentrations commonly found in the lumen of the human colon, appear to be mediated through impaired utilization of butyrate by colonocytes. (55) Hydrogen

How to cite this article: Rose S, Strombom A. Ulcerative Colitis – prevention and treatment with a plant-based diet. Adv Res Gastroentero Hepatol, 2020;15(2): 555908.
DOI: 10.19080/ARGH.2020.15.555908

sulfide has been found to cause increased epithelial permeability, loss of barrier function, (56) cellular proliferation, (57) and histological changes in rat colons that are similar to those seen in humans with UC. (45) UC patients have significantly higher luminal concentrations of hydrogen sulfide than controls (58) and disease activity correlates with sulfide production rates. (44)

Vegetarians tend to have higher fiber intakes, (59) which could be metabolized by the colonic microbiota instead of amino acids, leading to a reduction in indoxyl sulfate and p-cresyl sulfate. This provides another mechanism to explain why vegetarian protein sources appear less detrimental than animal protein sources.

5. Clinical considerations

The goals of treatment are induction of remission followed by maintenance of remission in conjunction with steroid-free treatments in the long term management. (60)

Current practice recommends lifelong medication for relapse prevention in IBD. (61, 62, 15) Current medications used in the treatment of ulcerative colitis include aminosalicylates, corticosteroids, immunomodulators and biologics. Diet, however, is critically important. Although medication is needed in the active phase of ulcerative colitis, diet is generally more important than medication to maintain remission in the quiescent phase. (15) If a suitable diet is established as part of a changing lifestyle, medication ultimately may not be needed to maintain remission. (15)

A suitable diet should be high in prebiotics. Fortunately, prebiotics occur naturally in many plant foods, because they're components of nondigestible plant fibers. Some plant foods which are good sources of prebiotic fibers include chicory, garlic, leeks, onion, asparagus, and Jerusalem artichokes. They're also found in lesser amounts in bananas, whole wheat, yams, and sweet potatoes. Since the adequate intake for prebiotics is undefined, a diet that includes a diverse variety of high-fiber fruits and vegetables, especially foods high in prebiotics, has the most potential for obtaining sufficient amounts. (63)

Vitamin D deficiency is common in people with ulcerative colitis with the prevalence being higher than the general population. (64) Vitamin D deficiency may also be a contributing factor in the development of ulcerative colitis (65). Vitamin D as a therapeutic agent has shown promise in lowering relapse rates and bettering quality-of-life in ulcerative colitis patients. (66)

Vitamin D is a pleiotropic hormone with a diverse range of effects ranging from immune modulation to cell differentiation and intercellular adhesion. Several in vivo and in vitro studies have examined the role of vitamin D in immune-mediated diseases such as ulcerative colitis. (67, 68, 69). The consequences of vitamin D deficiency on the gastrointestinal tract include, but are not limited to, decreased colonic bacterial clearance (70) reduced expression of tight junctions in the intestinal epithelium (71) and elevated Th1-driven inflammation at the gut level (72).

There is growing evidence that vitamin D status may affect disease activity. As such, consideration should be given to screening and management of vitamin D deficiency in this patient group (73, 74). Testing for Vitamin D deficiency should be part of every ulcerative colitis workup.

Other lab work should include B12 and, for potentially anemic patients, hemoglobin. Both the mean corpuscular volume (MCV) and the mean

How to cite this article: Rose S, Strombom A. Ulcerative Colitis – prevention and treatment with a plant-based diet. Adv Res Gastroentero Hepatol, 2020;15(2): 555908.
DOI: 10.19080/ARGH.2020.15.555908

corpuscular hemoglobin concentration (MCHC) will also have values below the normal range for the laboratory performing the test. A colonoscopy can be performed as indicated.

The plant-based diet compares favorably with standard treatments. Treatment with a plant-based may take a little longer to become evident. Lab work should take this into account. It is also important to titrate the doses of medications as the treatment effects of a plant-based diet become evident. This is also the case if patients are being treated with antidiabetic, antihypertensive and anti-hypercholesterolemics concurrently.

6. Discussion

Ulcerative colitis is a lifelong illness that has a profound emotional and social impact on the affected patients. Treating ulcerative colitis can be frustrating for doctor and patient alike. The symptoms usually cause discomfort and many of the medications used to treat the disease have significant side effects. In addition, some of the medications are quite expensive resulting in a financial burden for the patient. Therefore, practicing prevention of this disease is particularly desirable.

If ulcerative colitis is accepted to be a lifestyle disease mainly caused, or exacerbated by a westernized diet, then current practice should move toward encouraging the patient to change their diet. A plant-based diet is naturally much higher in fiber than the average American diet, thus promoting the bacterial species in the gut that produce butyrate, resulting in lower inflammation.

A plant-based diet can significantly reduce the risk or relapse in ulcerative colitis patients, almost as effectively as the leading drug, Mesalamine. It can be used as a monotherapy or as an adjunct along with medications that are usually prescribed for ulcerative colitis patients.

Treating the ulcerative colitis patient with a plant-based diet has several advantages. It has no contraindications or adverse reactions, is affordable and can prevent and treat common comorbidities such as type 2 diabetes and coronary artery disease. It also reduces the risk of colon cancer, which is raised for long standing cases of ulcerative colitis patients.

Plant-based diets are no longer very unusual as they have become more popular in the general population in recent years. Given all of the benefits, the plant-based diet deserves a place among the physician's treatment options for ulcerative colitis.

References

1. Wilks S. (1859) Morbid appearances in the intestine of Miss Bankes. *Treating ulcerative colitis*. Vol 2: Med Times Gazette
2. Danese S, Fiocchi C. (2011) Ulcerative colitis. *N Engl J Med*. 365(18):1713-1725.
3. Truelove S, Witts L. (1955) Cortisone in ulcerative colitis; final report on a therapeutic trial. *Br Med J*. 2(4947):1041-1048.
4. Dignass A, Lindsay JO, Sturm A, Windsor A, Colombel J-F et al. (2012) Second European evidence-based consensus on the diagnosis and management of ulcerative colitis Part 2: Current management. *J Crohns Colitis*. 6(10):991-1030.
5. Ng S, Bernstein C, Vatn M, Lakatos P, Loftus E, et al. (2013) Geographical variability and environmental risk factors in inflammatory bowel disease. *Gut*.62(4):630–649.
6. Danese S, Sans M, Fiocchi C. (2004) Inflammatory bowel disease: the role of environmental factors. *Autoimmun Rev*.3(5):394-400.
7. Birrenbach T, Böcker U. (2004) Inflammatory bowel disease and smoking: a review of

How to cite this article: Rose S, Strombom A. Ulcerative Colitis – prevention and treatment with a plant-based diet. Adv Res Gastroentero Hepatol, 2020;15(2): 555908.
DOI: 10.19080/ARGH.2020.15.555908

epidemiology, pathophysiology, and therapeutic implications. *Inflamm Bowel Dis*.10(6):848-859.

8. Rutgeerts P, D'Haens G, Hiele M, Geboes K, Vantrappen G. (1994) Appendectomy protects against ulcerative colitis. *Gastroenterology*.106(5):1251-1253.
9. Hou J, Abraham B, El-Serag H. (2011) Dietary intake and risk of developing inflammatory bowel disease: a systematic review of the literature. *Am J Gastroenterol*.106(4):563-573.
10. Ge J, Han TJ, Liu J, Lo JS, Zhang XH, et al. (2015) Meat intake and risk of inflammatory bowel disease: A meta-analysis. *Turk J Gastroenterol*.26(6):492-497.
11. Reif S, Klein I, Lubin F, Farbstein M, Hallak A, Gilat T. (1997) Pre-illness dietary factors in inflammatory bowel disease. *Gut*.40(6):754-760.
12. Li F, Liu X, Wang W, Zhang D. (2015) Consumption of vegetables and fruit and the risk of inflammatory bowel disease: a meta-analysis. *Eur J Gastroenterol Hepatol*. 27(6):623-630.
13. Jowett SL, Seal CJ, Pearce MS, Phillips E, Gregory W, et al. (2004) Influence of dietary factors on the clinical course of ulcerative colitis: a prospective cohort study. *Gut*. 53(10):1479-1484.
14. Chiba M, Nakane K, Tsuj T, Tsuda S, Ishii H, et al. (2018) Relapse prevention in ulcerative colitis by plant-based diet through educational hospitalization: A single-group trial. *Perm J*. 22:17-167.
15. Kawakami A, Tanaka M, Nishigaki M, Naganuma M, Iwao Y, et al. (2013) Relationship between non-adherence to aminosalicylate medication and the risk of clinical relapse among Japanese patients with ulcerative colitis in clinical remission: A prospective cohort study. *J Gastroenterol*. 48(9):1006-1015.
16. Moum B, Ekbom A, Vatn M, Aadland E, Sauar J, et al. (1997) Clinical course during the 1st year after diagnosis in ulcerative colitis and Crohn's disease. Results of a large, prospective population-based study in southeastern Norway, 1990-93. *Scand J Gastroenterol*. 32(10):1005-1012.
17. Henriksen M, Jahnsen J, Lygren I, Sauar J, Kjellevold Ø, et al. (2006) Ulcerative colitis and clinical course: Result of a 5-year population-based follow-up study (the IBSEN study). *Inflamm Bowel Dis*. 12(7):543-550.
18. Höie O, Wolters F, Riis L, Aamodt G, Solberg C, et al. (2007) Ulcerative colitis: patient characteristics may predict 10-yr disease recurrence in a European-wide population-based cohort. *Am J Gastroenterol*. 102(8):1692-1701.
19. Solberg I, Lygren I, Jahnsen J, Aadland E, Høie O, et al. (2009) Clinical course during the first 10 years of ulcerative colitis: Results from a population-based inception cohort (IBSEN Study). *Scand J Gastroenterol*. 44(4):431-440.
20. Bebb JR, Scott BB. (2004) How effective are the usual treatments for ulcerative colitis? *Aliment Pharmacol Ther*. 20(2):143-149.
21. Magro F, Rodrigues A, Vieira AI, Portela F, Cremers I, et al. (2012) Review of the disease course among adult ulcerative colitis population-based longitudinal cohorts. *Inflamm Bowel Dis*. 18(3):573-583.
22. Kitano A, Okawa K, Nakamura S, Komeda Y, Ochiai K, et al. (2011) The long-term assessment of the patients with ulcerative colitis (> 10 years follow-up, mean followup 21.7 years). *[Article in Japanese; abstract in English] Journal of New Remedies & Clinics*. 60(7):1347-1355.
23. Michail S, Durbin M, Turner D, Griffiths A, Mack D, et al. (2012) Alterations in the gut microbiome of children with severe ulcerative colitis. *Inflamm Bowel Dis*. 18(10):1799–1808.
24. Van Loo J, Cummings J, Delzenne N, Englyst H, Franck A, et al. (1999) Functional food properties of non-digestible oligosaccharides: a consensus report from the ENDO project (DGXII AIRII-CT94-1095). *Br J Nutr*. 81(2):121-132.

How to cite this article: Rose S, Strombom A. Ulcerative Colitis – prevention and treatment with a plant-based diet. Adv Res Gastroentero Hepatol, 2020;15(2): 555908.
DOI: 10.19080/ARGH.2020.15.555908

25. Fernández-Bañares F, Hinojosa J, Sánchez-Lombraña L, Navarro E, Martínez-Salmerón J, et al. (1999) Randomized clinical trial of Plantago ovata seeds (dietary fiber) as compared with mesalamine in maintaining remission in ulcerative colitis. Spanish Group for the Study of Crohn's Disease and Ulcerative Colitis (GETECCU). *Am J Gastroenterol*. 94(2):427-433.

26. Tilg H, Kaser A. (2004) A Diet and relapsing ulcerative colitis: take off the meat? *Gut*. 53(10):1399–1401.

27. Lorenz R, Weber PC, Szimnau P, Heldwein W, Strasser T, et al. (1989) Supplementation with n-3 fatty acids from fish oil in chronic inflammatory bowel disease—a randomized, placebo-controlled, double-blind cross-over trial. *J Intern Med Suppl*. 225(S731):225-232.

28. Stenson WF, Cort D, Rodgers J, Burakoff R, DeSchryver-Kecskemeti K, et al. (1992) Dietary supplementation with fish oil in ulcerative colitis. *Ann Intern Med*. 116(8):609-614.

29. Hawthorne AB, Daneshmend TK, Hawkey CJ, Nelluzzi A, Everitt S, et al. (1992) Treatment of ulcerative colitis with fish oil supplementation: a prospective 12 month randomised controlled trial. *Gut*. 33(7):922–928.

30. Aslan A, Triadafilopoulos G. (1992) Fish oil fatty acid supplementation in active ulcerative colitis: a double-blind, placebo-controlled, cross-over study. *Am J Gastroenterol*. 87(4):432-437.

31. Greenfield S, Green A, Teare J, Jenkins A, Punchard N, et al. (1993) A randomized controlled study of evening primrose oil and fish oil in ulcerative colitis. *Aliment Pharmacol Ther*. 7(2):159-166.

32. Ungaro R, Mehandru S, Allen P, Peyrin-Biroulet L, Colombel J. (2017) Ulcerative colitis. *Lancet*. 389(10080):1756-1770.

33. Ramos G, Papadakis K. (2019) Mechanisms of Disease: Inflammatory Bowel Diseases. *Mayo Clin Proc*. 94(1):155-165.

34. Brown K, DeCoffe D, Molcan E, Gibson DL. (2012) Diet-induced dysbiosis of the intestinal microbiota and the effects on immunity and disease. *Nutrients*. 4(8):1095–1119.

35. Keshteli A, Madsen K, Dieleman L. (2019) Diet in the pathogenesis and management of ulcerative colitis; A review of randomized controlled dietary interventions. *Nutrients*. 11(7):E1498.

36. Khalili H, Chan, S, Lochhead P, Ananthakrishnan A, Hart A, et al. (2018) The role of diet in the aetiopathogenesis of inflammatory bowel disease. *Nat Rev Gastroenterol Hepatol*. 15(9):525-535.

37. Wong J. (2014) Gut microbiota and cardiometabolic outcomes: influence of dietary patterns and their associated components. *Am J Clin Nutr*. 100(Suppl 1):369S-77S.

38. Hur S, Kang S, Jung H, Kim S, Jeon H, et al. (2012) Review of natural products actions on cytokines in inflammatory bowel disease. *Nutr Res*. 32(11):801-16.

39. Romier B, Schneider Y, Larondelle Y, During A. (2009) Dietary polyphenols can modulate the intestinal inflammatory response. *Nutr Rev*. 67(7):363-78.

40. Biasi F, Astegiano M, Maina M, Leonarduzzi G, Poli G. (2011) Polyphenol supplementation as a complementary medicinal approach to treating inflammatory bowel disease. *Curr Med Chem*. 18(31):4851-65.

41. Roediger W, Moore J, Babidge W. (1997) Colonic sulfide in the pathogenesis and treatment of ulcerative colitis. *Dig Dis Sci*. 42:1571–1579.

42. Roediger W. (1998) Decreased sulphur amino-acid intake in ulcerative colitis. *Lancet*. 351:1555.

43. Chapman M, Grahn M, Boyle M, Hutton M, Rogers J, et al. (1994) Butyrate oxidation is impaired in the colonic mucosa of sufferers of quiescent ulcerative colitis. *Gut*. 35(1):73–76.

44. Pitcher M, Beatty E, Cummings J. (2000) The contribution of sulphate reducing bacteria and 5-aminosalicylic acid to faecal sulphide in

How to cite this article: Rose S, Strombom A. Ulcerative Colitis – prevention and treatment with a plant-based diet. Adv Res Gastroentero Hepatol, 2020;15(2): 555908.
DOI: 10.19080/ARGH.2020.15.555908

patients with ulcerative colitis. *Gut*. 46(1):64–72.

45. Christl S, Eisner H, Dusel G, Kasper H, Scheppach W. (1996) Antagonistic effects of sulphide and butyrate on proliferation of colonic mucosa: a potential role for these agents in the pathogenesis of ulcerative colitis. *Dig Dis Sci*. 41:2477–2481.
46. Suarez F, Furne J, Springfield J, Levitt M. (1998) Bismuth subsalicylate markedly decreases hydrogen sulfide release in the human colon. *Gastroenterology*.114(5):923–929.
47. Magee E, Richardson C, Hughes R, Cummings J. (2000) Contribution of dietary protein to sulphide production in the large intestine: an in vitro and a controlled feeding study in humans. *Am J Clin Nutr*. 72(6):1488-1494.
48. Richardson C, Magee E, Cummings J. (2000) A new method for the determination of sulphide in gastrointestinal contents and whole blood by microdistillation and ion chromatography. *Clin Chim Acta*. 293(1-2):115-125.
49. Florin T, Gibson G, Neale G, Cummings J. (1990) A role for sulfate reducing bacteria in ulcerative colitis? *Gastroenterology*. 98:A170.
50. Florin T, Neale G, Gibson G, Christl S, Cummings J. (1991) Metabolism of dietary sulphate: absorption and excretion in humans. *Gut*.32(7):766-773.
51. Florin T, Neale G, Goretski S, Cummings J. (1993) The sulfate content of foods and beverages. *J Food Composition Anal*. 6:140–151.
52. Geypens B, Claus D, Evenepoel P, Hiele M, Maes B, et al. (1997) Influence of dietary protein supplements on the formation of bacterial metabolites in the colon. *Gut*. 41(1):70-76.
53. Gibson G, Cummings J, Macfarlane G. (1988) Use of a three-stage continuous culture system to study the effect of mucin on dissimilatory sulfate reduction and methanogenesis by mixed populations of human gut bacteria. *Appl Environ Microbiol*. 54(11):2750–2755.
54. Magee E, Richardson C, Cummings J. (2001) Dietary precursors of sulphide in the human large intestine. *Proc Nutr Soc*. 60:16A.
55. Ohkusa T. (1985) Production of experimental ulcerative colitis in hamsters by dextran sulfate sodium and changes in intestinal microflora. *Jpn J Gastroenterol*. 82:1327–1336.
56. Roediger W, Duncan A, Kapaniris O, Millard S. (1993) Reducing sulfur compounds of the colon impair colonocyte nutrition: implications for ulcerative colitis. *Gastroenterology*. 104(3):802-809.
57. Ng W, Tonzetich J. (1984) Effect of hydrogen sulfide and methyl mercaptan on the permeability of oral mucosa. *J Dent Res*. 63(7):994-997.
58. Aslam M, Batten J, Florin T, Sidebotham R, Baron J, et al. (1992) Hydrogen sulphide induced damage to the colonic mucosal barrier in the rat. *Gut*. 33:S69.
59. Bammens B, Evenepoel P, Keuleers H, Verbeke K, Vanrenterghem Y. (2006) Free serum concentrations of the protein-bound retention solute p-cresol predict mortality in hemodialysis patients. *Kidney Int*. 69(6):1081-7.
60. Kornbluth A, Sachar D, Practice Parameters Committee of the American College of Gastroenterology. (2010) Ulcerative colitis practice guidelines in adults: American College Of Gastroenterology, Practice Parameters Committee. *Am J Gastroenterol*. 105(3):501-523.
61. Kane SV. (2007) Overcoming adherence issues in ulcerative colitis. *Gastroenterol Hepatol (N Y)*. 3(10):795–799.
62. Jackson C, Clatworthy J, Robinson A, Horne R. (2010) Factors associated non-adherence to oral medication for inflammatory bowel disease: A systematic review. *Am J Gastroenterol*. 105(3):525-539.
63. Coleman Collins S. (2014) Entering the world of prebiotics – are they a precursor to good gut health? *Today's Dietitian*. 16(12):12.

How to cite this article: Rose S, Strombom A. Ulcerative Colitis – prevention and treatment with a plant-based diet. Adv Res Gastroentero Hepatol, 2020;15(2): 555908.
DOI: 10.19080/ARGH.2020.15.555908

64. Fletcher J, Swift A. (2017) Vitamin D screening in patients with inflammatory bowel disease. *Gastrointest. Nurs.* 15:16–23.
65. Cantorna MT. (2006) Vitamin D and its role in immunology: Multiple sclerosis, and inflammatory bowel disease. *Prog Biophys Mol Biol.* 92(1):60-64.
66. Del Pinto R, Pietropaoli D, Chandar A, Ferri C, Cominelli F. (2015) Association between inflammatory bowel disease and vitamin D deficiency: a systematic review and meta-analysis. *Inflamm Bowel Dis.* 21(11):2708-2717.
67. Ardizzone S, Cassinotti A, Trabattoni D, Manzionna G, Rainone V, et al. (2009) Immunomodulatory effects of 1,25-dihydroxyvitamin D3 on TH1/TH2 cytokines in inflammatory bowel disease: an in vitro study. *Int J Immunopathol Pharmacol.* 22(1):63-71.
68. Di Rosa M, Malaguarnera G, De Gregorio C, Palumbo M, Nunnari G, et al. (2012) Immunomodulatory effects of vitamin D3 in human monocyte and macrophages. *Cell Immunol.* 280:36–43.
69. Cantorna M, Munsick C, Bemiss C, Mahon B. (2000) 1,25-Dihydroxycholecalciferol prevents and ameliorates symptoms of experimental murine inflammatory bowel disease. *J Nutr.* 130(11):2648-2652.
70. Lagishetty V, Misharin A, Liu N, Lisse T, Chun R, et al. (2010) Vitamin D deficiency in mice impairs colonic antibacterial activity and predisposes to colitis. *Endocrinology.* 151(6):2423-2432.
71. Kong J, Zhang Z, Musch M, Ning G, Sun J, et al. (2008) Novel role of the vitamin D receptor in maintaining the integrity of the intestinal mucosal barrier. *Am J Physiol Gastrointest Liver Physiol.* 294(1):G208-G216.
72. Cantorna M, Zhu Y, Froicu M, Wittke A. (2004) Vitamin D status, 1,25-dihydroxyvitamin D3, and the immune system. *Am J Clin Nutr.* 80(6 Suppl):1717S-1720S.
73. Bancil A, Poullis A. (2015) The Role of Vitamin D in Inflammatory Bowel Disease. *Healthcare (Basel).* 3(2):338–350.
74. Rose S, Strombom A. (2019) Ensuring adequate vitamin D status for patients on a plant-based diet. *Ortho & Rheum Open Access J.* 15(3):555913.

How to cite this article: Rose S, Strombom A. Ulcerative Colitis – prevention and treatment with a plant-based diet. Adv Res Gastroentero Hepatol, 2020;15(2): 555908.
DOI: 10.19080/ARGH.2020.15.555908

Advanced Research in Gastroenterology & Hepatology
ISSN: 2472-6400

Juniper Publishers
key to the Researchers

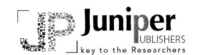

Review Article
Volume 14 Issue 4 – January 2020
DOI: 10.19080/ARGH.2020.14.555891

Adv Res Gastroenterol Hepatol

Gall Stones - Prevention with a Plant-Based Diet

Stewart Rose and Amanda Strombom*

Plant-Based Diets in Medicine, USA

Submission: December 12, 2019: **Published:** January 10, 2020

Corresponding Author: Amanda Strombom, Plant-based diets in Medicine, 12819 SE 38th St, #427, Bellevue, WA 98006, USA

Abstract

A plant-based diet has been shown to reduce the risk of cholesterol gall stones. This risk reduction is supported by the fact that vegetarians, and especially vegans, have a much lower prevalence of risk factors for cholesterol gallstones such as reduced risk of obesity, insulin resistance, Type 2 Diabetes and Crohn's disease.

Pregnant women are particularly susceptible to cholesterol gallstones due to the impact of weight gain, insulin resistance, leptin increases and hormonal changes. Since treatment for extreme hypercholesterolemia with medication during pregnancy is risky, a plant-based diet is indicated.

A plant-based diet excludes foods shown to increase the risk of cholesterol gallstones such as meat, poultry, fish along with the heme iron, saturated fat and dietary cholesterol which have been shown to increase cholesterol in gallstone disease patients. At the same time, a plant-based diet includes fruits, vegetables, whole grains, legumes rich with fiber along with mono and polyunsaturated oils, which have been shown to reduce the risk of cholesterol gallstones.

Keywords:

Gall Stones; Cholesterol gall stones; Obesity; Insulin resistance; Crohn's disease; Hypercholesterolemia; Polyunsaturated oils; Cholelithiasis; Cholecystitis; Pancreatitis; Gastrointestinal disease; Ascorbic acid; Gallbladder disease; Hepatitis C virus infection

1. Introduction

Gallstone disease constitutes a major health burden that has increased more than 20% over the last 3 decades. (1, 2, 3) The prevalence of gall stones (cholelithiasis) is about 10 to 15 percent of the population of the U.S., or well over 25 million people.

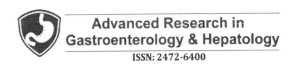

(1, 4) Nearly 1 million new cases of gallstone disease are diagnosed every year and approximately one quarter of these require treatment.

The burden of cholelithiasis and its complications, such as cholecystitis, pancreatitis, and cholangitis, are major public health problems. With an estimated 1.8 million ambulatory care visits each year, gallstone disease is a leading cause for hospital admissions related to gastrointestinal disease. (5) A 2006 study reported that more than 700,000 cholecystectomies were performed in the United States at a cost of $6.5 billion dollars annually. (6) Cholecystectomy is now the most common elective abdominal surgery performed in the United States. (7, 8, 9)

These numbers are likely an underestimate because laparoscopic cholecystectomy is often performed as a day procedure and thus not captured by hospital statistics that require overnight admission. Also not captured in the statistics is the pain of biliary colic that many patients experience.

2. Risk factors

Several studies, comparing those with gallstones versus those without, have shown that cholesterol gallstone formation is multifactorial. Some risk factors, such as ethnicity, genetics, advancing age, and female gender (including pregnancy) cannot be modified, whereas diet, BMI, Type 2 diabetes, and Crohn's Disease (plus excess alcohol consumption and cigarette smoking) can be modified. (4)

With regards to diet, studies have reported that the risk of gallstones was positively associated with intake of meat, excess calories, fat and saturated fat, but negatively associated with intake of vegetables and fiber. (10) Nutritional exposure to the western diet, i.e. increased intake of fat, refined carbohydrates and a decrease in fiber content, is a major risk factor for the development of gallstones. (10)

In Japan, postwar westernization has provided an example for the interplay between environment and disease. Since the late 1940's, the prevalence of gallstones in Tokyo has more than doubled. Moreover, there has been a change from pigment to cholesterol gallstones and the sex ratio has changed in favor of females. (11) This increase in gallstone incidence was associated with an increased fat intake and a decreased fiber content of the diet, and consequently was attributed to the westernization of the Japanese diet. (12)

When assessing the prevalence of gallstone disease, one must take into account that many people have gallstones but are asymptomatic. Approximately 20% become symptomatic after 10 years of follow up. (13) Comparing non-vegetarians to vegetarians, a study of both symptomatic and asymptomatic sonographically-confirmed cholelithiasis cases, found that the prevalence of gallstones was 1.9 time higher in non-vegetarians than in vegetarians. (14)

While most studies show a decreased risk of gall stones among vegetarians, one did not although this should be regarded with caution, since it runs counter to the greater weight of evidence. (15)

The lower risk that vegetarians seem to experience begs the question of which dietary factors are operational. A study of vegetarians examining this question, found that although the prevalence of gallstone disease was less than half that of non-vegetarians, there was no difference in the intake of macronutrients between the study and control groups. In this cross-sectional study, the prevalence of gallbladder disease (asymptomatic

How to cite this article: Rose S, Strombom A. Gall Stones – prevention with a plant-based diet. Adv Res Gastroentero Hepatol, 2020;14(3): 555891.
DOI: 10.19080/ARGH.2020.14.555891

gallstones or history of cholecystectomy) was significantly lower in vegetarians than omnivores (12% versus 25%). (16)

Heme iron, which is present in red meat, fish, and poultry, is highly bioavailable. In one large cohort study, a higher intake of heme iron was associated with a higher risk of gallstone disease, with a dose-response relation that was not accounted for by other potential risk factors. (17)

Another study, which looked not at total fat, but saturated fat versus mono- and poly-unsaturated fat, found that after adjustment for age and other potential risk factors, compared with men in the lowest quintile of dietary intake of long-chain saturated fats, the relative risk of gallstone disease for men in the highest quintile was 24% higher and the risk of cholecystectomy 41% higher than for omnivores. (18) Medium-chain saturated fatty acid and short-chain saturated fatty acid intake were unrelated to the risk. Short-chain saturated fats are found in the colon as the result of microbial action on dietary fiber, and medium-chain saturated fats occur naturally in plant foods, whereas long-chain fatty acids are primarily found in animal fats.

Complementing the above study was one that showed that polyunsaturated fats decrease the risk of gallstone formation by 18% for men in the highest quintile of dietary intake of cis unsaturated fats, compared with men in the lowest quintile. (19)

Consumption of vegetable protein is associated with a reduced risk of cholecystectomy. (20) In addition, adherence to a diet rich in fruit, vegetables, legumes, and olive oil has been associated with a reduction in cholecystectomy risk in women. (21, 22, 23)

Fiber decreases the transit time thereby lowering the risk of gall bladder disease and cholecystectomy in women. (24) In another study, women with the highest insoluble fiber intake had a 17% lowered risk of gallbladder surgery. (25) A study on the benefit of consuming nuts found that men consuming 5 or more ounces of tree nuts per week had a 30% lower risk of gallstone disease. (26)

Both obesity and insulin resistance are associated with gallbladder disease. (27, 28) BMI is a strong risk factor for gall bladder disease. (4) Vegetarians and vegans have significantly lower BMI's on average. A study of American vegetarians and vegans found that that vegetarians had a mean BMI of 25.7 and vegans a mean BMI of 23.6. (29) A European study found the average BMI of vegetarians and vegans to be 23.3 and 22.4 respectively for men and 22.8 and 21.8 for women. (30) A study of German vegans found an average BMI of 22.3. (31)

There is an increased risk of gallbladder disease among Type 2 diabetes patients. (27) Vegetarians, and even more so vegans, have less insulin resistance, and have a greatly reduced risk of T2DM. (32) This and their lower risk of obesity contribute to their lower risk of gallstones.

The prevalence of gallstones in patients with Crohn disease ranges from 13% to 34% in different studies, accounting for a total of about 700 patients. (33) However, the risk of Crohn's disease has been found to be reduced by 70% in female and 80% in male young people following a nearly vegetarian diet. (34)

As a result of this, vegetarians appear to have a lower risk of cholesterol gallstones because of their higher intake of fruits, vegetables, nuts, fiber and plant protein and also their lower BMI, risk of type 2 diabetes and Crohn's disease.

How to cite this article: Rose S, Strombom A. Gall Stones – prevention with a plant-based diet. Adv Res Gastroentero Hepatol, 2020;14(3): 555891.
DOI: 10.19080/ARGH.2020.14.555891

3. Pathogenesis

Cholesterol gallstone pathogenesis must be briefly considered to facilitate the presentation of risk factors. Cholesterol gallstones constitute more than 80% of stones in the Western world. Cholesterol gallstones, composed predominantly of cholesterol crystals, result from abnormalities in cholesterol metabolism. (12)

Four types of abnormalities have been considered to be responsible for cholesterol gallstone formation. The first and essential requirement is bile supersaturation in cholesterol.

The second abnormality is enhanced nucleation of cholesterol crystals. Mucin and its congeners, the major proteins, act as matrix molecules to hold cholesterol crystal aggregates together to form a stone. (12)

There also must be sufficient time for nucleation to occur, for crystals to form and grow to microliths, and for microliths to aggregate to form gallstones, hence gallbladder stasis is a contributing factor to gallstone formation. During overnight fasting, the gallbladder does not empty so that hours of storage occur in all individuals. (12)

Intestinal hypomotility has been recently recognized as a fourth primary factor in cholesterol lithogenesis. Having a longer exposure to intestinal micro-organisms, primary bile salts are in greater proportion deconjugated and dehydroxylated to more hydrophobic secondary bile salts. An increased proportion of the secondary bile acid deoxycholate, a potent down-regulator of the rate-limiting enzyme for bile acid biosynthesis, enhances cholesterol hypersecretion into bile. (12)

Excessive cholesterol secretion could result from defective conversion of cholesterol to bile acids, due to a low or relatively low activity of cholesterol 7α hydroxylase, the rate limiting enzyme for bile acid biosynthesis and cholesterol elimination. (35) Ascorbic acid, found in many fruits and vegetables reduces lithogenic risk in adults in that it influences α hydroxylase activity in the bile. (10)

Cholesterol supersaturation, the essential requirement for cholesterol gallstone formation, might occur via excessive cholesterol biosynthesis (increased 3-hydroxy-3-methylglutaryl (HMG) coenzyme A (CoA) reductase activity). (35)

Hepatic metabolism of cholesterol in gall stone patients is hypothesized to be different than in normal patients. (36) In gallstone disease, a patient's cholesterol and bile acid homeostasis is significantly altered. As a patient's dietary cholesterol increases, biliary cholesterol secretion increases and bile acid synthesis and pool decrease. These are changes associated with cholesterol gallstone formation. (35, 37)

4. Gallstone Disease in Pregnancy

Epidemiological and clinical studies have found that gallstone prevalence is twice as high in women as in men at all ages in every population studied. In pregnancy in particular, the incidence of cholesterol gallstones is increased by strong risk factors including obesity, serum leptin and extreme hypercholesterolemia.

The incidence rates of biliary sludge (a precursor to gallstones) and gallstones are up to 30% and 12%, respectively, during pregnancy and postpartum, and gallbladder disease is the most common non obstetrical cause of maternal hospitalization in the first year postpartum. (38, 39). Between 1% and 3% of pregnant women undergo cholecystectomy due to clinical symptoms or complications within the first year postpartum.

How to cite this article: Rose S, Strombom A. Gall Stones – prevention with a plant-based diet. Adv Res Gastroentero Hepatol, 2020;14(3): 555891.
DOI: 10.19080/ARGH.2020.14.555891

During the period of a normal, healthy pregnancy, the body undergoes substantial hormonal, immunological, and metabolic changes. (40, 41, 42, 43, 44) Some of these alterations become risk factors contributing to the formation of cholesterol gallstones in pregnant women, including weight gain, insulin resistance, and an altered gut microbiota. (40, 45, 46, 47, 48, 49, 50, 51) Insulin resistance is a risk factor for incident gallbladder sludge and stones during pregnancy, even after adjustment for body mass index. (52, 53, 54)

Increased estrogen levels during pregnancy induce significant metabolic changes in the hepatobiliary system, including the formation of cholesterol supersaturated bile and sluggish gallbladder motility, two factors enhancing cholelithogenesis. During pregnancy, bile becomes lithogenic because of a significant increase in estrogen levels, which lead to hepatic cholesterol hypersecretion and biliary lithogenicity. In addition, increased progesterone concentrations impair gallbladder motility function, with the resulting increase in fasting gallbladder volume and bile stasis. Such abnormalities greatly promote the formation of biliary sludge and gallstones. Because plasma concentrations of female sex hormones, especially estrogen, increase linearly with the duration of gestation, the risk of gallstone formation becomes higher in the third trimester of pregnancy. (40)

Serum leptin is a strong predictor of incident gallbladder disease in pregnant women. (55) However, a plant-based diet has been shown to lower leptin levels. (56)

Pre pregnancy obesity is a strong risk factors for pregnancy-associated gallbladder disease. (55) Those following a plant-based diet have, on average, a lower BMI thus reducing their risk of pre pregnancy obesity which is a strong risk factor for gall stone disease. (32) Prescribing a prenatal plant-based diet for prophylaxis is therefore indicated.

Prevention of gallstone disease is especially important in pregnancy when cholecystectomy is more problematic and medication can carry risks. At present extreme hypercholesterolemia is not treated during pregnancy, partly due to the absence of established normal parameters for pregnancy, as well as clinicians' uncertainty as to the significance of elevated levels for a limited time period. HMG CoA-reductase inhibitors (statins), which are the most commonly used drugs to treat high cholesterol outside of pregnancy, are contraindicated. (57)

With established pregnancy-specific reference values, extreme maternal hypercholesterolemia could be identified and monitored. Due to recognized adverse effects of very high cholesterol on the pregnancy and the fetus, intervention with a cholesterol-lowering diet may be necessary and prove beneficial. (57)

A plant-based diet has been shown to lower the risk of obesity, reduce leptin and eliminate cholesterol from the diet, thus reducing serum cholesterol during pregnancy without the risk that drug treatment may entail. (58) The American Academy of Nutrition and Dietetics position statement on plant-based diets confirms their safety during pregnancy and lactation and that they may confer additional health advantages. (59)

5. Gallstone disease in vegetarians

While the risk of cholelithiasis is lower in vegetarians, a study looked at the risk factors that remained among vegetarians themselves. Risk factors useful for predicting cholelithiasis in vegetarians are age and total bilirubin level in men, and age, BMI, and alcohol consumption in women. Just as interesting is some indication of those factors which weren't risk factors in this study. Many previously identified risk factors for the general population do not seem to apply to vegetarians. The study revealed that diabetes mellitus, coronary artery disease, cerebral vascular accident, chronic renal failure, hepatitis C virus infection, and lipid abnormalities were not associated with cholelithiasis in male and female vegetarians. This finding may be explained by the protective effect of vegetarian diets, according to the authors. (36)

Counseling patients who are already vegetarian should focus on modifiable risk factors, such as BMI and alcohol consumption, to reduce their risk still further. Some research has focused on determining which dietary factors account for the lower risk vegetarians have of gallstone disease. One study found that men consuming 5 or more ounces of tree nuts per week had a significantly lower risk of gallstone disease. (26) In another study, those consuming the most fruits and vegetables were 21% less likely than those with the lowest intake to require cholecystectomy. (23)

6. Discussion

While a plant-based diet cannot treat gallstones that have already formed, considering the scale of gallstone disease, the possibility of preventing about half the cases is very significant. It is particularly valuable as a way of reducing the risk of gallstones during pregnancy, when pharmaceutical methods are not possible. The plant-based diet can also prevent and treat common comorbidities such as type 2 diabetes, obesity and coronary artery disease. It has no adverse reactions and has no contraindications.

References:

1. Shaffer EA. (2005) Epidemiology and risk factors for gallstone disease: has the paradigm changed in the 21st century? *Curr Gastroenterol Rep* 7(2):132-140.
2. Sandler RS, Everhart JE, Donowitz M, et al. (2002) The burden of selected digestive diseases in the United States. *Gastroenterology* 122(5):1500-1511.
3. Everhart JE, Ruhl CE. (2009) Burden of digestive diseases in the United States part I: overall and upper gastrointestinal diseases. *Gastroenterology* 136(2):376-386.
4. Stinton LM, Shaffer EA. (2012) Epidemiology of gallbladder disease: Cholelithiasis and cancer. *Gut Liver* 6(2):172–187.
5. Shaheen N, Hansen R, Morgan D, et al. (2006) The burden of gastrointestinal and liver diseases, 2006. *Am J Gastroenterol* 101(9):2128-2138.
6. Shaffer EA. (2006) Epidemiology of gallbladder stone disease. *Best Pract Res Clin Gastroenterol* 20(6):981–996.
7. Everhart JE, Khare M, Hill M, Maurer KR. (1999) Prevalence and ethnic differences in gallbladder disease in the United States. *Gastroenterology* 117(3):632-639.
8. Kang J-, Ellis C, Majeed A, et al. (2003) Gallstones–an increasing problem: a study of hospital admissions in England between 1989/1990 and 1999/2000. *Aliment Pharmacol Ther* 17(4):561-569.
9. Russo MW, Wei JT, Thiny MT, et al. (2004) Digestive and liver diseases statistics, 2004. *Gastroenterology* 126(5):1448-1453.
10. Elkhateeb YAMM, Alghannam TM, Alkhamali SA. (2019) Gallbladder Stone Disease and its Relation to Dietary Intake. *Acta Scientific Gastrointestinal Disorders* 2(3).
11. Kameda H, Ishihara F, Shibata K, Tsukie E. (1984) Clinical and nutritional study on gallstone disease in Japan. *Jpn J Med* 23(2):109-113.

How to cite this article: Rose S, Strombom A. Gall Stones – prevention with a plant-based diet. Adv Res Gastroentero Hepatol, 2020;14(3): 555891.
DOI: 10.19080/ARGH.2020.14.555891

12. Acalovschi M. (2001) Cholesterol gallstones: from epidemiology to prevention. *Postgrad Med J* 77(906):221–229.
13. Attili AF, DeSantis A, Capri R, Repice AM, Maselli S. (1995) The natural history of gall-stones: the GREPCO experience. The GREPCO Group. *Hepatology* 21(3):655-660.
14. Pixley F, Wilson D, McPherson K, Mann J. (1985) Effect of vegetarianism on development of gall stones in women. *Br Med J (Clin Res Ed)* 291(6487):11-12.
15. McConnell T, Appleby P, Key T. (2017) Vegetarian diet as a risk factor for symptomatic gallstone disease. *Eur J Clin Nutr* 71(6):731–735.
16. Pixley F, Mann J. (1988) Dietary factors in the aetiology of gall stones: a case control study. *Gut* 29(11):1511–1515.
17. Tsai CJ, Leitzmann MF, Willett WC, Giovannucci EL. (2007) Heme and non-heme iron consumption and risk of gallstone disease in men. *Am J Clin Nutr* 85(2):518-522.
18. Tsai CJ, Leitzmann M, Willett W, Giovannucci E. (2008) Long-chain saturated fatty acids consumption and risk of gallstone disease among men. *Ann Surg* 247(1):95-103.
19. Tsai CJ, Leitzmann M, Willett W, Giovannucci E. (2004) The effect of long-term intake of cis unsaturated fats on the risk for gallstone disease in men: A prospective cohort study. *Ann Intern Med* 141(7):514-522.
20. Tsai CJ, Leitzmann MF, Willett WC, Giovannucci EL. (2004) Dietary protein and the risk of cholecystectomy in a cohort of US women: the Nurses' Health Study. *Am J Epidemiol* 160(1):11-8.
21. Barré A, Gusto G, Cadeau C, Carbonnel F, Boutron-Ruault M. (2017) Diet and Risk of Cholecystectomy: A Prospective Study Based on the French E3N Cohort. *Am J Gastroenterol* 112(9):1448-1456.
22. Nordenvall C, Oskarsson V, Wolk A. (2018) Fruit and vegetable consumption and risk of cholecystectomy: a prospective cohort study of women and men. *Eur J Nutr* 57(1):75–81.
23. Tsai CJ, Leitzmann MF, Willett WC, Giovannucci EL. (2006) Fruit and vegetable consumption and risk of cholecystectomy in women. *Am J Med* 119(9):760–767.
24. Tsai CJ, Leitzmann MF, Willett WC, Giovannucci EL. (2004) Long-term intake of dietary fiber and decreased risk of cholecystectomy in women. *Am J Gastroenterol* 99(7):1364-1370.
25. Hillemeier C. (1995) An overview of the effects of dietary fiber on gastrointestinal transit. *Pediatrics* 96(5 Pt 2):997-999.
26. Tsai CJ, Leitzmann MF, Hu FB, Willett WC, Giovannucci EL. (2004) A prospective cohort study of nut consumption and the risk of gallstone disease in men. *Am. J. Epidemiol* 160(10):961–968.
27. Aune D, Vattena LJ. (2016) Diabetes mellitus and the risk of gallbladder disease: A systematic review and meta-analysis of prospective studies. *J Diabetes Complications* 30(2):368-373.
28. Aune D, Norat T, Vatten LJ. (2015) Body mass index, abdominal fatness and the risk of gallbladder disease. *Eur J Epidemiol* 30(9):1009-1019.
29. Tonstad S, Butler T, Yan R, Fraser G. (2009) Type of Vegetarian Diet, Body Weight, and Prevalence of Type 2 Diabetes. *Diabetes Care* 32(5):791–796.
30. Bradbury K, Crowe F, Appleby P, Schmidt J, RC T, et al. (2014) Serum concentrations of cholesterol, apolipoprotein A-I, and apolipoprotein B in a total of 1 694 meat-eaters, fish-eaters, vegetarians, and vegans. *Eur J Clin Nutr* 68(2):178-183.
31. Waldmann A, Koschizke J, Leitzmann C, Hahn A. (2005) German vegan study: diet, life-style factors, and cardiovascular risk profile. *Annuls of Nutrition and Metabolism* 49(6):366-72.
32. Strombom A, Rose S. (2017) The prevention and treatment of Type II Diabetes Mellitus

with a plant-based diet. *Endocrin Metab Int J* 5(5):00138.

33. Fraquelli M, Losco A, Visentin S, et al. (2001) Gallstone disease and related risk factors in patients with Crohn disease: analysis of 330 consecutive cases. *Arch Intern Med* 161(18):2201-2204.
34. Rose S, Strombom A. (2018) Crohn's disease prevention and treatment with a plant-based diet. *Adv Res Gastroentero Hepatol* 9(1).
35. Kern F. (1994) Effects of dietary cholesterol on cholesterol and bile acid homeostasis in patients with cholesterol gallstones. *J Clin Invest* 93(3):1186–1194.
36. Chen YC, Chiou C, Lin MN, Lin CL. (2014) The prevalence and risk factors for gallstone disease in Taiwanese vegetarians. *PLoS One* 9(12).
37. Greenberger N, Paumgartner G. (2008) Diseases of the Gallbladder and Bile Ducts. In: Fauci AS, Braunwald E, Kasper DL, et al., eds. *Harrison's Principles of Internal Medicine*. 17th ed: McGraw-Hill Professional.
38. Ko C. (2006) Risk factors for gallstone-related hospitalization during pregnancy and the postpartum. *Am J Gastroenterol* 101(10):2263-2268.
39. Lydon-Rochelle M, Holt VL, Martin DP, Easterling TR. (2000) Association between method of delivery and maternal rehospitalization. *JAMA* 283(18):2411-2416.
40. deBari O, Wang TY, Liu M, Paik CN, Portincasa P, Q.Wang D. (2014) Cholesterol cholelithiasis in pregnant women: pathogenesis, prevention and treatment. *Ann Hepatol* 13(6):728-745.
41. Newbern D, Freemark M. (2011) Placental hormones and the control of maternal metabolism and fetal growth. *Curr Opin Endocrinol Diabetes Obes* 18(6):409-416.
42. Murphy VE, Smith R, Giles WB, Clifton VL. (2006) Endocrine regulation of human fetal growth: the role of the mother, placenta, and fetus. *Endocr Re* 27(2):141-169.
43. Barbour LA, McCurdy CE, Hernandez TL, Kirwan JP, Catalano PM, Friedman JE. (2007) Cellular mechanisms for insulin resistance in normal pregnancy and gestational diabetes. *Diabetes Care* 30(Suppl 2):S112-119.
44. Lain K, Catalano P. (2007) Metabolic changes in pregnancy. *Clin Obstet Gynecol* 50(4):938-948.
45. Zavalza-Gómez AB, Anaya-Prado R, Rincón-Sánchez AR, Mora-Martínez JM. (2008) Adipokines and insulin resistance during pregnancy. *Diabetes Res Clin Pract* 80(1):8-15.
46. Mor G, Cardenas I. (2011) The Immune System in Pregnancy: A Unique Complexity. *Am J Reprod Immunol* 63(6):425–433.
47. Jamieson DJ, Theiler RN, Rasmussen SA. (2006) Emerging infections and pregnancy. *Emerg Infect Dis* 12(11):1638-1643.
48. Koren O, Goodrich JK, Cullender TC, et al. (2012) Host remodeling of the gut microbiome and metabolic changes during pregnancy. *Cell* 150(3):470-480.
49. Ko CW, Beresford SAA, Schulte SJ, Lee SP. (2008) Insulin resistance and incident gallbladder disease in pregnancy. *Clin Gastroenterol Hepatol* 6(1):76-81.
50. Collado MC, Isolauri E, Laitinen K, Salminen S. (2008) Distinct composition of gut microbiota during pregnancy in overweight and normal-weight women. *Am J Clin Nutr* 88(4):894-899.
51. DiCianni G, Miccol R, Volpe iL, Lencioni C, DelPrato S. (2003) Intermediate metabolism in normal pregnancy and in gestational diabetes. *Diabetes Metab Res Rev* 19(4):259-270.
52. Gielkens HAJ, Lama WF, Coenraad M, et al. (1998) Effect of insulin on basal and cholecystokinin-stimulated gallbladder motility in humans. *J Hepatol* 28(4):595-602.
53. Haffner SM, Diehl AK, Mitchell BD, Stern MP, Hazuda HP. (1990) Increased prevalence of clinical gallbladder disease in subjects with non-insulin-dependent diabetes mellitus. *Am J Epidemiol* 132: 327-335.

How to cite this article: Rose S, Strombom A. Gall Stones – prevention with a plant-based diet. Adv Res Gastroentero Hepatol, 2020;14(3): 555891.
DOI: 10.19080/ARGH.2020.14.555891

54. Ruhl CE, Everhart JE. (2000) Association of diabetes, serum insulin, and C-peptide with gallbladder disease. *Hepatology* 31(2):229-303.

55. Ko CW, Beresford SAA, Schulte SJ, Matsumoto AM, Lee SP. (2005) Incidence, natural history, and risk factors for biliary sludge and stones during pregnancy. *Hepatology* 41(2):359-365.

56. Kahleova H, Matoulek M, Malinska H, Oliyarnik O, Kazdova L, et al. (2011) Vegetarian diet improves insulin resistance and oxidative stress markers more than conventional diet in subjects with Type 2 diabetes. *Diabet Med* 28(5):549-59.

57. Bartels Ä, O'Donoghue K. (2011) Cholesterol in pregnancy: a review of knowns and unknowns. *Obstet Med* 4(4):147–151.

58. Rose S, Strombom A. (2018) A comprehensive review of the prevention and treatment of heart disease with a plant-based diet. *J Cardiol & Cardiovas Ther* 12(5):555847.

59. Melina V, Craig W, Levin S. (2016) Position of the academy of nutrition and dietetics: vegetarian diets. *J Acad Nutr Diet* 116(12):1970-80.

How to cite this article: Rose S, Strombom A. Gall Stones – prevention with a plant-based diet. Adv Res Gastroentero Hepatol, 2020;14(3): 555891.
DOI: 10.19080/ARGH.2020.14.555891

Advanced Research in Gastroenterology & Hepatology
ISSN: 2472-6400

Juniper Publishers
key to the Researchers

Mini Review

Volume 14 Issue 2 - December 2019

DOI: 10.19080/ARGH.2019.14.555884

Adv Res Gastroenterol Hepatol

Diverticular Disease risk reduced with a Plant-Based Diet

Stewart D Rose and Amanda J Strombom*

Plant-Based Diets in Medicine, USA

Submission: November 22, 2019: **Published:** December 05, 2019

***Corresponding Author:** Amanda Strombom, Plant-Based Diets in Medicine, 12819 SE 38th St, #427, Bellevue, WA 98006, USA

Abstract

By age 60, two-thirds of all Americans will develop diverticulosis, and a significant percentage will go on to develop acute diverticulitis. Epidemiological studies show that the risk of diverticulitis is reduced significantly, the less red meat, refined grains and high fat dairy are consumed, and the more fruits, vegetables and whole grains are included in the diet.

The prevalence of diverticular disease in vegetarians was found to be 27% less and for vegans was 72% less than for meat eaters. Dietary fiber is an independent risk factor, reducing the risk by 41% for those consuming the most fiber, so one reason vegetarians, and especially vegans, have lower rates of diverticular disease may be their higher fiber intake. They also have a lower incidence of other risk factors such as obesity and hypertension. The properties of plant foods (the phytonutrients they contain) and the healthier and less inflammatory intestinal flora that vegetarians and especially vegans have, also contribute significantly to their reduced incidence of diverticulosis and diverticulitis and its complications.

The clinical implications of the research so far indicate a plant-based, or vegan diet, emphasizing high fiber, especially insoluble fiber, should be prescribed for all patients at risk of diverticular disease.

Keywords:

Diverticulitis; Diverticulosis; Fiber; Vegan; Vegetarian; Western diet

1. Introduction

By age 60, two-thirds of all Americans will have developed diverticulosis. (1) A significant percentage of patients with diverticulosis will go on to develop acute diverticulitis. This imposes a significant burden on healthcare systems, resulting in greater than 300,000 admissions per year with an estimated annual cost of $3 billion. (2) There is considerable evidence that a high fiber, plant-based diet is effective at reducing the risk of this painful condition.

The western diet, high in red meat, refined grains, and high-fat dairy, and a prudent diet, high in fruits, vegetables, and whole grains, were compared for risk of diverticulitis. The highest quintile of Western dietary pattern score had a 55% greater risk of diverticulitis compared to the lowest quintile. Even within the prudent diet group, high prudent diet scores were associated with decreased risk of diverticulitis of 26%. (3)

Another study compared with men in the lowest quintile of total red meat consumption to men in the highest quintile. The latter had an increased risk of diverticulitis of 58%.[4] A case control study and two large-scale prospective cohort studies found that frequent consumption of red meat is a risk factor for diverticular disease or for hospitalization as a result of diverticular disease. (5, 6, 7)

In 1979, a research article in the British journal, the Lancet, reported that the prevalence of diverticular disease in vegetarians was almost one third that of meat eaters. It was noted in this study that vegetarians had a mean intake of fiber of 42 gm/day compared to 21 gm/day for meat eaters. (8) In a more recent study, vegetarians were found to be at a 30% decreased risk of diverticulosis compared with omnivores. (9)

In a more detailed British study, the relative risk of diverticular disease was found to be 27% less for vegetarians and 72% less for vegans compared to meat eaters. (10) Dietary fiber was also determined to be an independent factor, reducing the relative risk of diverticular disease by 41% for those consuming the most. Other important variables were obesity, hypertension, cigarette smoking, hormone replacement therapy and oral contraceptives.

One of the reasons vegetarians, and especially vegans, have lower rates of diverticular disease may be their higher fiber intake, and a lower incidence of other risk factors such as obesity and hypertension. (11) It may also be reasonably hypothesized that the properties of plant foods (the phytonutrients they contain) and the healthier and less inflammatory intestinal flora that vegetarians and especially vegans have, contribute significantly to their reduced incidence of diverticulosis and diverticulitis and its complications. (12)

While one study showed a smaller association between fiber and diverticulosis, (13) its results should be regarded with caution partly because of its methodology and partly because of the greater weight of evidence showing an association between dietary fiber is very well established. (5, 6, 14)

A lack of dietary fiber is firmly anchored in the literature as the most important lifestyle associated risk factor for the development of diverticulosis as well as diverticular disease. (15, 16) There is agreement that there are considerable benefits of fiber for the management of other diseases and overall health; we therefore should continue to recommend fiber as part of a healthy diet. (17, 18)

The notion that individuals with diverticular disease should avoid nuts, seeds, corn, and popcorn are based on the hypothesis that their

How to cite this article: Rose SD, Strombom AJ. Diverticular disease risk reduced with a plant-based diet. Adv Res Gastroentero Hepatol, 2019;14(2): 555884.
DOI: 10.19080/ARGH.2019.14.555884

fragments could impact and obstruct a diverticulum, thereby causing diverticulitis or a diverticular hemorrhage. However, a large prospective documented an inverse relationship between nut and popcorn consumption and the risk of diverticulitis. Furthermore, no associations were observed between corn consumption and diverticulitis or between nut, corn, or popcorn consumption and diverticular hemorrhage or uncomplicated diverticulosis. (19)

2. Discussion

The etiology for diverticular disease may be more complicated than once thought. However, the clinical implications of the research so far indicates that a plant-based, or vegan, diet that emphasizes high fiber, especially insoluble fiber, would be indicated, and should be prescribed for all patients at risk of diverticular disease. (20)

References

1. Floch M, Bina I. (2004) The natural history of diverticulitis: fact and theory. *J Clin Gastroenterol*. 38(5 Suppl 1):S2-S7.
2. Agarwal A, Karanjawala B, Maykel J, Johnson E, Steele S. (2014) Routine colonic endoscopic evaluation following resolution of acute diverticulitis: Is it necessary? *World J Gastroenterol*. 20(35):12509–12516.
3. Strate L, Keeley B, Cao Y, Wu K, Giovannucci E, et al. (2017) Western Dietary Pattern Increases, Whereas Prudent Dietary Pattern Decreases, Risk of Incident Diverticulitis in a Prospective Cohort Study. *Gastroenterology*.152(5):1023-1030.
4. Cao Y, Strate L, Keeley B, Tam I, Wu K, et al. (2018) Meat intake and risk of diverticulitis among men. *Gut*. 67(3):466-472.
5. Aldoori W, Giovannucci E, Rimm E, Wing A, Trichopoulos D, et al. (1994) A prospective study of diet and the risk of symptomatic diverticular disease in men. *Am J Clin Nutr*. 60(5):757–764.
6. Aldoori W, Giovannucci E, Rockett H, Sampson L, Rimm E, et al. (1998) A Prospective Study of Dietary Fiber Types and Symptomatic Diverticular Disease in Men. *J Nutr*.128(4):714–719.
7. Manousos O, Day N, Tzonou A, Papadimitriou C, Kapetanakis A, et al. (1985) Diet and other factors in the aetiology of diverticulosis: an epidemiological study in Greece. *Gut*. 26(6):544–549.
8. Gear J, Ware A, Fursdon P, Mann J, Nolan D, et al. (1979) Symptomless diverticular disease and intake of dietary fibre. *Lancet*. 1(8115):511-514.
9. Peery A, Sandler R, Ahnen D, Galanko J, Holm A, et al. (2013) Constipation and a low-fiber diet are not associated with diverticulosis. *Clin Gastroenterol Hepatol*. 11(12):1622-1627.
10. Crowe F, Appleby P, Allen N, Key T. (2011) Diet and risk of diverticular disease in Oxford cohort of European Prospective Investigation into Cancer and Nutrition (EPIC): prospective study of British vegetarians and non-vegetarians. *BMJ*. 343:d4131.
11. Yeo L, Tseng T, Chen W, Kao T, Wu L, et al. (2019) Hypertension control and risk of colonic diverticulosis. *Therap Adv Gastroenterol*. 12:1756284819855734.
12. Kim M, Hwang S, Park E, Bae J. (2013) Strict vegetarian diet improves the risk factors associated with metabolic diseases by modulating gut microbiota and reducing intestinal inflammation. *Environ Microbiol Rep*. 5(5):765-775.
13. Barroso A, Quigley E. (2015) Diverticula and Diverticulitis: Time for a Reappraisal. *Gastroenterol Hepatol (N Y)*. 11(10):680–688.
14. Böhm S. (2015) Risk Factors for Diverticulosis, Diverticulitis, Diverticular Perforation, and Bleeding: a plea for more subtle history taking. *Viszeralmedizin*. 31(2):84-94.

How to cite this article: Rose SD, Strombom AJ. Diverticular disease risk reduced with a plant-based diet. Adv Res Gastroentero Hepatol, 2019;14(2): 555884.
DOI: 10.19080/ARGH.2019.14.555884

15. Böhm S. (2010) *Divertikelkrankheit*. Bremen: Uni-Med.

16. Strate L. (2012) Lifestyle factors and the course of diverticular disease. *Dig Dis*. 30(1):35-45.

17. Burgell R, Muir J, Gibson P. (2013) Pathogenesis of Colonic Diverticulosis: Repainting the Picture. *Clin Gastroenterol Hepatol*. 11(12):1628–1630.

18. Floch M. (2014) Is there really anything new on dietary fiber in colonic diverticular disease? *Clin Gastroenterol Hepatol*. 12:1200–1201.

19. Strate L, Liu Y, Syngal S, Aldoori W, Giovannucci E. (2008) Nut, Corn, and Popcorn Consumption and the Incidence of Diverticular Disease. *JAMA*. 300(8):907-914.

20. Aldoori W, Ryan-Harshman M. (2002) Preventing diverticular disease. Review of recent evidence on high-fibre diets. *Can Fam Physician*. 48:1632-1637.

How to cite this article: Rose SD, Strombom AJ. Diverticular disease risk reduced with a plant-based diet. Adv Res Gastroentero Hepatol, 2019;14(2): 555884.
DOI: 10.19080/ARGH.2019.14.555884

Orthopedics and Rheumatology
Open Access Journal
ISSN: 2471-6804

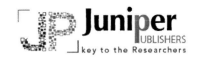

Juniper Publishers
key to the Researchers

Review Article
Volume 13 Issue 1 - October 2018
DOI: 10.19080/OROAJ.2018.13.555852

Orth & Rheum Open Access J

Rheumatoid Arthritis: Prevention and Treatment with a Plant-Based Diet

Stewart Rose* and Amanda Strombom

Plant-Based Diets in Medicine, USA

Submission: September 26, 2018; Published: October 05, 2018

Correspondence Author: Stewart Rose, Plant-Based Diets in Medicine, 12819 SE 38th St, #427, Bellevue, WA 98006, USA

Abstract

Rheumatoid arthritis has no cure, so long term treatment is indicated. An individual's dietary choices greatly influence the progression of chronic autoimmune rheumatic diseases. This review shows that the plant-based diet has good scientific evidence of safety and efficacy for both prevention and treatment of rheumatoid arthritis. Studies have shown significant improvements in specific symptoms, such as number of tender joints, Ritchie's articular index, number of swollen joints, pain score, duration of morning stiffness, grip strength, and improved laboratory values such as sed rate (ESR), C-reactive protein, and rheumatic factor. Patients placed on a plant-based diet also have a beneficial shift in intestinal microbiota, which correlates with clinical improvement. With respect to prevention, those following a plant-based diet experience a reduction in risk of rheumatoid arthritis by about 50%.

RA patients should be advised that a plant-based diet that includes appropriate amounts of carbohydrate, especially dietary fiber, is important for maintaining the symbiosis of intestinal flora, which could be beneficial for preventing autoimmunity. As disease severity worsens, individuals with RA may experience functional decline that can impact dietary intake. New healthy plant-based convenience foods are a good choice for such patients.

Treatment with a plant-based diet is affordable for the patient, has no adverse reactions and no contraindications, and it can be combined with any of the standard treatments. For mild cases it may suffice as a monotherapy. For moderate and severe cases, it may serve as an adjunct, allowing dosage reductions thus lessening the costs and side effects.

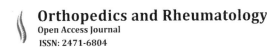

Keywords:
Rheumatoid Arthritis; Autoimmunity; Rheumatic; Plant-based diet; Vegan; Vegetarian; Intestinal flora; Microbiota; Dietary fiber; Dietary modification

1. Introduction

Rheumatoid arthritis (RA) is a chronic systemic inflammatory disease of unknown etiology. There is no cure, so long term treatment is indicated. Medication-based therapies comprise several classes of agents, including nonsteroidal anti-inflammatory drugs (NSAIDs), non-biologic and biologic disease modifying anti-rheumatic drugs (DMARDs), immunosuppressants, and corticosteroids. Other standard treatments include physical therapy and surgery.

Surveys have shown that a substantial proportion of people with RA will try complementary and alternative interventions, perhaps reflecting the lack of complete satisfaction with conventional approaches, and also a desire to help themselves. (1) In 1989, Arthritis Care noted that more than 50% of the Arthritis Care members who were surveyed, had invested in "unorthodox medicines, substances, or treatments (including diets), during the prior six months". (2)

Today, with increased access to health care information has come a growing demand for safe, cost-effective and easy to administer therapies. While a number of purported treatments have questionable or no research behind them, one of these so-called "unorthodox treatments" does. An individual's dietary choices can greatly influence the progression and manifestation of chronic autoimmune rheumatic diseases. In light of these effects, it makes sense that the search for additional therapies to attenuate such diseases would include investigations into dietary modifications. (3)

Dietary interventions have a widespread appeal for both patients as well as clinicians due to factors including affordability, accessibility, and presence of scientific evidence that demonstrates substantial benefits in reducing disease symptoms such as pain, joint stiffness, swelling, tenderness and associated disability with disease progression. (4)

2. Epidemiology

There have been few studies on the risk of RA in relation to vegetarian status. However, one good-sized study showed that non-vegetarian women had a 57% increased risk of RA, and semi-vegetarians an increased risk of 16%, when compared with vegetarian women. Non-vegetarian men showed an increased risk of 50% and semi-vegetarian men an increased risk of 14%. (5) These results are especially notable considering that the non-vegetarians in this study already had a relatively low consumption of meat.

3. Interventional studies

Many doctors have anecdotally noted an association between the consumption of animal-derived foods, especially meat, and Rheumatoid Arthritis. (6)

A meta-study on RA looked at studies on the effects of short-term modified fasting followed subsequently with plant-based diets lasting at least three months. The pooling of these studies showed a statistically and clinically significant beneficial long-term effect. Thus available evidence suggests that fasting followed by vegetarian diets might be useful in the treatment of RA. (7)

How to cite this article: Rose S, Strombom A. Rheumatoid arthritis – prevention and treatment with a plant-based diet. Ortho & Rheum Open Access J 2018; 13(1): 555852.
DOI: 10.19080/OROAJ.2018.13.555852

The effect of a one-year study on RA patients of brief (7-10 day) modified fasting, followed first by a vegan diet and then by a vegetarian diet was assessed in a randomized, single blind controlled trial. After four weeks, the diet group showed a significant improvement in the number of tender joints, Ritchie's articular index, number of swollen joints, pain score, duration of morning stiffness, grip strength, erythrocyte sedimentation rate, C reactive protein, white blood cell count, and a health assessment questionnaire score. The improvements were still present at the end of one year. A significant drop in the levels of intestinal Proteus Mirabilis was observed. (8)

In a follow-up study of the same patients two years later, pain score, duration of morning stiffness, Stanford Health Assessment Questionnaire index, number of tender joints, Ritchie's articular index, number of swollen joints, ESR and platelet count all maintained their improvement in patients who were responders. Interestingly, most patients who were originally in the vegetarian group, but switched back to their usual diet, reported an increase in disease symptoms after intake of meat. (9)

A separate one-year study of RA patients placed on a vegetarian diet, and focusing on clinical laboratory values, showed significant improvements in leukocyte count, IgM, RF (Rheumatic Factor), and the complement components C3 and C4, along with patient symptoms. (10)

It usually takes several months for a plant-based diet to reach full effect in RA. However, one study showed improvements in pain, joint swelling, severity in morning stiffness and limitation in function in only 4 weeks. There were also non-significant trends in the reduction of C-reactive protein and Rheumatic factor. Based on the results of other studies, these might have become significant with further time. (11)

Studies have noted a link between vegan diets and protection against other autoimmune diseases. For example, an analysis of an Adventist cohort found that a vegan diet, but not a vegetarian diet, was associated with a lower risk of hypothyroid disease. (12)

Several researchers have examined the role of gut bacteria in RA disease activity. (13, 14, 15, 16, 17) Researchers Ling and Hänninen tested subjects on both a conventional Western diet and a vegan diet for one month, in order to determine the shift in intestinal flora. They found that four fecal hydrolytic enzymes, associated with toxic and inflammatory products, diminished during consumption of the vegan diet. However, these changes in fecal urease, choloylglycine hydrolase, β-glucuronidase and β-glucosidase, disappeared within two weeks of resuming a conventional diet. The authors attribute these reductions in fecal enzymes not only to the activity of bacteria during the dietary shift, but also to the high fiber content of the vegan diet which can affect fecal weight, transit time and bacterial metabolism. (18)

RA patients have been found to have higher levels of Proteus mirabilis antibodies, when compared with healthy controls or subjects with other diseases. The subjects from the vegetarian diet study had a significantly lower mean antibody level against Proteus mirabilis, which was correlated significantly with the measured decrease in disease activity. (19) This suggests that the improvement in RA disease activity may be related to the effects of the vegan diet on the presence of gut bacteria, such

How to cite this article: Rose S, Strombom A. Rheumatoid arthritis – prevention and treatment with a plant-based diet. Ortho & Rheum Open Access J 2018; 13(1): 555852.
DOI: 10.19080/OROAJ.2018.13.555852

as Proteus mirabilis, and the body's response to such bacteria.

The possibility that a vegan diet can induce a rapid change in gut profile was supported by studies of rheumatoid arthritis patients, in which a one-month switch to a vegan diet was sufficient to significantly alter the fecal microflora, as determined by stool sample gas-liquid chromatography profiles of bacterial cellular fatty acids. (20, 21)

Peltonen et al. conducted a study of RA patients and found a significant change in intestinal flora after a one-year shift from a conventional diet to a vegan and then a lactovegetarian diet. They also noted a significant difference between the fecal flora of test subjects in the high improvement group and the low improvement group, suggesting a direct connection between gut profiles and levels of disease activity. (22)

To further test the role of diet-induced changes in levels of various intestinal flora on rheumatoid arthritis activity, 43 RA patients were randomly assigned to either a raw vegan diet rich in lactobacilli, or an omnivorous diet. After one month, there was a significant change in the fecal flora of the 18 subjects in the vegan diet group who completed the study; no such change was found in the omnivore control group. Importantly, the vegan diet also induced a decrease in disease activity in some of the RA patients, leading the authors to conclude that changes in the intestinal flora are associated with diet-induced changes in disease activity. (20)

Kjeldsen-Kragh et al. followed upon their work by putting rheumatoid arthritis patients on a fast followed by 3.5 months of a vegan diet, followed by a 9-month lactovegetarian diet. (23) Subjects in the vegan then vegetarian diet group improved significantly over those maintained on an omnivorous diet. Similar to other studies, the authors found that subjects' fecal flora during times of clinical improvement differed significantly from times of no or minor improvements. Others have found that a raw vegan diet rich in lactobacilli and fiber decreased symptoms of rheumatoid arthritis, suggesting that the probiotic lactobacilli, among other components of a raw vegan diet, may be helpful to RA patients. (24, 25, 26) One way that these bacteria are helpful is that they regulate the T cell phenotype and T cell mediated immunity. (27)

Caution is warranted in interpreting bacteriologic studies on vegan diets and RA. Although diet-induced modification in intestinal flora, and an associated reduction in inflammation severity, may be a contributing factor to the improvements seen in RA patients, it is important to note that other features of a vegan diet have been credited with alleviating RA symptoms among vegan diet adherents. These include an increase in fruit, vegetable and fiber intake, a reduction in saturated fat and caloric intake, improved antioxidant levels, weight loss, and a reduction in food allergies and intolerances. (28, 29, 17)

It has been observed that vegetarians consume enough foods naturally containing salicylates to have an anti-inflammatory effect. The presence of salicylate in the blood of patients placed on a vegetarian diet was found at concentrations that are known to inhibit the transcription of COX 2, a key inflammatory enzyme in various pathologies. An emphasis on those foods highest in salicylate might enhance the therapeutic effect of a plant-based diet and warrants further investigation. (30)

The low-fat vegan diet and diets rich in unsaturated fat (such as plant-based oils) or probiotics have positive effects at alleviating pain and on

How to cite this article: Rose S, Strombom A. Rheumatoid arthritis – prevention and treatment with a plant-based diet. Ortho & Rheum Open Access J 2018; 13(1): 555852.
DOI: 10.19080/OROAJ.2018.13.555852

inflammation markers. (31) There was much hope for the role for Omega 3 fatty acids from fish oil. However, clinical studies on supplementation of ω-3 fatty acids have not supported the expectations. (32, 33, 34, 35, 36, 37)

4. Reduction of risk of Coronary Artery Disease (CAD)

Patients with rheumatoid arthritis (RA) have increased cardiovascular disease and mortality. (38, 39, 40) Several recent studies indicate an increased prevalence not only of cardiovascular disease (CVD) but also of atherosclerosis as determined by ultrasound tomography of carotid arteries. (38, 41, 42) The underlying mechanisms causing this increased risk are not wholly clarified but inflammation and disease duration are suggested to be of importance. (43, 44, 45, 46)

One study investigated the effects of a vegan diet, in patients with rheumatoid arthritis (RA), on the blood lipids: oxidized low-density lipoprotein (oxLDL) and on natural atheroprotective antibodies against phosphorylcholine (anti-PCs). The study examined the effects of intervention using a gluten-free vegan diet on patients with active RA. They were randomly assigned to either a vegan diet or a well-balanced non-vegan diet for one year. The gluten-free vegan diet induced significantly lower body mass index (BMI), low density lipoprotein (LDL), ox LDL, total cholesterol, and higher anti-PC IgM than control diet. Triglycerides and high-density lipoprotein did not change, since this was not a low fat vegan diet. Therefore a vegan diet in patients with RA induces changes that are potentially atheroprotective and anti-inflammatory, including decreased LDL and oxLDL levels, and raised anti-PC IgM and IgA levels. (47)

5. Clinical Considerations

Rheumatoid arthritis (RA) afflicts approximately 1.5 million American adults and is a major cause of disability. As disease severity worsens, individuals with RA may experience functional decline that can impact dietary intake. The diet quality of many individuals with RA needs improvement and may be related to functional disability associated with RA. Healthcare providers should encourage individuals with RA to meet dietary guidelines and maintain a healthy diet. Moreover, healthcare providers should be aware of the potential impacts of functional disability on diet quality in individuals with RA. (48)

Patients with rheumatoid arthritis often have trouble preparing foods that require manual dexterity and strength. These patients should be counseled to purchase the new healthy plant-based convenience foods that are now widely available. These foods are usually higher in fiber and lower in sugar, fat, sodium and calories than ordinary convenience foods. (49)

RA patients should be advised that a plant-based diet that includes appropriate amounts of carbohydrate, especially dietary fiber, is important for maintaining the symbiosis of intestinal flora, which could be beneficial for preventing autoimmunity. (27)

Active participation of the patient and family in the design and implementation of the therapeutic program helps ensure compliance, as does explaining the rationale for dietary treatment.

This treatment may be sufficient as a monotherapy in mild cases, or can be used as an adjunct to standard treatments in moderate and severe cases. Dosages may be able to be titrated down as the clinical effects of the diet manifest themselves.

How to cite this article: Rose S, Strombom A. Rheumatoid arthritis – prevention and treatment with a plant-based diet. Ortho & Rheum Open Access J 2018; 13(1): 555852.
DOI: 10.19080/OROAJ.2018.13.555852

6. Discussion

Optimal care of patients with rheumatoid arthritis consists of an integrated approach that includes both pharmacologic and non-pharmacologic therapies. Medications have side effects which must be managed and are costly to the patient. Some of the non-pharmacologic treatments are available for this disease include physical therapy and surgery. (50) A plant-based diet should be added to this list.

Studies show that not only is a plant-based diet safe and efficacious for the prevention and treatment of Rheumatoid Arthritis, it has several advantages in its favor. It has no adverse effects, no contraindications, and it's very affordable for the patient. It can be combined with any standard treatment, and is likely to synergize treatments effects with them. It is safe in the long term, and has been shown to reduce the risk of comorbidities, such as coronary artery disease, in rheumatoid arthritis patients.

Further research should focus on the most effective dietary elements within plant-based diets.

References

1. Ernst E. (2004) Musculoskeletal conditions and complementary/alternative medicine. *Best Practice & Research Clinical Rheumatology* 18(4):539–556.
2. Darlington L. (1991) Dietary therapy for arthritis. *Rheumatic Disease Clinics of North America* 17(2):273-286.
3. Dahan S, Segal Y, Shoenfeld Y. (2017) Dietary factors in rheumatic autoimmune diseases: a recipe for therapy? *Nat Rev Rheumatol J* 13(6):348-358.
4. Khanna S, Jaiswal K, Gupta B. (2017) Managing Rheumatoid Arthritis with Dietary Interventions. *Front Nutr* 4:52.
5. Fraser G. (1999) Associations between diet and cancer, ischemic heart disease, and all-cause mortality in non-Hispanic white California Seventh-day Adventists. *American Journal of Clinical Nutrition* 70(3):532s-538s.
6. Kutlu A, Oztürk S, Taşkapan O, Onem Y, Kiralp MZ, et al. (2010) Meat-induced joint attacks, or meat attacks the joint: rheumatism versus allergy. *Nutrition in Clinical Practice* 25(1):90-91.
7. Müller H, de Toledo F, Resch K. (2001) Fasting followed by vegetarian diet in patients with rheumatoid arthritis: a systematic review. *Scandinavian Journal of Rheumatology* 30(1):1-10.
8. Kjeldsen-Kragh J, Haugen M, Borchgrevink C, et al. (1991) Controlled trial of fasting and one-year vegetarian diet in rheumatoid arthritis. *The Lancet*.338(8772):899-902.
9. Kjeldsen-Kragh J, Haugen M, Borchgrevink C, Førre O. (1994) Vegetarian diet for patients with rheumatoid arthritis–status: two years after introduction of the diet. *Clinical Rheumatology* 13(3):475-482.
10. Kjeldsen-Kragh J, Mellbye O, Haugen M, Mollnes TE, Hammer HB, et al. (1995) Changes in laboratory variables in rheumatoid arthritis patients during a trial of fasting and one-year vegetarian diet. *Scandinavian Journal of Rheumatology* 24(2):85-93.
11. McDougall J, Bruce B, Spiller G, Westerdahl J, McDougall, M. (2002) Effects of a very low-fat, vegan diet in subjects with rheumatoid arthritis. *Journal of Alternative and Complementary Medicine*. 8(1):71-75.
12. Tonstad S, Nathan E, Oda K, Fraser G. (2013) Vegan Diets and Hypothyroidism. *Nutrients*. 5(11):4642-4652.
13. Hazenberg M, Klasen I, Kool J, Ruseler-van Embden JG, Severijnen AJ. (1992) Are intestinal bacteria involved in the etiology of rheumatoid arthritis? Review article. *APMIS*. 100(1):1-9.
14. 14. Deighton C, Gray J, Bint A, Walker DJ. (1992) Anti-Proteus antibodies in rheumatoid arthritis same-sexed sibships. *British Journal of Rheumatology*. 31(4):241-245.

How to cite this article: Rose S, Strombom A. Rheumatoid arthritis – prevention and treatment with a plant-based diet. Ortho & Rheum Open Access J 2018; 13(1): 555852.
DOI: 10.19080/OROAJ.2018.13.555852

15. Ebringer A, Ptaszynska T, Corbett M, Wilson C, Macafee Y et al. (1985) Antibodies to Proteus in Rheumatoid Arthritis. *The Lancet*. 326(8450):305–307.

16. Rogers P, Hassan J, Bresnihan B, Feighery C, Whelan A. (1988) Antibodies to Proteus in rheumatoid arthritis. *British Journal of Rheumatology*. 27 Suppl 2:90-94.

17. Glick-Bauer M, Yeh MC. (2014) The Health Advantage of a Vegan Diet: Exploring the Gut Microbiota Connection. *Nutrients*. 6(11):4822-4838.

18. Ling W, Hänninen O. (1992) Shifting from a conventional diet to an uncooked vegan diet reversibly alters fecal hydrolytic activities in humans. *Journal of Nutrition*. 122(4):924-930.

19. Kjeldsen-Kragh J, Rashid T, Dybwad A, Ebringer A. (1995) Decrease in anti-Proteus mirabilis but not anti-Escherichia coli antibody levels in rheumatoid arthritis patients treated with fasting and a one year vegetarian diet. *Annals of the Rheumatic Diseases*. 54(3):221-224.

20. Peltonen R, Nenonen M, Helve T, Hänninen O, Toivanen P, et al. (1997) Faecal microbial flora and disease activity in rheumatoid arthritis during a vegan diet.. *British Journal of Rheumatology*. 36(1):64-68.

21. Peltonen R, Ling W, Hänninen O, Eerola E. (1992) An uncooked vegan diet shifts the profile of human fecal microflora: Computerized analysis of direct stool sample gas-liquid chromatography profiles of bacterial cellular fatty acids. *Applied and Environmental Microbiology*. 58(11):3660-3666.

22. Peltonen R, Kjeldsen-Kragh J, Haugen M, Eerola E. (1994) Changes of faecal flora in rheumatoid arthritis during fasting and one-year vegetarian diet. *British Journal of Rheumatology*. 33(7):638-643.

23. Kjeldsen-Kragh J. (1999) Rheumatoid arthritis treated with vegetarian diets. *American Journal of Clinical Nutrition*. 70(3 Suppl):594s-600s.

24. Nenonen M, Helve T, Rauma A, Hänninen OO. (1998) Uncooked, lactobacilli-rich, vegan food and rheumatoid arthritis. *British Journal of Rheumatology*. 37(3):274-281.

25. Hänninen O, Rauma A, Kaartinen K, Nenonen M. (1999) Vegan diet in physiological health promotion. *Acta Physiologica Hungarica*. 86(3-4):171-180.

26. Hänninen O, Kaartinen K, Rauma A, Nenonen M, Törrönen R, et al. (2000) Antioxidants in vegan diet and rheumatic disorders. *Toxicology*. 155(1-3):45-53.

27. Masuko K. (2018) A Potential Benefit of "Balanced Diet" for Rheumatoid Arthritis. *Front Med (Lausanne)*. 5:141.

28. Smedslund G, Byfuglien M, Olsen S, Hagen K. (2010) Effectiveness and safety of dietary interventions for rheumatoid arthritis: A systematic review of randomized controlled trials.. *Journal of the American Dietetic Assoc*. 110(5):727-35.

29. Hafström I, Ringertz B, Spångberg A, von Zweigbergk L, Brannemark S, et al. (2001) A vegan diet free of gluten improves the signs and symptoms of rheumatoid arthritis: The effects on arthritis correlate with a reduction in antibodies to food antigens. *Rheumatology (Oxford)*. 40(10):1175-1179.

30. Blacklock C, Lawrence J, Wiles D, Malcolm EA, Gibson IH, et al. (2001) Salicylic acid in the serum of subjects not taking aspirin. Comparison of salicylic acid concentrations in the serum of vegetarians, non-vegetarians, and patients taking low dose aspirin. *Journal of Clinical Pathology*. 54(7):553-555.

31. Badsha H. (2018) Role of Diet in Influencing Rheumatoid Arthritis Disease Activity. *Open Rheumatol J*. 12:19-28.

32. Haugen M, Fraser D, Forre O. (1999) Diet therapy for the patient with rheumatoid arthritis? *Rheumatology (Oxford)*. 38(11):1039-1044.

33. Pullman-Mooar S, Laposata M, Lem D, Holman RT, Leventhal LJ, et al. (1990) Alteration of

cellular fatty acid profile and the production of eicosanoids in human monocytes by gamma-linolenic acid. *Arthritis and Rheumatism*. 33(10):1526-1533.

34. Kremer J, Jubiz W, Michalek A, Rynes RI, Bartholomew LE, et al. (1987) Fish-Oil Fatty Acid Supplementation in Active Rheumatoid Arthritis: A Double-Blinded, Controlled, Crossover Study. *Annals of Internal Medicine*. 106(4):497-503.
35. Tate G, Mandell B, Laposata M, Ohliger D, Baker DG, et al. (1989) Suppression of acute and chronic inflammation by dietary gamma linolenic acid. *Journal of Rheumatology*. 16(6):729-734.
36. Endres S, Ghorbani R, Kelley V, Georgilis K, Lonnemann G, et al. (1989) The effect of dietary supplementation with n-3 polyunsaturated fatty acids on the synthesis of interleukin-1 and tumor necrosis factor by mononuclear cells. *New England Journal of Medicine*. 320(5):265-271.
37. Kjeldsen-Kragh J, Lund J, Riise T, Finnanger B, Haaland K, et al. (1992) Dietary omega-3 fatty acid supplementation and Naproxen treatment in patients with rheumatoid arthritis. *Journal of Rheumatology*. 19(10):1531-1536.
38. Frostegård J. (2005) Atherosclerosis in patients with autoimmune disorders. *Arteriosclerosis, Thrombosis and Vascular Biology*. 25(9):1776-85.
39. Solomon D, Karlson E, Rimm E, Cannuscio CC, Mandi LA, et al. (2003) Cardiovascular morbidity and mortality in women diagnosed with rheumatoid arthritis. *Circulation*. 107(9):1303-1307.
40. Wolfe F, Freundlich B, Straus W. (2003) Increase in cardiovascular and cerebrovascular disease prevalence in rheumatoid arthritis. *Journal of Rheumatology*. 30(1):36-40.
41. Park Y, Ahn C, Choi H, Lee SH, In BH, et al. (2002) Atherosclerosis in rheumatoid arthritis: morphologic evidence obtained by carotid ultrasound. *Arthritis and Rheumatism*. 46(7):1714-9.
42. Jonsson S, Backman C, Johnson O, Karp K, Lundström E, et al. (2001) Increased prevalence of atherosclerosis in patients with medium term rheumatoid arthritis. *Journal of Rheumatology*. 28(12):2597-2602.
43. Del Rincón I, Williams K, Stern M, Freeman GL, O'Leary DH, et al. (2003) Association between carotid atherosclerosis and markers of inflammation in rheumatoid arthritis patients and healthy subjects. *Arthritis and Rheumatism*. 48(7):1833-1840.
44. Nagata-Sakurai M, Inaba M, Goto H, Kumeda Y, Furumitsu Y, et al. (2003) Inflammation and bone resorption as independent factors of accelerated arterial wall thickening in patients with rheumatoid arthritis. *Arthritis and Rheumatism*. 48(11):3061-3067.
45. Wållberg-Jonsson S, Cvetkovic J, Sundqvist K, Lefvert AK, Rantapää-Dahlqvist S. (2002) Activation of the immune system and inflammatory activity in relation to markers of atherothrombotic disease and atherosclerosis in rheumatoid arthritis. *Journal of Rheumatology*. 29(5):875-882.
46. Del Rincón I, O'Leary D, Freeman G, Escalante A. (2007) Acceleration of atherosclerosis during the course of rheumatoid arthritis. *Atherosclerosis*. 195(2):354-360.
47. Elkan A, Sjöberg B, Kolsrud B, Ringertz B, Hafström I, Frostegård J, et al. (2008) Gluten-free vegan diet induces decreased LDL and oxidized LDL levels and raised atheroprotective natural antibodies against phosphorylcholine in patients with rheumatoid arthritis: a randomized study. *Arthritis Research & Therapy*. 10(2):R34.
48. Berube L, Kiely M, Yazici Y, Woolf K. (2017) Diet quality of individuals with rheumatoid arthritis using the Healthy Eating Index (HEI)-2010. *Nutr Health*. 23(1):17-24.
49. Mizukami Y, Matsui T, Tohma S, Masuko K. (2017) Distinct patterns of dietary intake in

How to cite this article: Rose S, Strombom A. Rheumatoid arthritis – prevention and treatment with a plant-based diet. Ortho & Rheum Open Access J 2018; 13(1): 555852.
DOI: 10.19080/OROAJ.2018.13.555852

different functional classes of patients with rheumatoid arthritis. *Top Clin Nutr*. 32(2):141-151.

50. National Collaborating Centre for Chronic Conditions (UK). (2009) Rheumatoid Arthritis: National Clinical Guideline for Management and Treatment in Adults. *London: Royal College of Physicians (UK)*.

Orthopedics and Rheumatology
Open Access Journal
ISSN: 2471-6804

Juniper PUBLISHERS key to the Researchers

Review Article
Volume 15 Issue 3 - December 2019
DOI: 10.19080/OROAJ.2019.15.555914

Orth & Rheum Open Access J

Osteoarthritis Prevention and Treatment with a Plant-Based Diet

Stewart Rose* **and Amanda Strombom**

Plant-Based Diets in Medicine, USA

Submission: November 14, 2019; **Published:** December 03, 2019

***Corresponding author:** Stewart Rose, Plant-Based Diets in Medicine, 12819 SE 38th St, #427, Bellevue, WA 98006, USA

Abstract

The prevalence of osteoarthritis is increasing not only because of longer life expectancy but also because of the modern lifestyle, in particular physical inactivity and diets low in plant foods and rich in saturated fats, which promote chronic low-grade inflammation and obesity.

No proven disease-modifying or structure-modifying drugs for osteoarthritis are currently known. Consequently, pharmacologic treatment is directed at symptom relief. However, a whole food plant-based diet (WFPBD) has been shown to reduce the symptoms of osteoarthritis by reducing risk factors such as obesity, metabolic syndrome and Type II Diabetes.

In an interventional study, a whole food plant-based diet was associated with a significant reduction in pain compared to an ordinary omnivorous diet, with statistically significant pain reduction seen as early as two weeks after initiation of dietary modification. Within the plant-based diet, several specific phytonutrients have been shown to reduce the symptoms and severity of osteoarthritis and can be considered active ingredients.

Treating patients with a plant-based diet has the advantage of having no contraindications or adverse reactions and can be combined with any standard treatment. It also has the advantage of treating common comorbidities such as type 2 diabetes and coronary artery disease.

Keywords:

BMI; Diabetes; Inflammation; Metabolic syndrome; Phytonutrients; Plant-based diet; Obesity; Osteoarthritis

Abbrevations:

BMI: Body Mass Index; NRF2: Nuclear Factor Erythroid 2-related factor 2; OA Osteoarthritis; PQQ: Pyrroloquinoline Quinone; SFN: Sulforaphane; SIRT6: Sirtuin 6 T2DM Type 2 Diabetes Mellitus; WFPBD: Whole Food Plant Based Diet

1. Introduction

The prevalence of osteoarthritis is increasing not only because of longer life expectancy but also because of the modern lifestyle, in particular physical inactivity and diets low in plant foods and rich in saturated fats, which promote chronic low-grade inflammation and obesity. (1)

Osteoarthritis is believed to be a very complex multifactorial disease. It's a degenerative disease characterized by low grade inflammation in cartilage and synovium, resulting in the loss of joint structure and progressive deterioration of cartilage. Inflammation is one of the major drivers of the progression of osteoarthritis. Although the disease can be dependent on genetic and epigenetic factors, sex, ethnicity, lubricin level, apoptosis and age, it is also associated with obesity and being overweight, dietary factors, sedentary lifestyle and sport injuries. (2)

2. Epidemiology

Vegetarians have a lower risk of osteoarthritis. One study showed that even light meat consumption once a week increased the risk of osteoarthritis by 31% in women and 19% in men, compared to vegetarians. (3)

Obesity is the greatest modifiable risk factor for osteoarthritis (OA). (4, 5, 6) Coggon et al. reported that subjects with a BMI greater than 30 kg/m^2 were 6.8 times more likely to develop knee OA than normal weight control subjects. (7) A recent meta-analysis reported that the pooled odds ratio for developing OA was 2.63 for obese subjects compared to normal weight control subjects. (8)

Vegetarians and vegans have significantly lower BMIs on average. A study of American vegetarians and vegans found that that vegetarians had a mean BMI of 25.7 and vegans a mean BMI of 23.6. (9) A European study found the average BMI of vegetarians and vegans to be 23.3 and 22.4 respectively for men and 22.8 and 21.8 for women. (10) A study of German vegans found an average BMI of 22.3. (11) A study of vegetarian children found that they too had lower BMI's than their meat-eating counterparts with an average BMI of 17.3 in ages 6 to 11 and average of 20.0 ages 12-18. (12) One study found the risk of being overweight or obese is 65% less for vegans and 46% less for vegetarians. (13)

High body mass index (BMI) is a well-established risk factor for Type 2 Diabetes Mellitus (T2DM). T2DM increases the risk of development of severe osteoarthritis, necessitating arthroplasty independent of age and BMI. Diabetics face about double the risk of severe osteoarthritis suggesting that there is a strong metabolic component in the pathogenesis of osteoarthritis. (14)

Metabolic factors are important for the development of osteoarthritis, as suggested by the following lines of evidence:

1. The association between obesity and OA extends beyond weight-bearing joints, suggesting that this link is not solely based on mechanical factors. (15)

How to cite this article: Rose S, Strombom A. Osteoarthritis prevention and treatment with a plant-based diet. Ortho & Rheum Open Access J 2019; 15(3): 555914.
DOI: 10.19080/OROAJ.2019.15.555914

2. Metabolic syndrome is significantly more common among subjects with than without OA. (16, 17)

Two lines of experimental evidence may help to explain the link between type 2 diabetes and OA:

- chondrocytes express the GLUT/SLC2A, and high blood glucose levels shift the synthesis pattern of chondrocytes from type II collagen to reactive oxygen species, potentially mediating cartilage destruction. (18, 19, 20)
- Advanced glycosylation end products, elicited by sustained hyperglycemia, can stimulate chondrocyte expression of proinflammatory and prodegenerative proteins via the receptor for advanced glycosylation end products. (21, 22, 23)

Vegetarians have a 56% reduced risk of metabolic syndrome. (24) Vegetarian and vegans also have a substantially lower risk of Type 2 Diabetes. The consumption of meat and the increase in risk of T2DM in a dose dependent manner has been established since at least 1985. (25) More recently, a large, well-regarded study showed that semi-vegetarians reduced their risk of T2DM by 38%, pesco vegetarians by 51%, vegetarians by 61% and vegans by 78%. This indicates a dose-response relationship between risk reduction and amount of plant foods in the diet. (26) Therefore, it follows that those following a plant-based diet would have a lower risk of osteoarthritis, because of their lower BMI and lower risk of type 2 diabetes.

3. Intervention

Individuals diagnosed with arthritis can take steps to improve their diet quality as a possible route to reduce arthritis symptoms and maintain a healthy body weight. (27) In an interventional study, a whole food plant-based diet was associated with a significant reduction in pain compared to an ordinary omnivorous diet, with statistically significant pain reduction seen as early as two weeks after initiation of dietary modification. (28) The primary mechanism by which diet reduces subjective pain may be as a result of normalization of the fatty acid profile and reduction in exposure to inflammatory protein precursors. (28)

The plant-based dietary profile (low fat, high fiber) can lead to a diet that is less energy dense and so results in a significant reduction in caloric intake. Despite reductions in calorie intake, the WFPB diet is associated with increased nutrient density as well as increased concentrations of several vitamins and trace minerals. Therefore, the WFPB diet group may have taken in fewer calories than the treated group while encouraged to eat to satiety without calorie counting. The reduction in mean body weight was achieved with no attempt to limit calorie intake in this study. (28)

While not a fully plant-based diet, the Mediterranean Diet is high in plant foods and low in meat. In one study the Mediterranean Diet was associated with better quality of life and decreased pain and disability in patients with osteoarthritis. (29)

3.1 Specific phytonutrients and their mechanisms

Several phytonutrients have been shown to reduce the symptoms of osteoarthritis. Dietary phytonutrients (phytochemicals) are found in plant-based foods such as fruits, vegetables and grains, and may be categorized in a nested hierarchical manner with many hundred individual phytochemicals identified to date. (30) Phytonutrients

How to cite this article: Rose S, Strombom A. Osteoarthritis prevention and treatment with a plant-based diet. Ortho & Rheum Open Access J 2019; 15(3): 555914.
DOI: 10.19080/OROAJ.2019.15.555914

are "bioactive compounds" that have the ability to interact with one or more compounds in living tissue, resulting in an effect on human health. (31) Exploring dietary phytochemical intake from foods may complement current dietary strategies for the management of osteoarthritis. (32)

Cyanidin is the major component of anthocyanins commonly found in plant foods. Increasing evidence has shown that cyanidin exhibits anti-inflammatory effects in a variety of diseases. Cyanidin is a rare Sirtuin 6 (SIRT6 or Sirt6) activator. SIRT6 is a stress responsive protein deacetylase and mono-ADP ribosyltransferase enzyme encoded by the SIRT6 gene. (33) SIRT6 functions in multiple molecular pathways related to aging, including DNA repair, telomere maintenance, glycolysis and inflammation. (33) Cyanidin could inhibit the NF-κB pathway in IL-1β-stimulated human osteoarthritic chondrocytes and its effect may to some extent depend on SIRT6 activation, suggesting that cyanidin may exert a protective effect through regulating the Sirt6/NF-κB signaling axis. Moreover, an in vivo study also showed that cyanidin ameliorated the development of osteoarthritis in surgical destabilization of the medial meniscus in mouse osteoarthritic models. (34)

Sulforaphane (SFN), a phytonutrient found in broccoli, has been reported to regulate signaling pathways relevant to chronic diseases. SFN inhibits the expression of key metalloproteinases implicated in osteoarthritis, independently of Nrf2, and blocks inflammation at the level of NF-κB to protect against cartilage destruction in vitro and in vivo. (35)

Pyrroloquinoline quinone (PQQ) is a compound found ubiquitously in plants, many simple and single cell eukaryotes (e.g., yeast), and certain bacteria. (36) Certain foods such as green peppers, cabbage, spinach, papaya and kiwi fruit have higher levels of PQQ. (37) Accumulating evidence suggests that oxidative stress plays an important role in the progression of osteoarthritis, and PQQ is considered a strong antioxidant. (38) Supplementation largely prevented these alterations in mice. Articular surfaces were maintained, while the thickness of articular cartilage and the abundance of cartilage matrix protein were also positively affected. (38)

Supplementation with **vitamin D** over four years was associated with significantly less progression of knee joint abnormalities. Given the observational nature of this study, future longitudinal randomized controlled trials of vitamin D supplementation are warranted. (39)

Dietary polyphenols have been studied for their anti-inflammatory properties and potential anabolic effects on the cartilage cells. Blueberries are widely consumed and are high in dietary polyphenols, therefore regular consumption of blueberries may help improve osteoarthritis. (40) The findings of one study shows that daily incorporation of whole blueberries may reduce pain, stiffness, and difficulty to perform daily activities, while improving gait performance, and would therefore improve quality of life in individuals with symptomatic knee osteoarthritis. (40)

A study showed that strawberries may have significant analgesic and anti-inflammatory effects in obese adults with established knee osteoarthritis. (41) Another study showed that strawberries lowered TNF-α, and lipid peroxidation products in obese adults with knee osteoarthritis. (42)

How to cite this article: Rose S, Strombom A. Osteoarthritis prevention and treatment with a plant-based diet. Ortho & Rheum Open Access J 2019; 15(3): 555914.
DOI: 10.19080/OROAJ.2019.15.555914

4. Discussion

Osteoarthritis is a chronic disease. While several medications have shown efficacy in reducing the symptoms, their daily use in the long term can be problematic. However, a plant-based diet can help treat the symptoms without long term problems, and with long term benefits for osteoarthritic symptoms and common comorbidities such coronary artery disease. There are no contraindications or adverse reactions to the treatment of osteoarthritis with a plant-based diet.

A vegetarian diet lowers the risk of osteoarthritis. "As well as treating those who already have the condition, you need to be able to tell healthy people how to protect their joints into the future," study author Dr. Ian Clark, at the University of East Anglia in Norwich, U.K, said in a statement. "There is currently no way to prevent the disease pharmaceutically and you cannot give healthy people drugs unnecessarily, so this is where diet could be a safe alternative."

For those already with osteoarthritis a whole food plant-based diet reduces the symptoms of osteoarthritis. Even diets that were mostly plant-based showed some effect on symptoms. While there are still a large number to investigate, several phytonutrients and plant foods have already shown efficacy in reducing the symptoms of osteoarthritis. Understanding the effect of dietary phytochemical intake from foods on osteoarthritis and its long-term outcomes may inform public health strategies for osteoarthritis prevention and management, reducing healthcare costs globally.

References:

1. Biver E, Berenbaum F, Valdes A, Araujo de Carvalho I, Bindels L, et al. (2019) Gut microbiota and osteoarthritis management: An expert consensus of the European society for clinical and economic aspects of osteoporosis, osteoarthritis and musculoskeletal diseases (ESCEO). *Ageing Res Rev*. 55: 100946.
2. Musumeci G, Aiello F, Szychlinska M, DiRosa M, Castrogiovanni P, et al. (2015) Osteoarthritis in the XXIst century: risk factors and behaviours that influence disease onset and progression. *Int J Mol Sci*. 16(3): 6093-6112.
3. Hailu A, Knutsen , Fraser G.(2006) Associations between meat consumption and the prevalence of degenerative arthritis and soft tissue disorders in the adventist health study, California U.S.A. *J Nutr Health Aging*. 10(1):7-14.
4. Anandacoomarasamy A, Caterson I, Sambrook P, Fransen M, March L. (2008) The impact of obesity on the musculoskeletal system. *Int J Obes (Lond)*. 32(2):211–222.
5. Spector T, Hart D, Doyle D. (1994) Incidence and progression of osteoarthritis in women with unilateral knee disease in the general population: the effect of obesity. *Ann Rheum Dis*. 53(9):565-568.
6. Szoeke C, Dennerstein L, Guthrie J, Clark M, Cicuttini F. (2006) The relationship between prospectively assessed body weight and physical activity and prevalence of radiological knee osteoarthritis in postmenopausal women. *J Rheumatol*. 33(9):1835-1840.
7. Coggon D, Reading I, Croft P, McLaren M, Barrett D, et al. (2001) Knee osteoarthritis and obesity. *Int J Obes Relat Metab Disord*. 25(5):622-627.
8. Blagojevic M, Jinks C, Jeffery A, Jordan K. (2010) Risk factors for onset of osteoarthritis of the knee in older adults: a systematic review and meta-analysis. *Osteoarthritis Cartilage*. 18(1):24-33.
9. Tonstad S, Butler T, Yan R, Fraser G. (2009) Type of Vegetarian Diet, Body Weight, and Prevalence of Type 2 Diabetes. *Diabetes Care*. 32(5):791–796.

How to cite this article: Rose S, Strombom A. Osteoarthritis prevention and treatment with a plant-based diet. Ortho & Rheum Open Access J 2019; 15(3): 555914.
DOI: 10.19080/OROAJ.2019.15.555914

10. Bradbury K, Crowe F, Appleby P, Schmidt J, RC T, et al. (2014) Serum concentrations of cholesterol, apolipoprotein A-I, and apolipoprotein B in a total of 1 694 meat-eaters, fish-eaters, vegetarians, and vegans. *Eur J Clin Nutr*. 68(2):178-183.
11. Waldmann A, Koschizke J, Leitzmann C, Hahn A. (2005) German vegan study: diet, life-style factors, and cardiovascular risk profile. *Ann Nutr Metab*. 49(6):366-72.
12. Haddad E, Tanzman J. (2003) What do vegetarians in the United States eat? *Am J Clin Nutr*. 78(3):626S-632S.
13. Newby P, Tucker K, Wolk A. (2005) Risk of overweight and obesity among semivegetarian, lactovegetarian, and vegan women. *Am J Clin Nutr*. 81(6):1267-74.
14. Schett G, Kleyer A, Perricone C, Sahinbegovic E, Iagnocco A, et al. (2013) Diabetes is an independent predictor for severe osteoarthritis: results from a longitudinal cohort study. *Diabetes Care*. 36(2):403-409.
15. Pottie P, Presle N, Terlain B, Netter P, Mainard D, et al. (2006) Obesity and osteoarthritis: more complex than predicted! *Ann Rheum Dis*. 65(11):1403-1405.
16. Puenpatom R, Victor T. (2009) Increased prevalence of metabolic syndrome in individuals with osteoarthritis: an analysis of NHANES III data. *Postgrad Med*. 121(6):9-20.
17. Cimmino M, Cutolo M. (1990) Plasma glucose concentration in symptomatic osteoarthritis: a clinical and epidemiological survey. *Clin Exp Rheumatol*. 8(3):251-257.
18. Shikhman A, Brinson D, Valbracht J, Lotz M. (2001) Cytokine regulation of facilitated glucose transport in human articular chondrocytes. *J Immunol*. 167(12):7001-7008.
19. Rosa S, Gonçalves J, Judas F, Mobasheri A, Lopes C, et al. (2009) Impaired glucose transporter-1 degradation and increased glucose transport and oxidative stress in response to high glucose in chondrocytes from osteoarthritic versus normal human cartilage. *Arthritis Res Ther*. 11(3): R80.
20. Henrotin Y, Bruckner P, Pujol J. (2003) The role of reactive oxygen species in homeostasis and degradation of cartilage. *Osteoarthritis Cartilage*. 11(10):747-755.
21. Steenvoorden M, Huizinga T, Verzijl N, Bank R, Ronday H, et al. (2006) Activation of receptor for advanced glycation end products in osteoarthritis leads to increased stimulation of chondrocytes and synoviocytes. *Arthritis Rheum*. 54(1):253-263.
22. Loeser R, Yammani R, Carlson C, Chen H, Cole A, et al. (2005) Articular chondrocytes express the receptor for advanced glycation end products: Potential role in osteoarthritis. *Arthritis Rheum*. 52(8):2376-2385.
23. Verzijl N, DeGroot J, Zaken CB, Brau-Benjamin O, Maroudas A, et al. (2002) Crosslinking by advanced glycation end products increases the stiffness of the collagen network in human articular cartilage: A possible mechanism through which age is a risk factor for osteoarthritis. *Arthritis Rheum*. 46(1):114-123.
24. Rizzo N, Sabaté J, Jaceldo-Siegl K, Fraser G. (2011) Vegetarian dietary patterns are associated with a lower risk of metabolic syndrome: the adventist health study 2. *Diabetes Care*. 34(5):1225-7.
25. Snowdon D, Phillips R. (1985) Does a vegetarian diet reduce the occurrence of diabetes? *Am J Public Health*. 75(5):507-12.
26. Fraser G. (2009) Vegetarian diets:what do we know of their effects on common chronic diseases? *Am J Clin Nutr*. 5:1607S-1612S.
27. Comee L, Taylor C, Nahikian-Nelms M, Ganesan L, Krok-Schoen J. (2019) Dietary patterns and nutrient intake of individuals with rheumatoid arthritis and osteoarthritis in the United States. *Nutrition*. 67-68: 110533.
28. Clinton C, O'Brien S, Law J, Renier C, Wendt M. (2015) Whole-Foods Plant-Based Diet Alleviates the Symptoms of Osteoarthritis. *Arthritis*.2015: 708152.

How to cite this article: Rose S, Strombom A. Osteoarthritis prevention and treatment with a plant-based diet. Ortho & Rheum Open Access J 2019; 15(3): 555914.
DOI: 10.19080/OROAJ.2019.15.555914

29. Veronese N, Stubbs B, Noale M, Solmi M, Luchini C, et al. (2016) Adherence to the Mediterranean diet is associated with better quality of life: data from the Osteoarthritis Initiative. *Am J Clin Nutr*. 104(5):1403-1409.
30. Probst Y, Guan V, Kent K. (2017) Dietary phytochemical intake from foods and health outcomes: a systematic review protocol and preliminary scoping. *BMJ Open*. 7(2):e013337.
31. Biesalski H, Dragsted L, Elmadfa I, Grossklaus R, Müller M, et al. (2009) Bioactive compounds: definition and assessment of activity. *Nutrition*. 25(11-12):1202-1205.
32. Guan V, Mobasheric A, Probst Y. (2019) A systematic review of osteoarthritis prevention and management with dietary phytochemicals from foods. *Maturitas*. 122:35-43.
33. Frye R. (2000) Phylogenetic classification of prokaryotic and eukaryotic Sir2-like proteins. *Biochem Biophys Res Commun*. 273(2):793-798.
34. Jiang C, Sun Z, Hu J, Jin Y, Guo Q, et al. (2019) Cyanidin ameliorates the progression of osteoarthritis via the Sirt6/NF-κB axis in vitro and in vivo. *Food Funct*. 10(9):5873-5885.
35. Davidson R, Jupp O, deFerrars R, Kay C, Culley K, et al. (2013) Sulforaphane Represses Matrix-Degrading proteases and protects cartilage from destruction in vitro and in vivo. *Arthritis Rheum*. 65(12):3130–3140.
36. Jonscher K, Rucker R. (2019) Pyrroloquinoline Quinone Its Profile, Effects on the Liver and Implications for Health and Disease Prevention. In: Watson R, Preedy V, eds. *Dietary Interventions in Liver Disease: Foods, Nutrients, and Dietary Supplements*: Academic Press.
37. Kumazawa T, Sato K, Seno H, Ishii A, Suzuki O. (1995) Levels of pyrroloquinoline quinone in various foods. *Biochem J*. 307(Pt 2):331-333.
38. Qin R, Sun J, Wu J, Chen L. (2019) Pyrroloquinoline quinone prevents knee osteoarthritis by inhibiting oxidative stress and chondrocyte senescence. *Am J Transl Res*. 11(3):1460-1472.
39. Joseph G, McCulloch C, Nevitt M, Neumann J, Lynch J, et al. (2019) Associations between Vitamin C and D Intake and Cartilage Composition and Knee Joint Morphology over 4 years: Data from the Osteoarthritis Initiative. *Arthritis Care Res (Hoboken)*. doi: 10.1002/acr.24021.
40. Du C, Smith A, Avalos M, South S, Crabtree K, et al. (2019) Blueberries Improve Pain, Gait Performance, and Inflammation in Individuals with Symptomatic Knee Osteoarthritis. *Nutrients*. 11(2): E290.
41. Schell J, Scofield R, Barrett J, Kurien B, Betts N, et al. (2017) Strawberries Improve Pain and Inflammation in Obese Adults with Radiographic Evidence of Knee Osteoarthritis. *Nutrients*. 9(9): E949
42. Basu A, Kurien B, Tran H, Byrd B, Maher J, et al. (2018) Strawberries decrease circulating levels of tumor necrosis factor and lipid peroxides in obese adults with knee osteoarthritis. *Food Funct*. 9(12):6218-6226.

How to cite this article: Rose S, Strombom A. Osteoarthritis prevention and treatment with a plant-based diet. Ortho & Rheum Open Access J 2019; 15(3): 555914.
DOI: 10.19080/OROAJ.2019.15.555914

Orthopedics and Rheumatology
Open Access Journal
ISSN: 2471-6804

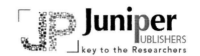

Juniper Publishers
key to the Researchers

Mini Review
Volume 15 Issue 2 - November 2019
DOI: 10.19080/OROAJ.2019.15.555910

Orth & Rheum Open Access J

Treating Fibromyalgia with a Plant-Based Diet

Stewart Rose* **and Amanda Strombom**

Plant-Based Diets in Medicine, USA

Submission: November 22, 2019; **Published:** November 27, 2019

Corresponding author: Amanda Strombom, Plant-Based Diets in Medicine,
12819 SE 38th St, #427, Bellevue, WA 98006, USA

Abstract

Fibromyalgia is a difficult disease to treat. Many patients do not have a good quality of life and cannot maintain normal daily activity with currently prescribed treatments, so new treatments are called for.

Three interventional studies have shown significant improvements by treating patients with a vegetarian diet. Patients experience an increase in well-being, a reduction in pain, and a reduction in cardiovascular risk factors such as obesity and total serum cholesterol.

Plant-based diets have demonstrated efficacy for treating fibromyalgia while lowering cardiovascular risk factors and reducing exacerbating factors such high BMI and common comorbidities. Often the efficacy is as good and, in some cases, better than standard treatment. The plant-based diet has the advantage of having no side effects and no contraindications. This allows it to be easily integrated with other treatments.

Keywords:

Cardiovascular disease; Fibromyalgia; Muscle pain; Neuropathic pain; Oxidative stress; Plant-based diet; Vegetarian diet

1. Introduction

As the physician will already know, fibromyalgia is a disease which is often very difficult to treat. Fully efficacious treatments for fibromyalgia remain elusive which can be frustrating for both the patient and the clinician. (1) These patients do not have a good quality of life and cannot maintain normal daily activity with currently prescribed treatments. Hence, many fibromyalgia patients inquire about dietary interventions. (2)

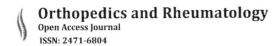

Among the different hypotheses for its etiologic pathophysiology, oxidative stress has been

suggested as one of the possibilities. (2) In fact, recent studies have shown some evidences demonstrating that oxidative stress is associated with clinical symptoms in fibromyalgia patients. (3, 4) High oxidative stress is associated with neuropathic and muscle pain in fibromyalgia patients. (5) It therefore makes sense for vegetarian diets to have some beneficial effects, probably due to the increase in antioxidant intake. (2, 3)

2. Interventional Studies

Three interventional studies have shown significant improvements from treating patients with a vegetarian diet:

An interventional study on the effect of a vegetarian diet on fibromyalgia patients showed a significant decrease in serum peroxides indicating an improved antioxidant status. The results also showed that a vegetarian diet had a significantly beneficial effect on plasma fibrinogen concentration, and on the serum levels of several lipoprotein-related coronary risk factors. Most importantly, 70% of patients reported increased well-being and reduced pain. (6) Also important was the improvement in cardiovascular risk factors, considering that a recent study showed that fibromyalgia patients have double the risk of coronary artery disease. (7)

A 7-month long interventional study of treating fibromyalgia with a vegetarian diet yielded significant results. The mean fibromyalgia impact questionnaire (FIQ) score decreased 46%. Significant improvements were seen in shoulder pain at rest and after motion, abduction range of motion of shoulder, flexibility, chair test, and 6-minute walk. At 7 months, responders' Quality of Life scores for all scales except bodily pain were no longer statistically different from the norms for adults aged 45-54. (8)

A 3-month interventional study with a plant-based diet resulted in significant improvements in visual analogue scale of pain, joint stiffness, quality of sleep, Health assessment questionnaire, General health questionnaire, and a rheumatologist's own questionnaire. Overweight patients experienced a significant reduction in body mass index and in total serum cholesterol. (9)

3. Discussion

The plant-based diet has the advantage of having no side effects and no contraindications. This allows it to be easily integrated with other treatments. It also safe in the long term, which is very important since fibromyalgia is considered incurable. At least one of its mechanisms of action appears to be its antioxidant action, but there are likely to be others as well that should be researched.

Lifestyle treatments such as increased exercise and sleep hygiene are already recommended to most patients, along with cognitive behavioral therapy. The therapeutic use of a plant-based diet fits right in with these recommendations. Patients should be advised that it will take a couple of months until the full effects of the diet are made evident.

References

1. Okifuji A, Gao J, Bokat C, Hare B. (2016) Management of fibromyalgia syndrome in 2016. *Pain Management*. 6(4):383-400.
2. Arranz L, Canela M, Rafecas M. (2010) Fibromyalgia and nutrition, what do we know? *Rhematology International*. 30(11):1417-27.
3. Russell I, Jon X, Yangming H, et al. (2009) Serum Hydrogen Peroxide Levels Are Elevated

How to cite this article: Rose S, Strombom A. Treating fibromyalgia with a plant-based diet. Ortho & Rheum Open Access J 2019; 15(2): 555910.
DOI: 10.19080/OROAJ.2019.15.555910

in Fibromyalgia Syndrome. *Arthritis and Rheumatism*. 60 Suppl 10:92.

4. Cordero M, Cano-García F, Alcocer-Gómez E, et al. (2012) Oxidative stress correlates with headache symptoms in fibromyalgia: coenzyme Q_{10} effect on clinical improvement. *PLoS One*. 7(4):e35677.
5. Cordero M, de Miguel M, Sánchez Alcázar J. (2012) The Role of Oxidative Stress and Mitochondrial Dysfunction in the Pathogenesis of Fibromyalgia. In: Wilke WS, ed. *New Insights into Fibromyalgia*. Vol Chapter 5: InTech.
6. Høstmark A, Lystad E, Vellar O, et al. (1993) Reduced plasma fibrinogen, serum peroxides, lipids, and apolipoproteins after a 3-week vegetarian diet. *Plant Foods for Human Nutrition*. 43(1):55-61.
7. Tsai P, Fan Y, Huang C. (2015) Fibromyalgia is associated with coronary heart disease: a population-based cohort study. *Regional Anesthesia and Pain Medicine*. 40(1):37-42.
8. Donaldson M, Speight N, Loomis S. (2001) Fibromyalgia syndrome improved using a mostly raw vegetarian diet: an observational study. *BMC Complementary Alternative Medicine*. 1:7.
9. Kaartinen K, Lammi K, Hypen M. (2000) Vegan diet alleviates fibromyalgia symptoms. *Scandinavian Journal of Rheumatology*. 29(5):308-13.

How to cite this article: Rose S, Strombom A. Treating fibromyalgia with a plant-based diet. Ortho & Rheum Open Access J 2019; 15(2): 555910.
DOI: 10.19080/OROAJ.2019.15.555910

Journal of
Gynecology and Women's Health
ISSN 2474-7602

Juniper Publishers
key to the Researchers

Review Article
Volume 18 Issue 2 - February 2020
DOI: 10.19080/JGWH.2020.18.555985

J Gynecol Women's Health

Managing the Nutritional Requirements of Vegetarian and Vegan Mothers during Pregnancy

Amanda Strombom* and Stewart Rose

Plant-Based Diets in Medicine, USA

Submission: January 31, 2020; **Published:** February 06, 2020

***Corresponding author:** Amanda Strombom, Plant-Based Diets in Medicine,
12819 SE 38th St, #427, Bellevue, WA 98006, USA

Abstract

Vegan pregnant women have a lower-than-average rate of cesarean delivery, less postpartum depression, and lower neonatal and maternal mortality. Well-planned plant-based diets have been confirmed as safe during pregnancy and lactation, as well as conferring additional health advantages. However, vegan diets that are highly restricted in calories and nutrients may give birth to infants whose weights are significantly lower than expected, so it's important for physicians to know how to manage such pregnancies.

Vegetarians and vegans have significantly lower BMIs, on average, and a lower risk of hypothyroidism, which are the most significant risk factors for Gestational Diabetes Mellitus. They also have a lower risk of pre-eclampsia and gallstone disease. Comorbidities such as chronic kidney disease and hypercholesterolemia can be effectively treated with a plant-based diet. Fear that the risk of the birth defect hypospadias was increased by following a vegetarian diet have proved unwarranted.

Protein intake of vegan women should be increased by 10% while pregnant, and they should be encouraged to consume a wide variety of plant-based foods. Adequate sources of Omega 3 fats, calcium, iodine, vitamins B12 and D must be ensured, and a multi-micronutrient supplement tablet containing the recommended daily allowance (RDA) of several vitamins and minerals is recommended.

A plant-based diet offers significant advantages in reducing complications of pregnancy as well as treating comorbidities such as Type II diabetes. While attention to vitamin B12 and other nutrients, when indicated, is important, a vegan pregnancy is not very different from the more common pregnancies.

Keywords:
Birth defects; Birthweight; Gestational diabetes; Lactation; Plant-based; Pre-eclampsia; Pregnancy; Pregnant; Vegan; Vegetarian

1. Introduction

Although often framed in terms of lacking, vegan diets are actually rich in a wide variety of foods: grains, legumes (including soy and its derivatives), vegetables, fruits, nuts and seeds, vegetable fats, and herbs and spices (1, 2). The American Academy of Nutrition and Dietetics position statement on plant-based diets confirms their safety during pregnancy and lactation and that they may confer additional health advantages. (1) Vegan pregnant women have a lower-than-average rate of cesarean delivery, less postpartum depression, and lower neonatal and maternal mortality, with no complications or negative outcomes that are higher than average. (3, 4, 5)

Both maternal malnutrition and overnutrition are associated with subsequent diabetes in the offspring. Pregnancy represents a window of opportunity for health care providers to change dietary patterns toward habits that will be healthier for the individual now, as well as impacting the mother and child in the future. (6)

A growing number of people are choosing to be vegetarians and vegans in the United States. According to a survey conducted by Vegetarian Times there are about 7.3 million vegetarians in United States. Of those about 1 million are vegan. (7) These numbers are likely to rise especially with the increased availability of meat substitutes. It's important for the physician to know how to manage their pregnancies.

2. Birthweight concerns for vegetarian mothers

Several studies have looked at the birthweight of infants born to vegetarian mothers. Five studies showed a lower birthweight in the children of vegetarian mothers. (8, 9, 10, 11, 12) However the result was significant in only one study. (8) Conversely, birthweight and length were higher in children of vegetarian mothers in two studies. (13, 14)

Results of all these studies are affected by country, ethnicity, socioeconomic status, and other health related behaviors such as smoking and access to prenatal care. (15, 16) This is a crucial issue also reflected in the different social patterns in rich, western countries, in which vegan–vegetarian diets are often chosen in the quest for a healthier lifestyle, compared with low income countries, in which the nutritional deficits may be linked to forced limitations in the availability of food. (17)

One study found that significantly higher birthweight (mean 99g) above that of non-vegetarians, and involved a community of Seventh-Day Adventists. (14) This is notable because, as a group, Seventh-day Adventists follow a healthy lifestyle. The difference in this study was therefore most likely related to diet.

Another study showed that the birthweight of children of vegan mothers is lower than that of the omnivorous mothers' children, but the values of this anthropometric parameter were all within the accepted range. No significant difference has emerged from the comparison for the length,

How to cite this article: Rose S, Strombom A. Managing the nutritional requirements of vegetarian and vegan mothers during pregnancy. J Gynecol Women's Health. 2020: 18(2): 555985.
DOI: 10.19080/JGWH.2020.18.555985

cranial circumference and BMI at birth between the vegan group and the omnivorous group. (18)

Vegan diets that are highly restricted in calories and nutrients, in contrast to well-planned vegan diets, give birth to infants whose weights are significantly lower than expected. (12) Concerns about vegan diets during pregnancy, breastfeeding, infancy, and childhood arose in the past (17, 19, 20), but this was due to the fact that although being categorized as "vegan", the investigated subjects were following highly restrictive diets, not respecting all the criteria required to define the diet as being well-planned.

3. Risk of Gestational Diabetes

Observational studies show consistent evidence that increased BMI and hypothyroidism are the strongest risk factors for Gestational Diabetes Mellitus (GDM). (21) Vegetarians and vegans have significantly lower BMIs on average. A study of American vegetarians and vegans found that that vegetarians had a mean BMI of 25.7 and vegans a mean BMI of 23.6. (22) A European study found the average BMI of vegetarians and vegans to be 23.3 and 22.4 respectively for men and 22.8 and 21.8 for women. (23) A study of German vegans found an average BMI of 22.3. (24)

While vegan diets are associated with lower body weight, which may protect against hypothyroidism, a lower risk of hypothyroidism among vegans exists even after controlling for BMI and potential demographic confounders. One study showed that following a vegan diet tended to be associated with a 22% reduced risk of hypothyroidism, although statistical significance was not quite attained. (25)

A high intake of fiber during pregnancy also seems to be particularly beneficial in preventing GDM. Indeed, maternal diets characterized by low intakes of fiber and a high glycemic load seem to be associated with an increased risk of GDM, In particular, an increment of 10 g/day in total fiber intake was found to be associated with a 26% risk reduction in GDM and an increment of 5 g/day in cereal or fruit fiber intake was associated with a 23% or 26% reduction in GDM, respectively. (26) The vegetarian diet was also associated with a lower incidence of excessive gestational weight gain. (27)

Higher intake of animal protein, in particular red meat, was significantly associated with a greater risk of GDM. Several major food sources of animal protein, such as red meat, were positively associated with the risk of GDM. (28) In particular, a meat-centered diet was associated with significantly higher GDM risk in parous and obese women (29)

By contrast, higher intake of vegetable protein, specifically nuts, was associated with a significantly lower risk. Substitution of vegetable protein for animal protein was associated with a lower risk of GDM. (30)

4. Risk of Gallstones

The incidence rates of biliary sludge (a precursor to gallstones) and gallstones are up to 30% and 12%, respectively, during pregnancy and postpartum, and gallbladder disease is the most common non obstetrical cause of maternal hospitalization in the first year postpartum. (31, 32). Prevention of gallstone disease is especially important during pregnancy, as cholecystectomy is problematic and medication can carry risks.

In pregnancy, the incidence of cholesterol gallstones is increased by strong risk factors including obesity, serum leptin and extreme hypercholesterolemia. A plant-based diet has been shown to lower the risk of obesity, reduce leptin and eliminate cholesterol from the diet, thus reducing serum cholesterol and therefore gallstone risk during pregnancy without the risk that drug treatment may entail. (33)

5. Risk of Pre-eclampsia

Vegans may have a lower risk of preeclampsia. The risk of preeclampsia in the general population is about 3%. However, in a study of 775 vegan pregnancies, only one case of preeclampsia was noted, (4) giving a rate of only about .01%. Other less specific studies have shown decreased risk with higher consumptions of fruits and vegetables. In a Norwegian study, women with high scores on a dietary pattern characterized by vegetables, plant foods, and vegetable oils, were at 28% decreased risk of preeclampsia for the highest tertile vs. the lowest tertile. (34)

This could be related to the theory that the risk of preeclampsia is directly associated with a high consumption of fat and sugar and a low intake of fiber, since plant-based dietary patterns generally provide low amounts of fat and sugar and higher quantities of fiber (35). One study showed that the highest quartile of soluble fiber intake reduced the risk of preeclampsia by 70% and insoluble fiber by 65% compared to the lowest quartile. (36)

6. Risk of Birth Defects

Early concerns were expressed about the birth defect hypospadias (a congenital malformation in which the opening of the penile urethra occurs on the ventral side of the penis) in association with vegetarian diets. However, this has turned out to be unwarranted according to a large study. (37)

Other concerns raised over the use of soy phytoestrogens also seem to be unwarranted. According to one study, a higher intake of some phytoestrogens was associated with reduced risks of delivering infants with hypospadias, even after adjustment for several covariates. This finding applied to overall intake of phytoestrogens as well as intake of specific phytoestrogens, so phytoestrogens may actually be protective of hypospadias. (38)

Pregnant women following a well-planned plant-based diet, being naturally higher in folate, may have a reduced risk of an infant being born with spina bifida or aencephaly. (39) In contrast, a western diet (including high intake of meat) was shown to increase by around 2-fold the risk of offspring with orofacial cleft palate. (40)

7. Pregnant with Chronic Kidney Disease

Using the most recent classification system, 3% of women of childbearing age are affected by Chronic Kidney Disease (CKD). (41, 42) For these women, the risk of an adverse pregnancy rises very significantly, even in stage 1. (43) Despite vast improvements in fetal outcomes, pregnancy in women with CKD is fraught with hazards; worsening renal function and complications such as pre-eclampsia and premature delivery are common. (44)

During the pregnancy of a patient with CKD, the amount of protein in the diet must be balanced between the goal of diminishing hyperfiltration and increasing metabolic needs of pregnancy. (45) Due to the fact that pregnancy induces hyperfiltration, diets with restricted amount of protein should

How to cite this article: Rose S, Strombom A. Managing the nutritional requirements of vegetarian and vegan mothers during pregnancy. J Gynecol Women's Health. 2020: 18(2): 555985.
DOI: 10.19080/JGWH.2020.18.555985

be beneficial in this group of patients. (46, 47) Vegan or vegetarian supplemented low-protein diets in pregnant women with stages 3–5 CKD reduce the risk of small-for-gestational-age babies, without detrimental effects on kidney function or proteinuria in the mother. (48)

CKD during pregnancy presents a clinical challenge, especially considering the paucity of therapeutic tools available in pregnant women. One study investigated the feasibility of supplemented vegetarian low-protein diets in pregnancy, as a "rescue treatment" for severe CKD and or proteinuria. (46) None of the 11 patients needed renal replacement therapy within the 6 months before delivery. No patient complained of side effects, nor developed hyperkalemia or hypercalcaemia. All babies were well at 1 month post delivery, and 7.5 years later. (46) A supplemented vegetarian low-protein diet (0.6–0.7 g/kg per day) turned out to be sufficient for the maintenance of satisfactory nutritional status during the pregnancy and after delivery, even in breast-feeding women. (49)

For pregnant women with focal segmental glomerulosclerosis, a study showed that a moderately protein restricted, keto analogue supplemented, plant-based diet helped control proteinuria. (50)

Another study reviewed the results obtained over 15 years of treating pregnant women with CKD on moderately restricted plant-based low-protein diets. It confirms that such a diet is a safe option in the management of pregnant CKD patients. (51) A trend towards better preserved fetal growth was observed.

These results indicate that the treatment of pregnant CKD women on moderately restricted plant-based low-protein diet is a safe option in the management of pregnant CKD.

8. Clinical considerations during pregnancy and lactation on a vegan diet

Appropriately planned vegetarian, including vegan, diets are healthful, nutritionally adequate, and may provide health benefits for the prevention and treatment of certain diseases. These diets are appropriate for all stages of the life cycle, including during pregnancy and lactation. (1)

Protein intakes should be increased by 10% in vegan pregnant and lactating women, compared with non-pregnant adult vegetarians. (2, 52, 53) Additional servings of grains, protein-rich plant foods (legumes, soy milk, soy yogurt, tofu, tempeh, and meat analogs based on wheat or soy protein) and nuts and seeds should be consumed by vegan women during the second and third trimester of pregnancy and during breastfeeding to meet these increased protein requirements. (53)

The patient should be advised to consume large amounts and a wide variety of plant foods, emphasizing the intake of whole or minimally processed foods: a vegan diet can be nutritionally adequate when meeting the calorie requirements from a variety of nutrient-dense foods, mainly unprocessed, belonging to all the plant food groups.

It is recommended that the amount of vegetable fats be limited, as suggested by the Dietary Reference Intakes (DRIs), in order to limit excess calories and not displace more nutrient-dense foods. However, DHA plays an important role in pregnancy and lactation. Infants of vegetarian mothers appear to have lower cord and plasma DHA than do infants of nonvegetarians although the functional significance of this is not known. (9, 13) Vegetable fats should therefore be chosen carefully, in order to consume good sources of omega-3 fatty acids such as walnuts, ground chia seeds and flax seeds (which can be converted to DHA) and monounsaturated oils, while avoiding trans fats and tropical oils (coconut, palm, and palm kernel oils), to emphasize the efficiency of the omega-3 metabolic pathway. DHA supplements made from microalgae are available and can be a supplement for patients when indicated. Note that during infancy and early childhood, fats should not be limited but should still be carefully chosen. (2, 53, 54)

Adequate amounts of calcium should be consumed, and vitamin D status should be checked. Additional calcium can be obtained by increasing the intakes of calcium-rich foods from plant sources. Conversely, since a plant-based diet cannot provide adequate amounts of vitamin D, the recommendations for vitamin D are the same as for the general population. (2, 53, 54)

Adequate amounts of vitamin B12 are essential, as deficiency increases the risk of neural tube defects in the infant. (55) The intake of a reliable source of vitamin B12 is fundamental to a well-planned vegetarian diet, as vitamin B12 status can be compromised, over time, in all vegetarian subjects who do not supplement it. (2, 53, 54) Since B12 deficiency can occur during pregnancy regardless of the type of diet, because of store depletion due to higher demands (56), the use of a specific vitamin B12 supplement represents the most reliable way or ensuring an adequate B12 status during vegan pregnancy. (57)

Increased caloric and nutrient intakes are recommended to meet the demands of the rapidly growing fetus and the increased physiological requirements of the mother, especially for folate, iron, iodine, and copper. (58, 59) Although nutrient intakes should preferably come from a variety of food sources, it is possible that pregnant women and those of childbearing age won't meet their needs for some nutrients through diet alone. (60, 61) As such, prenatal dietary supplements are generally recommended during pregnancy (62, 63) and were used by about 75% of pregnant women in a nationally representative US sample. (60)

However, prenatal dietary supplements provide variable nutrient content and the number of nutrients included in dietary supplement formulations is not standard. (62) Concerns exist of excessive intakes of some nutrients during pregnancy, especially folic acid and vitamin A, (64, 65) while low intake of iron and iodine in reproductive-aged US women has also been of concern. (66) Thus, ensuring that pregnant and reproductive-aged women have adequate, but not excessive, dietary intakes is crucial during this critical life stage. (67)

A multimicronutrient supplement tablet containing the recommended daily allowance (RDA) for pregnancy of several vitamins and minerals: vitamin A, vitamin B1, vitamin B2, niacin, vitamin B6, vitamin B12, folic acid, vitamin C, vitamin D, vitamin E, iron, copper, selenium, and zinc, should be prescribed. (68)

The patient should be questioned about their sources of iodine, such as iodized salt and seaweed. If these are lacking in their diet then a prenatal supplement containing iodine is important.

One advantage of a plant-based diet is that it can prevent and treat comorbidities. When comorbidities are present, it is important to titrate any medications when initiating a plant-based diet as the effects of the plant-based diet becomes evident.

How to cite this article: Rose S, Strombom A. Managing the nutritional requirements of vegetarian and vegan mothers during pregnancy. J Gynecol Women's Health. 2020: 18(2): 555985.
DOI: 10.19080/JGWH.2020.18.555985

9. Ensuring good quality breast milk

The breast milk of vegetarian women is similar in composition to that of nonvegetarians and is nutritionally adequate. Commercial infant formulas should be used if infants are not breastfed or are weaned before 1 year of age. Soy formula is the only option for non-breastfed vegan infants. Other preparations including regular soymilk, rice milk, and homemade formulas should not be used to replace breast milk or commercial infant formula. (69)

The period of lactation is extremely important for growing patterns of infants and the effectiveness of breastfeeding depends on maternal nutritional status. A lack of macro- and micronutrient intake during lactation may lead to the reduction of micronutrients and energy content in breast milk that could potentially lead to severe illness in the breastfed infant. (70)

Breast milk of vegan women following well-planned vegan diets including a reliable source of vitamin B12 provides adequate nutrition for their breastfed infants. (53) According to one study, 20% of study participants were classified as having low breast-milk vitamin B-12 concentrations (<310 pmol/L), independent of maternal diet pattern. (57) In this study, 85% of participants categorized as having low vitamin B-12 were taking vitamin B-12 supplements at doses in excess of the RDA, which suggests that more research is needed to determine breast-milk adequacy values. (57) Milk from breastfeeding vegan mothers provides adequate vitamin B12 in infants only if vegan mothers are supplementing with B12 sufficiently larger than the recommended amounts. (57) Given the safety of vitamin B12 supplements, (71) large amounts should ensure sufficiency.

Although containing 100% of the RDA for vitamin B12, common pre- and postnatal multivitamins have been negatively associated with low B12 concentration in breastmilk of vegan women, because only a fraction of the B12 they provide is absorbed. (2, 56) Pregnant and lactating vegan mothers should be encouraged to take an individual B12, not multivitamin, supplement and to dissolve it under the tongue or chew it slowly in order to increase absorption. (2, 57)

Breast milk DHA is lower in vegans and lacto-ovo-vegetarians than in nonvegetarians (72, 73) Because of DHA's beneficial effects on gestational length, infant visual function, and neurodevelopment, pregnant and lactating vegetarians and vegans should choose the DHA precursor linolenic acid in their diet (ground flaxseed, ground chia seeds, walnuts, canola oil, soybean oil), food sources of DHA (foods fortified with DHA-rich microalgae) or use a microalgae-derived DHA supplement (74, 75). Supplementation with ALA, a DHA precursor, in pregnancy and lactation may not be sufficient to increase infant DHA levels or breast milk DHA concentration. (76, 77)

10. Discussion

A plant-based diet offers significant advantages in reducing complications of pregnancy. It also provides a safe and effective treatment for comorbidities that are happening earlier in life such as Type II diabetes, extreme hypercholesterolemia, and auto-immune diseases such as hypo and hyperthyroidism, plus it helps prevent gallstones to which pregnant women are more susceptible. The American Academy of Nutrition and Dietetics position statement on plant-based diets confirms their safety during pregnancy and lactation, and that they may confer additional health advantages.

How to cite this article: Rose S, Strombom A. Managing the nutritional requirements of vegetarian and vegan mothers during pregnancy. J Gynecol Women's Health. 2020: 18(2): 555985.
DOI: 10.19080/JGWH.2020.18.555985

Supplementation with vitamin B12 is essential, since deficiency increases the risk of neural tube defects. Some vegan women resist vitamin B12 supplementation out of philosophical objections. They seem to want to show that a plant-based diet is sufficient by itself, and they misunderstand that since vitamin B12 is synthesized by soil bacteria, it is our modern hygiene practices (scrupulously washing our vegetables) that results in less Vitamin B12 being absorbed by those not consuming animal products. It is likely that if more women following a plant-based diet, as a group, ensured adequate vitamin B12 and iodine intake, their health advantages in pregnancy would be even greater than they already are.

However, while attention to vitamin B12 and other nutrients is important, a vegan pregnancy is not very different from the more common pregnancies, while conferring considerable benefits.

References

1. Melina V, Craig W, Levin S. (2016) Position of the Academy of Nutrition and Dietetics: Vegetarian Diets. *J Acad Nutr Diet*. 116(12):1970-1980.
2. Agnoli C, Baroni L, Bertini I, Ciappellano S, Fabbri A, et al. (2017) Position paper on vegetarian diets from the working group of the Italian Society of Human Nutrition. *Nutr Metab Cardiovasc Dis*. 27(12):1037-1052.
3. Gaskin IM. (2002) *Spiritual Midwifery*. Summertown (TN): Book Publishing Company.
4. Carter J, Furman T, Hutcheson H. (1987) Preeclampsia and reproductive performance in a community of vegans. *South Med J*. 80(6):692-697.
5. Aronson D. (2007) Advice for Vegan Mothers-to-Be — Nine Months of Proper Nutrition. *Today's Dietitian*. 12 :38.
6. Jovanovic L. (2004) Nutrition and pregnancy: the link between dietary intake and diabetes. *Curr Diab Rep*. 4(4):266-272.
7. Vegetarian Times Editors. (2008) Vegetarianism In America. *VEGETARIAN TIMES*. Apr issue.
8. Wen X, Justicia-Linde F, Kong K, Zhang C, Chen W, et al. (2013) Associations of diet and physical activity with the three components of gestational weight gain. *Am J Epidemiol*. 11(Suppl):S1–S181.
9. Reddy S, Sanders TAB, Obeid O. (1994) The influence of maternal vegetarian diet on essential fatty acid status of the newborn. *Eur J Clin Nutr*. 48(5):358-368.
10. Ward RJ, Abraham R, McFadyen IR, Haines AD, North WR, et al. (1988) Assessment of trace metal intake and status in a Gujerati pregnant Asian population and their influence on the outcome of pregnancy. *Br J Obstet Gynaecol*. 95(7):676-682.
11. Campbell-Brown M, Ward RJ, Haines AP, North WR, McFadyen IR, et al. (1985) Zinc and copper in Asian pregnancies–is there evidence for a nutritional deficiency? *Br J Obstet Gynaecol*. 92(9):875-885.
12. Thomas J, Ellis F. (1977) The health of vegans during pregnancy. *Proc Nutr Soc*. 36(1):46A.
13. Lakin V, Haggarty P, Abramovich D, Ashton J, Moffat C, et al. (1998) Dietary intake and tissue concentration of fatty acids in omnivore, vegetarian and diabetic pregnancy. *Prostaglandins Leukot Essent Fatty Acids*. 59(3):209-220.
14. Fønnebø V. (1994) The healthy Seventh-Day Adventist lifestyle: what is the Norwegian experience? *Am J Clin Nutr*. 59(5 Suppl):1124S-1129S.
15. Tofail F, Persson LÅ, Arifeen SE, Hamadani JD, Mehrin F, et al. (2008) Effects of prenatal food and micronutrient supplementation on infant development: a randomized trial from the Maternal and Infant Nutrition Interventions, Matlab (MINIMat) study. *Am J Clin Nutr*. 87(3):704–711.

How to cite this article: Rose S, Strombom A. Managing the nutritional requirements of vegetarian and vegan mothers during pregnancy. J Gynecol Women's Health. 2020: 18(2): 555985.
DOI: 10.19080/JGWH.2020.18.555985

16. McDonald EC, Pollitt E, Mueller W, Hsueh AM, Sherwin R. (1981) The Bacon Chow study: maternal nutrition supplementation and birth weight of offspring. *Am J Clin Nutr*. 34(10):2133–2144.
17. Piccoli G, Clari R, Vigotti F, Leone F, Attini R, et al. (2015) Vegan-vegetarian diets in pregnancy: danger or panacea? A systematic narrative review. *BJOG*. 122(5):623-633.
18. Ferrara P, Sandullo F, Ruscio FD, Franceschini G, Peronti B, et al. (2019) The impact of lacto-ovo-/lacto-vegetarian and vegan diets during pregnancy on the birth anthropometric parameters of the newborn. *J Matern Fetal Neonatal Med*. 1-7.
19. Schürmann S, Kersting M, Alexy U. (2017) Vegetarian diets in children: a systematic review. *Eur J Nutr*. 56(5):1797-1817.
20. Richter M, Boeing H, Grünewald-Funk D, Heseker H, Kroke A, et al. (2016) Vegan diet. *Position of the German Nutrition Society (DGE) Ernahrungs Umschau*. 63:92–102.
21. Giannakou K, Evangelou E, Yiallouros P, Christophi C, Middleton N, et al. (2019) Risk factors for gestational diabetes: An umbrella review of meta-analyses of observational studies. *PLoS One*. 14(4):e0215372.
22. Tonstad S, Butler T, Yan R, Fraser G. (2009) Type of Vegetarian Diet, Body Weight, and Prevalence of Type 2 Diabetes. *Diabetes Care*. 32(5):791–796.
23. Bradbury K, Crowe F, Appleby P, Schmidt J, Travis R, et al. (2014) Serum concentrations of cholesterol, apolipoprotein A-I, and apolipoprotein B in a total of 1694 meat-eaters, fish-eaters, vegetarians, and vegans. *European Journal of Clinical Nutrition*. 68(2):178-183.
24. Waldmann A, Koschizke J, Leitzmann C, Hahn A. (2005) German vegan study: diet, life-style factors, and cardiovascular risk profile. *Annuls of Nutrition and Metabolism*. 49(6):366-72.
25. Tonstad S, Nathan E, Oda K, Fraser G. (2013) Vegan diets and hypothyroidism. *Nutrients*. 2013;5(11):4642–4652.
26. Zhang C, Liu S, Solomon CG, Hu FB. (2006) Dietary fiber intake, dietary glycemic load, and the risk for gestational diabetes mellitus. *Diabetes Care*.29:2223–2230.
27. Streuling I, Beyerlein A, Rosenfeld E, Schukat B, Kries Rv. (2011) Weight gain and dietary intake during pregnancy in industrialized countries – a systematic review of observational studies. *J Perinat Med*. 39(2):123-129.
28. Zhang C, Schulze MB, Solomon CG, Hu FB. (2006) A prospective study of dietary patterns, meat intake and the risk of gestational diabetes mellitus. *Diabetologia*. 49:2604–2613.
29. Schoenaker DAJM, Soedamah-Muthu SS, Callaway LK, Mishra GD. (2015) Pre-pregnancy dietary patterns and risk of gestational diabetes mellitus: results from an Australian population-based prospective cohort study. *Diabetologia*. 58(12):2726-2735.
30. Bao W, Bowers K, Tobias DK, Hu FB, Zhang C. (2013) Prepregnancy Dietary Protein Intake, Major Dietary Protein Sources, and the Risk of Gestational Diabetes Mellitus. *Diabetes Care*. 36(7):2001-2008.
31. Ko C. (2006) Risk factors for gallstone-related hospitalization during pregnancy and the postpartum. *Am J Gastroenterol*. 101(10):2263-2268.
32. Lydon-Rochelle M, Holt VL, Martin DP, Easterling TR. (2000) Association between method of delivery and maternal rehospitalization. *JAMA*. 283(18):2411-2416.
33. Rose S, Strombom A. (2018) A comprehensive review of the prevention and treatment of heart disease with a plant-based diet. *J Cardiol & Cardiovas Ther*. 12(5):555847.
34. Brantsæter AL, Haugen M, Samuelsen S, Torjusen H, Trogstad L, et al. (2009) A dietary pattern characterized by high intake of vegetables, fruits, and vegetable oils Is associated with reduced risk of preeclampsia in nulliparous pregnant Norwegian women. *J Nutr*. 139(6):1162–1168.

How to cite this article: Rose S, Strombom A. Managing the nutritional requirements of vegetarian and vegan mothers during pregnancy. J Gynecol Women's Health. 2020: 18(2): 555985.
DOI: 10.19080/JGWH.2020.18.555985

35. Frederick I, Williams M, Dashow E, Kestin M, Zhang C, et al (2005) Dietary fiber, potassium, magnesium and calcium in relation to the risk of preeclampsia. *J Reprod Med*. 50:332–344.
36. Qiu C, Coughlin KB, Frederick IO, Sorensen TK, Williams MA. (2008) Dietary Fiber Intake in Early Pregnancy and Risk of Subsequent Preeclampsia. *Am J Hypertens*. 21(8):903–909.
37. Carmichael S, Ma C, Feldkamp M, Munger R, Olney R, et al. (2012) Nutritional factors and hypospadias risks. *Paediatr Perinat Epidemiol*. 26(4):353-360.
38. Carmichael SL, Cogswell ME, Ma C, Gonzalez-Feliciano A, Olney R, et al. (2013) Hypospadias and Maternal Intake of Phytoestrogens. *Am J Epidemiol*. 178(3):434–440.
39. Centers for Disease Control and Prevention (CDC). (2004) Spina bifida and anencephaly before and after folic acid mandate–United States, 1995-1996 and 1999-2000. *MMWR Morb Mortal Wkly Rep*. 53(17):362-365.
40. Vujkovic M, Ocke MC, van der Spek PJ, Yazdanpanah N, Steegers EA, et al. (2007) Maternal Western dietary patterns and the risk of developing a cleft lip with or without a cleft palate. *Obstet Gynecol*. 110(2 Pt 1):378-384.
41. Piccoli GB, Attini R, Vasario E, Conijn A, Biolcati M, et al. (2010) Pregnancy and chronic kidney disease: a challenge in all CKD stages. *Clin J Am Soc Nephrol*. 5(5):844-855.
42. Cabiddu G, Castellino S, Gernone G, Santoro D, Moroni G, et al. (2016) A best practice position statement on pregnancy in chronic kidney disease: the Italian Study Group on Kidney and Pregnancy. *J Nephrol*. 29(3):277-303.
43. Piccoli GB, Fassio F, Attini R, Parisi S, Biolcati M, et al. (2012) Pregnancy in CKD: whom should we follow and why? *Nephrol Dial Transplant*. 27(Suppl 3): iii111–iii118.
44. Vellanki K. (2013) Pregnancy in chronic kidney disease. *Adv Chronic Kidney*. 20(3):223-228.
45. Gluba-Brzózka A, Franczyk B, Rysz J. (2017) Vegetarian Diet in Chronic Kidney Disease-A Friend or Foe. *Nutrients*. 9(4):pii: E374.
46. Piccoli GB, Attini R, Vasario E, Gagliotí P, Piccoli E, et al. (2011) Vegetarian supplemented low-protein diets. A safe option for pregnant CKD patients: report of 12 pregnancies in 11 patients. *Nephrol Dial Transplant*. 26(1):196-205.
47. Brenner B, Lawler E, Mackenzie H. (1996) The hyperfiltration theory: a paradigm shift in nephrology. *Kidney Int*. 49(6):1774-1777.
48. Piccoli GB, Leone F, Attini R, Parisi S, Fassio F, et al. (2014) Association of low-protein supplemented diets with fetal growth in pregnant women with CKD. *Clin J Am Soc Nephrol*. 9(5):864-873.
49. Zaldivar MC, Peixoto A. (2003) CKD series: cardiovascular risk reduction in patients with chronic kidney disease. *Hosp Physician*. 39:29-35, 50.
50. Attini R, Leone F, Montersino B, Fassio F, Minelli F, et al. (2017) Pregnancy, Proteinuria, Plant-Based Supplemented Diets and Focal Segmental Glomerulosclerosis: A Report on Three Cases and Critical Appraisal of the Literature. *Nutrients*. 9(7): pii: E770.
51. Attini R, Leone F, Parisi S, Fassio F, Capizzi I, et al. (2016) Vegan-vegetarian low-protein supplemented diets in pregnant CKD patients: fifteen years of experience. *BMC Nephrol*. 17(1):132.
52. Kniskern MA, Johnston CS. (2011) Protein dietary reference intakes may be inadequate for vegetarians if low amounts of animal protein are consumed. *Nutrition*. 27(6):727-730.
53. Baroni L, Goggi S, Battaglino R Berveglieri M, Fasan I, et al. (2019) Vegan Nutrition for Mothers and Children: Practical Tools for Healthcare Providers. *Nutrients*. 11(1):5.
54. Baroni L. (2015) Vegetarianism in Food-Based Dietary Guidelines. *Int. J. Nutr.* 2:49–74.
55. 55. Molloy A, Kirke P, Troendle J, Burke H, Sutton M, et al. (2009) Maternal vitamin B12 status and risk of neural tube defects in a population with high neural tube defect

How to cite this article: Rose S, Strombom A. Managing the nutritional requirements of vegetarian and vegan mothers during pregnancy. J Gynecol Women's Health. 2020: 18(2): 555985.
DOI: 10.19080/JGWH.2020.18.555985

prevalence and no folic acid fortification. *Pediatrics*. 123(3):917-23.

56. Balcı YI, Ergin A, Karabulut A, Polat A, Doğan M, et al. (2014) Serum vitamin B12 and folate concentrations and the effect of the Mediterranean diet on vulnerable populations. *Pediatr Hematol Oncol*. 31(1):62-67.
57. Pawlak R, Vos P, Shahab-Ferdows S, Hampel D, Allen LH, et al. (2018) Vitamin B-12 content in breast milk of vegan, vegetarian, and nonvegetarian lactating women in the United States. *Am J Clin Nutr.*108(3):525-531.
58. Institute of Medicine Food Nutrition Board. (2006) *Dietary Reference Intakes: The Essential Guide to Nutrient Requirements*. Washington, DC: The National Academies Press
59. Institute of Medicine (US) (1990) Committee on Nutritional Status During Pregnancy and Lactation. *Nutrition During Pregnancy: Part I Weight Gain: Part II Nutrient Supplements.* Washington, DC: National Academies Press
60. Branum AM, Bailey R, Singer BJ. (2013) Dietary supplement use and folate status during pregnancy in the United States. *J Nutr*. 143(4):486-492.
61. Picciano MF. (2003) Pregnancy and lactation: physiological adjustments, nutritional requirements and the role of dietary supplements. *J Nutr*. 133(6):1997S-2002S.
62. Marra MV, Bailey RL. (2018) Position of the Academy of Nutrition and Dietetics: Micronutrient Supplementation. *J Acad Nutr Diet*. 118(11):2162-2173.
63. Kominiarek MA, Rajan P. (2016) Nutrition recommendations in pregnancy and lactation. *Med Clin North Am*. 100(6):1199–1215.
64. Rader JI, Yetley EA. (2002) Nationwide folate fortification has complex ramifications and requires careful monitoring over time. *Arch Intern Med*. 162(5):608-609.
65. Yetley EA, Rader JI. (2004) Modeling the level of fortification and post-fortification assessments: U.S. experience. *Nutr Rev*. 62(6 Pt 2):S50-S59.
66. Gupta PM, Gahche JJ, Herrick KA, Ershow AG, Potischman N, et al. (2018) Use of Iodine-Containing Dietary Supplements Remains Low among Women of Reproductive Age in the United States: NHANES 2011-2014. *Nutrients*. 10(4):pii: E422.
67. Bailey RL, Pac SG, Fulgoni VL, Reidy KC, Catalano PM. (2019) Estimation of Total Usual Dietary Intakes of Pregnant Women in the United States. *JAMA Netw Open*. 2(6):e195967.
68. Pense J, Neher J, Kelsberg G. (2015) Micronutrient Supplementation During Pregnancy. *Am Fam Physician*. 92(3):222-223.
69. Craig W, Mangels A, American Dietetic Association. (2009) Position of the American Dietetic Association: vegetarian diets. *J Am Diet Assoc*. 109(7):1266-1282.
70. Sebastiani G, Barbero AH, Borrás-Novell C, Alsina Casanova M, Aldecoa-Bilbao V, et al. (2019) The Effects of Vegetarian and Vegan Diet during Pregnancy on the Health of Mothers and Offspring. *Nutrients*. 11(3):557.
71. Rose S, Strombom A. (2019) Ensuring adequate Vitamin B12 status on a plant-based diet. *Adv Res Gastroentero Hapatol*. 13(3):555862.
72. Weaver CM, Proulx WR, Heaney R. (1999) Choices for achieving adequate dietary calcium with a vegetarian diet. *Am J Clin Nutr*. 70(3 Suppl):543S-548S.
73. Sanders AB, Reddy S. (1992) The influence of a vegetarian diet on the fatty acid composition of human milk and the essential fatty acid status of the infant. *J Pediatr*. 120(4 Pt 2):S71-S77.
74. Messina V, Melina V, Mangels AR. (2003) A new food guide for North American vegetarians. *J Am Diet Assoc*. 103:771-775.
75. American Dietetic Association; Dietitians of Canada. (2003) Position of the American Dietetic Association and Dietitians of Canada: Vegetarian diets. *J Am Diet Assoc*. 103(6):748-765.
76. Slattery ML, Jacobs DR, Hilner JE, Caan B, Van Horn L, et al. (1991) Meat consumption and its

associations with other diet and health factors in young adults: the CARDIA study. *Am J Clin Nutr*. 54(5):930-935.

77. Tesar R, Notelovitz M, Shim E, Kauwell G, Brown J. (1992) Axial and peripheralbone density and nutrient intakes of postmeno-pausal vegetarian and omnivorous women. *Am J Clin Nutr*. 56(4):699–704.

How to cite this article: Rose S, Strombom A. Managing the nutritional requirements of vegetarian and vegan mothers during pregnancy. J Gynecol Women's Health. 2020: 18(2): 555985.
DOI: 10.19080/JGWH.2020.18.555985

Advanced Research in Gastroenterology & Hepatology
ISSN: 2472-6400

Juniper Publishers
key to the Researchers

Case Report
Volume 12 Issue 3 – February 2019
DOI: 10.19080/ARGH.2019.12.555837

Adv Res Gastroenterol Hepatol

Treating Crohn's Disease with a Plant-Based Diet – A Case Report

Stewart D Rose* **and Amanda J Strombom**

Plant-Based Diets in Medicine, USA

Submission: January 01, 2019; **Published:** February 13, 2019

***Corresponding author:** Stewart Rose, Plant-Based Diets in Medicine, 12819 SE 38th St, #427, Bellevue, WA 98006, USA

Abstract

Crohn's disease is notoriously difficult to treat and this patient was no exception. Patients are typically treated with a wide range of drugs, most of which have significant side effects, and surgery.

This is a case study of a 63-yr old male, who was first diagnosed with Crohn's disease in 1988. Over the past thirty years, he experienced persistent pain, chronic diarrhea and chronic fatigue. Extraintestinal manifestations included aphthous stomatitis, arthralgia especially in the knees and hips, eczema and uveitis. His comorbidities included shingles, exacerbated by immunosuppression, severe post herpetic neuralgia, and noise-induced hearing loss of both ears. The patient also has benign prostatic hypertrophy and diverticulosis.

Despite the full range of treatment, the patient remained with very significant symptoms, medication side effects and poor quality of life.

In May 2017, the patient chose to go on a plant-based diet. Within two months, significant improvements in symptoms resulted. After three months, the patient was able to discontinue all immunosuppressant drugs. After one year, the patient reports no symptoms requiring medications other than ranitidine 150mg 2x/day and loperamide 10mg/day needed for post op management of resections. Fatigue, pain, diarrhea and all extraintestinal manifestations have virtually been eliminated. The patient reports a very large improvement in quality of life.

Keywords:

Crohn's disease; Diarrhea; Fatigue; Pain; Plant-based diet; Vegetarian; Vegan

Abbreviations:

BMI: Body Mass Index; CDAI: Crohn Disease Activity Index; CRP: C-Reactive Protein; HDL: High Density Lipoprotein; LDL: Low Density Lipoprotein

1. Introduction

The current standard treatment for Crohn's disease involves medication to manage symptoms and induce remission, and when necessary, bowel resection. An epidemiological study found that the risk of Crohn's disease was reduced by 70% in females and 80% in males following a vegetarian diet. This suggested treating Crohn's disease with a plant-based diet. (1,2)

A well-designed interventional study published in 2010, using a semi-vegetarian diet, achieved a 100% remission rate at 1 year and 92% at 2 years. (1,3)

A more advanced study published in 2017 examined whether a substantial improvement of the relapse-free rate in Crohn's disease could be obtained by incorporating three recently developed concepts in medicine: biologics, a plant-based diet and window of opportunity. This was followed by maintenance of remission with a plant-based diet, rather than further use of biologics with or without immunosuppressants. (4) All patients in this study who completed the protocol achieved remission at week 6. Remission rates by intention-to-treat and per protocol analysis were 96% and 100%, respectively. Improvements were seen in biomarkers such as C-reactive protein (CRP) and Crohn Disease Activity Index (CDAI) and in mucosal healing. This study has shown that a plant-based diet can improve the efficacy of biologics such as infliximab. (4)

While research shows the efficacy of a plant-based diet in the treatment of Crohn's disease, few physicians currently employ it as a therapeutic modality. This treatment, if used appropriately, can save the patient medication side effects, surgery, extraintestinal manifestations and quite a bit of money. Here, we report on a case of a patient with longstanding Crohn's disease, successfully treated with a vegetarian diet.

2. Case Report

A 63-year old male patient was first diagnosed with Crohn's disease in 1988 at the age of 33 years old. Once diagnosed, he realized that symptoms had been present since his late teens.

Symptoms included persistent pain, chronic diarrhea and chronic fatigue. Crohn's disease may be complicated by extraintestinal manifestations in up to 40% of patients. (5) In this patient, extraintestinal manifestations included apthous stomatitis, arthralgia especially in the knees and hips, eczema and uveitis. The patient's medical history was otherwise unremarkable. He was normotensive and had a BMI within the acceptable range. Total cholesterol and ratio of HDL and LDL were within normal limits. Renal function was normal.

His comorbidities included shingles, exacerbated by immunosuppression, and severe post herpetic neuralgia (treated with block transforaminal steroid epidural and block lumbar epidural steroid), and noise-induced hearing loss of both ears. The patient had benign prostatic hypertrophy and diverticulosis.

The patient was initially treated with sulfasalazine and prednisone. This treatment was not fully effective. The patient complained that medication side effects were extreme irritability, greatly increased appetite with weight gain and trouble sleeping. His symptoms of Crohn's disease stabilized at a not very comfortable level with continued pain, occasional severe diarrhea and chronic, moderate fatigue.

How to cite this article: Rose S, Strombom A. Treating Crohn's disease with a plant-based diet – a case report. Adv Res Gastroentero Hepatol. 2019; 12(3): 555837.
DOI: 10.19080/ARGH.2019.12.555837

Later treatments included were azathioprine, mesalamine, metronidazole, infliximab (discontinued due to allergic reaction), pregabalin, certolizumab pegol, famotidine, and Budesonide. More recently, albuterol, fluticasone, ranitidine and loperamide were added. However, significant symptoms persisted, although attenuated, and the patient continued to have a poor quality of life.

Results of CT scan, MRI, flouriscopic and endoscopic examinations were consistent with Crohn's disease. Biopsy confirmed the diagnosis.

During the course of illness, surgeries were required to:

1. Relieve obstruction in the proximal duodenum and the gastric outlet.
2. Remove the cecum and appendix with reanastomosis
3. Resection of four severe obstructions along the jejunum and ileum
4. Resection of two of the obstructed sections along with the ileocecal valve
5. A cholecystectomy – extensive scarring was noted.

3. Results

In May 2017, the patient chose to go on a plant-based diet. Within two months, significant improvements in symptoms resulted. By August 2017, the patient was able to discontinue all immunosuppressant drugs.

After one year, the patient reports no symptoms requiring medications other than ranitidine 150mg 2x/day and loperamide 10mg/day needed for post op management of resections. Fatigue, pain, diarrhea and all extrainstestinal manifestations have virtually been eliminated. The patent reports a very large improvement in quality of life.

He reports currently eating primarily whole grains, beans, fruits, vegetables, tofu, and using plant-based milks. Over the past few months he has begun to eat fish, mostly white fleshed with some salmon, usually around 3-4 times per month, eggs once or twice per week, and has some dairy products, always cultured, never milk, and ice cream once a week or so. The fish does not cause any symptoms but the eggs and dairy cause some very mild discomfort on occasion.

4. Discussion

The results for this patient are in line with interventional studies. The safety and efficacy of a plant-based diet to treat Crohn's disease would seem quite advantageous. It has no contraindications and no adverse reactions. Therefore, it may be safely used as monotherapy, or combined with standard treatments.

Treatment with a plant-based diet also reduces the risk of common diseases that the Crohn's patient will face in common with all patients, such as coronary artery disease and type II diabetes mellitus.

Given the substantial advantages, more study is warranted. However, given its safety, the physician can institute therapy with a plant-based diet immediately.

References

1. Rose S, Strombom A. (2018) Crohn's disease prevention and treatment with a plant-based diet. Adv Res Gastroentero Hepatol 9(1).
2. D'Souza S, Levy E, Mack D, Israel D, Lambrette P, et al. (2008) Dietary patterns and risk for Crohn's disease in children. Inflamm Bowel Dis 14(3): p. 367-73.

How to cite this article: Rose S, Strombom A. Treating Crohn's disease with a plant-based diet – a case report. Adv Res Gastroentero Hepatol. 2019; 12(3): 555837.
DOI: 10.19080/ARGH.2019.12.555837

3. Chiba M, Abe T, Tsuda H, Sugawara T, Tsuda S, et al. (2010) Lifestyle-related disease in Crohn's disease: Relapse prevention by a semi-vegetarian diet. World J Gastroenterol 16(20): p. 2484–2495.

4. Chiba M, Tsuji T, Nakane K, Tsuda S, Ishii H, et al. (2017) Induction with Infliximab and a plant-based diet as first-line (IPF) therapy for Crohn disease: a single-group trial. Perm J 21: p. 17-009.

5. Williams H, Walker D, Orchard T. (2008) Extraintestinal manifestations of inflammatory bowel disease. Curr Gastroenterol Rep 10(6): p. 597-605.

How to cite this article: Rose S, Strombom A. Treating Crohn's disease with a plant-based diet – a case report. Adv Res Gastroentero Hepatol. 2019; 12(3): 555837.
DOI: 10.19080/ARGH.2019.12.555837

Orthopedics and Rheumatology
Open Access Journal
ISSN: 2471-6804

Juniper Publishers
key to the Researchers

Case Report
Volume 15 Issue 4 - December 2019
DOI: 10.19080/OROAJ.2019.15.555918

Orth & Rheum Open Access J

Treating Chronic Pain with a Plant-Based Diet – a Case Report

Stewart Rose and Amanda Strombom*

Plant-Based Diets in Medicine, USA

Submission: December 10, 2019; **Published:** December 18, 2019

***Corresponding author:** Amanda Strombom, Plant-Based Diets in Medicine, 12819 SE 38th St, #427, Bellevue, WA 98006, USA

Abstract

Treatment with a plant-based diet has already been shown to be safe and effective both for several pathologies with chronic pain as a symptom. Here we describe the case of a 41-year old male patient who had been injured at work in 2009 and suffered from pain and restricted range of motion in his lumbar spine and legs for three years.

During that time, he was treated with pain medications, including epidural steroid injections and a short course of opioids. The patient then underwent L4-L5 microdiscectomy followed by lumbar laminectomy and L5-S1 discectomy, fusion and was given a series of steroid epidural injections. However, he remained with very significant pain, limited range of motion and was unable to work.

The patient was then referred to a physical and rehabilitative physician who prescribed a plant-based diet. Recognizing that standard treatment did not achieve the results he hoped for, the patient was open to the idea and embraced it whole-heartedly. He was also encouraged to eliminate caffeine and alcohol, and to rely on water for hydration, and to start some gentle physical therapy. Within 2 weeks, the patient noticed a reduction of symptoms. Within a month he no longer experienced back pain and his range of motion was improving. He gradually lost 50 lbs and regained the ability to walk and stand straight. Within three months he was able to resume work. The patient was very satisfied with the role of the plant-based diet in relieving his symptoms and enabling him to resume a normal and productive life.

1. Introduction

Chronic pain, one of the most common reasons adults seek medical care, (1) has been linked to restrictions in mobility and daily activities, (2, 3) dependence on opioids, (4) anxiety and depression, (2) and poor perceived health or reduced quality of life. (2, 4)

Eight percent of U.S. adults (19.6 million) had high-impact chronic pain, with higher prevalence of both chronic pain and high-impact chronic pain reported among women, older adults, previously but not currently employed adults, adults living in poverty, and rural residents. (5)

Long term treatment with opioids has become a growing concern. Long term use of other medications often used as an adjunct can also be problematic. New treatments are needed for the treatment of chronic pain.

Consumption of a plant-based diet has shown positive improvements in chronic pain and function. (6)

A plant-based diet has been shown to be a safe and effective treatment in several specific pathologies which present with chronic pain as a symptom. This includes rheumatoid arthritis, (7) diabetic peripheral neuropathy, (8, 9) fibromyalgia, (10, 11, 12) and angina pectoris. (13)

2. Case Report

The patient, a 41-yr old male carpenter married with 2 dependent children, had been injured at work in December 2009. He was lifting something at work when he felt a sudden onset lumbar pain extending to the left lower limb.

His Range of Motion (ROM) at the lumbar spine was restricted in flexion to 65 degrees. He had a decreased left ankle jerk reflex, and decreased sensation at the lateral aspect of the left foot. An MRI showed a lumbar disc herniation at L4-L5.

At that time his BMI was 31.3, blood pressure was 148/88. A former smoker, he drank wine on occasion and consumed caffeine throughout the day. He had a family history of diabetes mellitus (father) and hypertension (mother). He was taking Lisinopril (10mg daily) and ibuprofen (800mg x 3 daily).

He was put on light duty at work, and tried physical therapy and increased medications. He was given a series of 3 epidural steroid injections, but these resulted in diminishing returns and his pain returned a month after last epidural.

In June 2010, he underwent L4-L5 microdiscectomy and a short course of opioids. He experienced initial improvement, but recurrent lumbar pain had returned by Sept 2010.

In October 2010, he underwent lumbar laminectomy and L5-S1 discectomy, but he continued to have post-operative pain and chronic radicular symptoms in both legs. An MRI showed degenerative changes in lumbar spine, with epidural fibrosis causing lateral recess stenosis L3-S1. A lumbar discography was performed and lumbar spinal fusion recommended.

In Jan 2011, he underwent posterior lumbar spinal fusion with pedicle screw instrumentation, but he experienced ongoing chronic pain despite the corrective surgery.

3. Results

In May 2012, he was referred to a physical and rehabilitative physician. At that time, he could not stand straight, could barely lift 15lbs, and experienced extreme 10/10 pain in spine and legs. He had gained additional 30lbs due to immobility.

How to cite this article: Rose S, Strombom A. Treating chronic pain with a plant-based diet – a case report. Ortho & Rheum Open Access J. 2019; 15(4): 555918.
DOI: 10.19080/OROAJ.2019.15.555918

The concept of plant-based anti-inflammatory diet was introduced to him and he was encouraged to drink water for hydration, and to restrict alcohol and caffeine to reduce neurotoxins. He started some gentle physical therapy. He was desperate for a solution, and so embraced the plant-based diet wholeheartedly.

Within two weeks, he noticed decreased radicular symptoms. By late June the patient had no back pain, and his range of motion had improved.

By July he was able to lift 100 lbs on an occasional basis. He gradually lost 50lbs of body fat, and was able to walk and stand straight, with full painless ROM.

By August he was interviewing for work and was able to return to work. He was enthusiastic about the role a plant-based diet (in conjunction with rehabilitation) had in treating his chronic pain.

4. Discussion

Treatment of chronic pain often includes opiates which carry the risk of addiction along with significant side effects. However, treatment with a plant-based diet is a low risk and low-cost option, with no adverse reactions and no contraindications, that can be very effective for several pathologies with pain as a major symptom. It's also a safe and efficacious treatment for comorbid diseases such as coronary artery disease and type II diabetes mellitus.

The physician should explain the benefits and offer guidance on implementing a plant-based diet to patients suffering from relevant chronic pain condition. This treatment can be used as a monotherapy or as an adjunct to standard treatment.

References

1. Schappert S, Burt C. (2006) Ambulatory care visits to physician offices, hospital outpatient departments, and emergency departments: United States, 2001-02. *Vital Health Stat 13* (159):1-66.
2. Gureje O, Von Korff M, Simon G, Gater R. (1998) Persistent pain and well-being: a World Health Organization Study in Primary Care. *JAMA* 280(2):147-151.
3. Smith B, Elliott A, Chambers W, Smith W, Hannaford P, Penny K. (2001) The impact of chronic pain in the community. *Fam Pract* 18(3):292-299.
4. Interagency Pain Research Coordinating Committee. (2016) *National Pain Strategy: a comprehensive population health-level strategy for pain*. Washington DC: US Department of Health and Human Services, National Institutes of Health.
5. Dahlhamer J, Lucas J, Zelaya C, et al. (2018) Prevalence of Chronic Pain and High-Impact Chronic Pain Among Adults — United States, 2016. *MMWR Morb Mortal Wkly Rep* 67:1001-1006.
6. Towery P, Guffey J, Doerflein C, Stroup K, Saucedo S, Taylor J. (2018) Chronic musculoskeletal pain and function improve with a plant-based diet. *Complement Ther Med* 40:64-69.
7. Rose S, Strombom A. (2018) Rheumatoid Arthritis – Prevention and Treatment with a Plant-Based Diet. *Orth & Rheum Open Access J* 13(1):555852.
8. Crane M, Sample C. (1994) Regression of Diabetic Neuropathy with Total Vegetarian (Vegan) Diet. *Journal of Nutritional Medicine* 4(4):431-9.
9. Strombom A, Rose S. (2017) The prevention and treatment of Type II Diabetes Mellitus with a plant-based diet. *Endocrin Metab Int J* 5(5):00138.
10. Høstmark A, Lystad E, Vellar O, et al. (1993) Reduced plasma fibrinogen, serum peroxides, lipids, and apolipoproteins after a 3-week vegetarian diet. *Plant Foods for Human Nutrition* 43(1):55-61.

How to cite this article: Rose S, Strombom A. Treating chronic pain with a plant-based diet – a case report. Ortho & Rheum Open Access J. 2019; 15(4): 555918.
DOI: 10.19080/OROAJ.2019.15.555918

11. Donaldson M, Speight N, Loomis S. (2001) Fibromyalgia syndrome improved using a mostly raw vegetarian diet: an observational study. *BMC Complementary Alternative Medicine* 1:7.

12. Kaartinen K, Lammi K, Hypen M. (2000) Vegan diet alleviates fibromyalgia symptoms. *Scandinavian Journal of Rheumatology* 29(5):308-13.

13. Rose S, Strombom A. (2018) A comprehensive review of the prevention and treatment of heart disease with a plant-based diet. *J Cardiol & Cardiovas Ther* 12(5):555847.

How to cite this article: Rose S, Strombom A. Treating chronic pain with a plant-based diet – a case report. Ortho & Rheum Open Access J. 2019; 15(4): 555918.
DOI: 10.19080/OROAJ.2019.15.555918

Cancer Therapy & Oncology
International Journal
ISSN: 2473-554X

Juniper PUBLISHERS key to the Researchers

Case Report
Volume 15 Issue 5 - February 2020
DOI: 10.19080/CTOIJ.2020.15.555922

Canc Therapy & Oncol Int J

Stage 3 Prostate Cancer Treated with a Plant-Based Diet – A Case Report

Stewart D Rose and Amanda J Strombom*

Plant-Based Diets in Medicine, USA

Submission: February 04, 2020; **Published:** February 20. 2020

***Correspondence Author:** Amanda Strombom, Plant-Based Diets in Medicine, 12819 SE 38th St, #427, Bellevue, WA 98006.

Abstract

Treatment of early-stage prostate cancer (with a Gleason score less than seven) with a plant-based diet has been studied, and efficacy noted even after 5 years. However, this is a case of a patient with Stage 3 prostate cancer, who chose to follow a plant-based diet after his diagnosis, and is still alive today, 32 years later, despite being given a prognosis of 10% 3-year survival.

The patient is a retired physician, who was given the best available treatment since his diagnosis in 1987. He also chose to follow a largely plant-based diet after his diagnosis, recognizing its potential for treating prostate cancer. He has outlasted all other patients with a similar diagnosis, who were given the same treatment at his major city-based hospital. He attributes this to his plant-based diet.

This is the first case we are aware of where a patient with stage III prostate cancer exceeded his prognosis for 32 years.

Keywords:

Case report, plant-based diet, prostate cancer, stage 3, vegetarian, vegan

1. Introduction

Treatment of early stage prostate cancer (with a Gleason score less than seven) with a plant based diet has been studied, and efficacy noted even after 5 years. (1) However, this is a case of a patient with Stage 3 prostate cancer, who chose to follow a plant-based diet after his diagnosis, and is still alive today, 32 years later, despite being given only a 10% chance of 3 year survival.

While this case is anecdotal, and a plant-based diet was combined with standard treatment, it joins a growing body of evidence that prostate cancer is responsive to treatment with a plant-based diet. The patient's longevity may also partially be the result of a plant-based diet preventing and treating common comorbidities such coronary artery disease, (2) Type 2 diabetes, (3) and renal failure. (4)

2. Case Report

The patient is a 91-year old male retired physician who specialized in Internal Medicine. In 1987, at the age of 59 he was diagnosed with Stage 3 prostate cancer that had metastasized to the lymph nodes in the pelvic region. The attending physician suggested that he quit his medical practice because the prognosis only gave him a 10% chance of 3-year survival. At the time of diagnosis, he had no other comorbidities and his weight was normal.

As a child, aged 8, he had had rheumatic fever. His doctor ordered numerous fluoroscopic exams during this time. The radiation exposure continued when, as a physician, he had a fluoroscope in his office. He found he was able to diagnose patients more quickly using this than sending the patient for an X-ray. Despite wearing a lead apron during these radiological procedures, he inevitably experienced some radiation exposure to his face and extremities.

As a busy physician he had rarely had time to think about his diet, and hurriedly consumed a low fiber diet of white bread, aged cheeses and sausages, and no raw vegetables. Looking back on it now, he feels this likely contributed to his developing prostate cancer.

2.1 Medical Treatment received

The patient first underwent lymphadenectomy. The prostate and testicles were treated with radiation, which made him very weak for several weeks. Medications taken since diagnosis to treat his prostate cancer were as follows:

- Lupron (leuprolide acetate) Taken until May 2014.
- Casadex – an antiandrogen. Taken until it was no longer effective.
- Diethylstilbestrol – discontinued due to gynecomastia and radiation treatment, and a deep vein thrombosis in his right leg.
- Ketoconezole – Taken until severe edema developed due to impaired renal function. His renal function improved after the ketoconazole was discontinued.
- Zytiga – combined *with prednisone.* Taken until October 2016, when it became ineffective.
- Xtandi – *Seems to be working currently, though the dose had to be lowered due to dizziness side effects.*

Over the years, the patient has switched from one medication to another as efficacy diminished and as others became available. Many of these medications gave him severe side effects. He has relied upon having his PSA monitored regularly, and has tracked the effectiveness of each medication on that basis. Aspirin and other non-steroidal anti-inflammatory drugs taken for arthritis pain resulted in gastric and esophageal ulcers. He now uses the herb turmeric and cannabidiol (CBD) as anti-inflammatories.

How to cite this article: Rose S, Strombom A. Stage 3 prostate cancer treated with a plant-based diet – a case report. Canc Therapy & Oncol Int J. 2020; 15(5): 555922.
DOI: 10.19080/CTOIJ.2020.15.555922

2.2 Dietary self-treatment

As he recovered from the initial radiation, he started to explore various alternative therapies, and was particularly drawn to the Macrobiotic diet. The patient started following the mainly vegetarian diet and has largely followed it ever since. Today he focuses on getting as much plant phytoestrogens as possible, plus the phytochemical sulforaphane, found in vegetables such as broccoli, so he consumes plenty of tofu, beans, mushrooms, and cruciferous vegetables.

However, due to the lack of good plant-based options in the retirement community where he currently lives, he finds it necessary to consume more fish and poultry than he would wish, but still avoids products from mammals – beef, pork, lamb.

Recently he has had a hip replacement and both knees have been replaced. He experiences some loss of balance as a result of this, and due to sarcopenia. He has belonged to a cancer support group for the past 30 years, where other patients were being treated with similar medications, but he has outlasted them all and is now the longest term survivor with metastatic prostate cancer in his major city-based hospital. He attributes this to his largely plant-based diet.

3. Discussion

This is an interesting case for several reasons. The patient is a former professor of internal medicine and so better informed than most patients. He was able to recognize the potential of a plant-based diet to treat his prostate cancer and assess its efficacy, and to consciously combine standard treatment with dietary treatment. He has outlived his prognosis for 32 years.

This case also points to the problem that many senior citizens face in obtaining healthy plant-based meals in residential communities. This is all the more problematic because diet is the number one risk factor for disease and disability in the United States.

References

1. Rose S, Strombom A. (2018) A plant-based diet prevents and treats prostate cancer. *Canc Therapy & Oncol Int J* 11(3):555813.
2. Rose S, Strombom A. (2018) A comprehensive review of the prevention and treatment of heart disease with a plant-based diet. *J Cardiol & Cardiovas Ther* 12(5):555847.
3. Strombom A, Rose S. (2017) The prevention and treatment of Type II Diabetes Mellitus with a plant-based diet. *Endocrin Metab Int J* 5(5):00138.
4. Rose S, Strombom A. (2019) A plant-based diet prevents and treats chronic kidney disease. *JOJ Uro & Nephron* 6(3):555687.

How to cite this article: Rose S, Strombom A. Stage 3 prostate cancer treated with a plant-based diet – a case report. Canc Therapy & Oncol Int J. 2020; 15(5): 555922.
DOI: 10.19080/CTOIJ.2020.15.555922

The Clinical Practice of Prescribing Plant-Based Diets

Stewart D Rose* **and Amanda J Strombom**

Plant-Based Diets in Medicine, USA

***Corresponding author:** Stewart Rose, Plant-Based Diets in Medicine, 12819 SE 38th St, #427, Bellevue, WA 98006, USA

1. Introduction

Consumers reported in focus groups that their family doctor is the health professional they expect to advise them on diet. (1) Their function is to treat or prevent disease in their patients. Doctors are trusted, so it is acceptable for the family doctor to talk about diet, even if it seems remote from the presenting symptom. (2)

Health care professionals should ask patients on a plant-based diet about their dietary practices and assess for possible nutrient deficiencies through physical examination, periodic serum monitoring and perhaps bone mineral density (BMD) monitoring. (3)

Research has documented the high rate of compliance by patients treated with a plant-based diet, especially when physicians explain the rationale behind the treatment and specifically prescribe it to their patients. (4) It has also been shown to have good compliance, even in parts of the country that traditionally have a very meat-centered diet. (5)

The importance of talking to patients about their diet cannot be overstated. In a National Health Interview survey, 24,275 patients were surveyed. Only 30% reported receiving health promotion advice, and yet 88% of those patients complied with the advice they were given. This led to 21% increased odds that patients who received and complied with the advice they were given reported an improved health status, compared with those who did not comply or were not advised. (6)

2. Talking about making dietary changes

One way to start the conversation with your patient about their nutrition status is to ask them to complete a Nutrition History Form at check in (see appendix of this chapter for sample form). (7) Alternatively, the patient could be asked to describe the previous or a typical day's eating pattern, with the physician listening attentively and asking questions to be able to gather information similar to the form.

From this information, the physician can identify areas in the dietary pattern where changes would be most beneficial to the patient. When discussing a patient's treatment plan, diet can be included as a viable and affordable option.

Some key frames that can be used to create motivation for change are the following: (8)

- Feedback: How unhealthy behaviors are harming the individual – based on interview and data.
- Responsibility: Emphasize that the patient has the responsibility and freedom to make the choice to change.
- Advice: Provide clear and direct advice about importance of making changes and suggest ways to accomplish them.

- Locus of control: Discuss different options and let patient decide which make most sense.
- Empathy: The patient needs to feel heard and their concerns understood
- Self-efficacy: Instill optimism and confidence in the patient, "you can do this!"

Examples of the types of questions that can motivate patients to make changes (9):

- Given your recent lab results, is there a specific lifestyle change you've been thinking about making?
- Would you be interested in hearing some of the changes others with this diagnosis make?
- On a scale from 1-10, how ready are you to make changes in your eating patterns?
- What benefits do you think you'll get from a healthier diet?
- What concerns do you have about eating healthier?
- If you were to change, what would it be like?
- What things stand in the way of taking your first step?
- What barriers might impede your success?
- How do you think you'll go about making changes?

The patient should be asked if they prepare their own meals. If not, they may rely on prepared or frozen meals, or may regularly eat at restaurants. A discussion on available plant-based options for meals, drinks and snacks is helpful.

For those patients where another family member prepares their meals, eliciting the support of those who do can be very helpful. (10) Further support can come from family and friends. The patient may gain greater support if they can explain to friends and family why they chose to be treated with a plant-based diet and what its advantages are.

Since the plant-based diet will be new to most patients, it is very helpful to write down dietary directions on stationary with doctor's name on it which will give it the feel of a prescription. This is what most patients are used to, and it can be shown to family and friends for help in implementation. Potential resources that could assist the patient in their transition can also be listed.

Charting the patient's current dietary status and agreed goals, and enlisting other health care practitioners on the patient's team to support and encourage the patient can help with compliance. If a dietitian with experience in the therapeutic use of a plant-based diet is available for referral, this may be an option for certain more complex cases.

Two potential strategies for treating patients with a plant-based diet are to counsel patients briefly at each regular visit, or to arrange a longer in-depth session with the patient. Five to ten minutes of each office visit can be used to gradually help the patient transition toward a plant-based, charting improvements as they become evident. This may be a good strategy for when the plant-based diet is prescribed as a prophylaxis.

Alternatively, it can be effective to spend one or two office visits thoroughly explaining the diet and working with the patient on the best implementation for them. This will facilitate a more immediate implementation of treatment with a plant-based diet. This may be more appropriate as an interventional treatment with patients already with a pathology.

3. Medication titration

The treatment effects of the plant-based diet often take longer than drug therapy to become evident. Six weeks are frequently necessary for improvements to be noted. Effectiveness also depends on how quickly and completely the patient is able to implement their dietary transition. Medications should be titrated as clinical improvements become evident. Lab work should be scheduled in accordance with the pace of clinical improvement.

Since the plant-based diet treats common comorbidities, titration of any medications prescribed to treat those pathologies will be necessary as well. Likewise, labs for these pathologies should be ordered on a schedule that keeps pace with the expected pace of clinical improvements of comorbidities.

Improvements of signs and symptoms often continue for a few months. Therefore, it may take some time to judge the full efficacy of treatment. Patients, often used to the faster action of drugs, should be informed that the treatment may take a little longer but is well worth the wait.

4. Discussion

Vegetarian and vegan diets and food are not as uncommon as they used to be. The sales and availability of meat and dairy substitutes are have grown enormously in recent years. These products make dietary changes much easier in most cases, and when combined with a diet composed of vegetables, whole grains, fruits, legumes and nuts they can be very healthy.

Many people struggle with copayments and have high deductibles. With rising health care costs, treatment with a plant-based diet can relieve financial stress on the patient. Patients should be informed that it may save them money both in the short and the long term.

We live in an age of advanced medical technology. These advances have alleviated much suffering and saved countless lives. They have an unquestioned place in modern medicine. However, this can sometimes lead towards a kind of technological tunnel vision on the part of the patient. Little notice may be taken of treatments that, such as a plant-based diet, while lacking in technological sophistication, are nevertheless safe and quite efficacious. Patients should be told that while it's a low tech treatment, it is still very effective.

As most physicians know, many patients these days attempt to gain health-related information and to treat themselves based upon what they read on the internet. Such information is often highly unreliable. (11) Most patients would rather get their health information and advice from their physicians, but turn to the internet when they can't. Therefore, to serve the best interests and needs of their patients, physicians should familiarize themselves with this treatment. Physicians should warn their patients that nutritional information gained on the internet may be very unreliable.

References

1. van Dillen S, Hiddink G, Koelen M, de Graaf C, van Woerkum C. (2003) Understanding nutrition communication between health professionals and consumers: development of a model for nutrition awareness based on qualitative consumer research. *Am J Clin Nutr* 77(4 Suppl):1065S-1072S.
2. Truswell A, Hiddink G, Blom J. (2003) Nutrition guidance by family doctors in a changing world: problems, opportunities, and future possibilities. *Am J Clin Nutr* 77(4):1089S-1092S.

3. Fields H, Ruddy B, Wallace M, Shah A, Millstine D, Marks L. (2016) How to monitor and advise vegans to ensure adequate nutrient intake. *J Am Osteo Assoc* 116(2):96-99.
4. Esselstyn CJ, Gendy G, Doyle J, Golubic M, Roizen M. (2014) A way to reverse CAD? *J Fam Pract* 63(7):356-364b.
5. Drozek D, Diehl H, Nakazawa M, Kostohryz T, Morton D, et al. (2014) Short-term effectiveness of a lifestyle intervention program for reducing selected chronic disease risk factors in individuals living in rural appalachia: a pilot cohort study. *Advances in Preventive Medicine* 2014:798184.
6. Ndetan H, Evans MBS, Felini M, Rupert R, Singh K. (2010) The health care provider's role and patient compliance to health promotion advice from the user's perspective: analysis of the 2006 National Health Interview Survey data. *J Manipulative Physiol Ther* 33(6):413-418.
7. Hark L, Deen D. (1999) Taking a Nutrition History: A Practical Approach for Family Physicians. *Am Fam Phys* 59(6):1521-1528.
8. Miller W, Sovereign G. (1989) The check-up: A model for early intervention in addictive behaviors. In: Miller W, Nathan P, Marlatt G, eds. *Addictive behaviors: Prevention and early intervention*. Lisse, Netherlands: Swets & Zeitlinger.
9. Rudd Center for Food Policy and Obesity. Motivational Interviewing for Diet, Exercise and Weight. *UConn Rudd Center for Food Policy & Obesity*.
10. Avery K, Donovan J, Horwood J, et al. (2014) The importance of dietary change for men diagnosed with and at risk of prostate cancer: a multi-centre interview study with men, their partners and health professionals. *BMC Family Practice* 15:81.
11. Schwartz K, Roe T, Northrup J, et al. (2006) Family Medicine Patients' Use of the Internet for Health Information: A MetroNet Study. *Journal of American Board of Family Medicine* 19(1):39-45.

Appendix: Sample Nutrition History Form

1. How many meals and snacks do you typically eat each day? Meals ________ Snacks ________
2. How many times a week do you typically eat the following meals away from home?
   Breakfast _______ Lunch ________ Dinner ________

   What types of eating places do you frequently visit? (Check all that apply)

   Fast-food _______ Diner/Cafeteria _______ Restaurant _______ Other ______
3. Do you follow any specific dietary pattern? Yes / No If yes, name or describe it:

   ____
4. On average, how many servings of fruit (eg. apple, bowl of strawberries) do you eat each day?
   Fresh fruit _______ Frozen fruit (eg. in smoothie) ________ Cooked fruit _______
5. On average, how many servings of vegetables/green salad do you eat each day? ___________
6. On average, how many servings of grains do you eat each day?
   (includes cereals, baked goods, bread, pasta, rice, oats, other grains) ___________

   What percentage of these are whole grain (eg. whole wheat, brown rice) ___________
7. At how many meals each week do you eat red meat (beef, lamb, veal) or pork? ___________
8. At how many meals each week do you eat processed meat (eg. bacon, salami) ___________
9. At how many meals each week do you eat chicken or turkey? ___________
10. At how many meals each week do you eat fish or shellfish? ___________
11. At how many meals each week do you eat meat or fish substitute products? ___________
12. At how many meals each week do you eat beans, lentils, tofu or tempeh? ___________
13. What types of beverages do you usually drink? How many cups of each do you drink in a day? ___________

Water	_______	<u>Milk</u>:		<u>Alcohol</u>:	
Juice	_______	Whole milk	______	Beer	_______
Soda	_______	1 or 2%	______	Wine	_______
Diet Soda	_______	Nonfat milk	______	Hard Liquor	_______
Sports drinks	_______	Soymilk	______		
Tea or iced tea	_______	Nut milk	______		
Coffee	_______				
Other drinks	_______				

Full Name: ____________________________________ Today's date: ______________

The Plant-Based Diet – What Physicians Need to Know

Stewart D Rose* and Amanda J Strombom

Plant-Based Diets in Medicine, USA

***Corresponding author:** Stewart Rose, Plant-Based Diets in Medicine, 12819 SE 38th St, #427, Bellevue, WA 98006, USA

1. Introduction

The plant-based diet includes vegetables, legumes, whole grains, fruits, tree nuts and seeds. The American Academy of Nutrition (formally the American Dietetic Association) has formally endorsed the plant-based diet as both nutritionally adequate for all phases of the life cycle, and as having all necessary nutrients except Vitamin B12 in their position paper. Their full statement is well worth reading:

> "It is the position of the Academy of Nutrition and Dietetics that appropriately planned vegetarian, including vegan, diets are healthful, nutritionally adequate, and may provide health benefits for the prevention and treatment of certain diseases. These diets are appropriate for all stages of the life cycle, including pregnancy, lactation, infancy, childhood, adolescence, older adulthood, and for athletes. Plant-based diets are more environmentally sustainable than diets rich in animal products because they use fewer natural resources and are associated with much less environmental damage. Vegetarians and vegans are at reduced risk of certain health conditions, including ischemic heart disease, type 2 diabetes, hypertension, certain types of cancer, and obesity. Low intake of saturated fat and high intakes of vegetables, fruits, whole grains, legumes, soy products, nuts, and seeds (all rich in fiber and phytochemicals) are characteristics of vegetarian and vegan diets that produce lower total and low-density lipoprotein cholesterol levels and better serum glucose control. These factors contribute to reduction of chronic disease. Vegans need reliable sources of vitamin B-12, such as fortified foods or supplements." (1)

There may be a health advantage of not consuming large amounts of very highly processed foods. Americans in general currently consume large amounts of these foods. Data from NHANES 2009–2010 suggests that Americans currently consume 60% of their calories from ultra-processed foods such as candy, sugared beverages, cakes, cookies, pizza, French fries, salty and sweet snacks, and desserts, with only 5% of calories from fruits and less than 1% from vegetables. (2)

While a patient on a plant-based diet typically consumes less processed foods, it is still wise for the physician to make sure they are not consuming vegan processed foods in excess. Using the term "whole-food plant-based diet" encourages the patient to focus both on plant-foods and on whole foods as opposed to highly processed foods. However, meat and dairy alternatives, while often processed, are valuable transition foods which maintain the texture and flavor of foods they are familiar with and support the patient socially by giving foods such as a veggie burger, which can help them feel more comfortable.

Nutrients present in various foods play an important role in maintaining the normal functions of the human body. The major nutrients present in foods include the macronutrients: carbohydrates, proteins, and lipids, plus vitamins, minerals and fiber. Besides these, there are some bioactive food components known as "phytonutrients" that play an important role in the prevention and treatment of disease. (3)

The following chart illustrates the macronutrients typically consumed by following the current government recommendations, known as MyPlate, compared to the macronutrients consumed on a whole foods plant-based diet: (4)

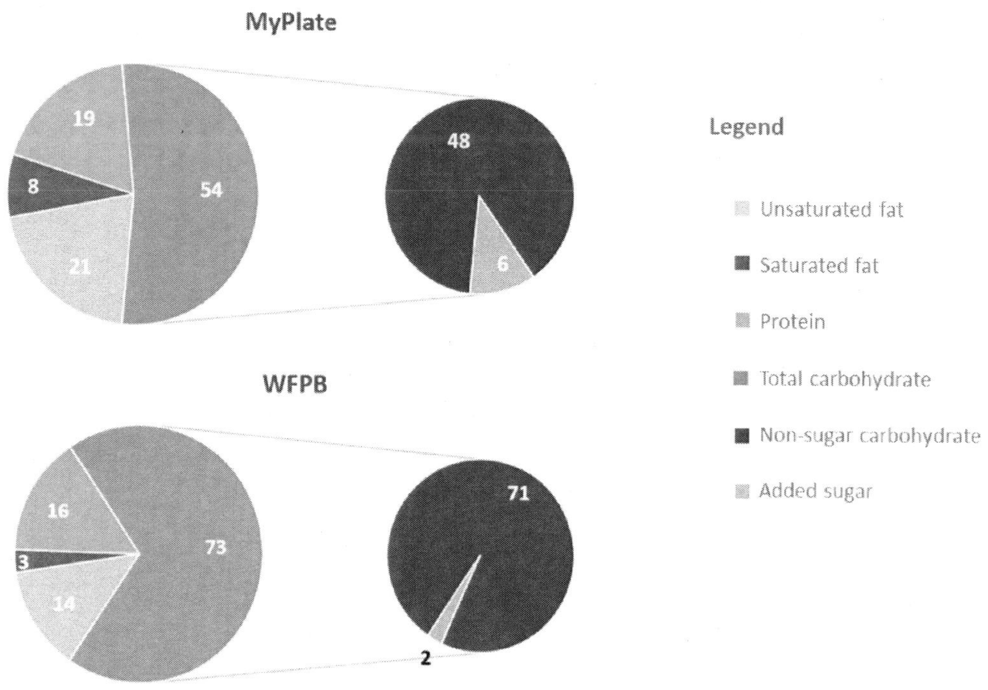

A whole food plant-based diet is commendable, and a well-planned vegan diet can be adequate to achieve proper nutrition. Individuals who adhere to WFBP meal plans have higher overall dietary quality as defined by the HEI-2015 score as compared to typical US intakes, with the exceptions of calcium for older women, and vitamins B12 and D without supplementation. (4) There are some nutrients of concern that the physician should take note of. These are Vitamin B12, vitamin D, calcium, iron, zinc and omega 3 fatty acids. These are addressed in more detail as separate articles in the nutrition chapter.

Adequate water is of course essential, and other water-based beverages such as tea are useful as well. Care should be taken to avoid heavily sugared beverages.

2. Protein

The concern that vegans, and particularly vegan athletes, may not consume an adequate amount and quality of protein is unsubstantiated. Vegetarian diets that include a variety of plant products provide the same protein quality as diets that include meat. (1) The amounts and proportions of amino acids consumed by vegans are typically more than sufficient to meet and exceed individual daily requirements, provided that a reasonable variety of foods are consumed and energy intake needs are being met. (5) In developed countries, plant proteins are typically mixed, especially in vegan diets, and total intake of protein usually exceeds the requirement. This results in intakes of all 20 amino acids that are more than sufficient to cover requirements. (5)

There is very little evidence at present regarding a marked difference in protein digestibility in humans. The more precise data collected so far in humans, assessing real (specific) oro-ileal nitrogen digestibility, has shown that the differences in the digestibility between plant and animal protein sources are only a few percent different. (6)

Several studies have shown the adequacy of protein intake among vegans. The EPIC-Oxford study showed that vegans had 13.1% of their Calories from protein yielding 64g. (7, 8) A French study showed vegans consuming 12.8 percent of the calories as protein for a total of 62g. (9) An American study of vegans showed 14.1% of Calories as protein resulting in an intake of 71gm of protein(10) and a Belgian study showed that vegans consumed 14.0% of their Calories as protein resulting an intake 82gm. (11) All these studies exceeded the RDA of greater than 10% Calories from protein or approximately 50gm.

The myth that plant proteins must be combined at every meal to be of any use to the body was popularized in the early 70's by the book *Diet for a Small Planet* by Frances Moore Lappé. The author has since been retracting the statement frequently. "In combating the myth that meat is the only way to get high-quality protein, I reinforced another myth," she said. Unfortunately, the protein combining myth has taken root in the public and even among a few doctors.

Combining two or more incomplete protein foods (those low in one or more essential amino acids), such as rice and beans, peanut butter and whole grain bread, tortillas with beans, and cooked beans with cornbread is not required in every meal, as long as variety is present over a day or two. (1) The reason for this lies in the pool of indispensable amino acids (IAAs) maintained by the body, (12, 13) that can be used to complement dietary proteins. The pool of amino acids come from four sources: (14, 15, 16)

- Enzymes secreted into the intestine to digest proteins.
- Intestinal cells sloughed off in the intestine.
- Intracellular spaces of the skeletal musculature
- Synthesis of amino acids by intestinal microflora.

Thus patients can consume, for example, beans at dinner and have a grain-based breakfast the next morning, and still have sufficient amino acids.

3. Carbohydrates

Carbohydrates play an important role in the human body. They act as an energy source, help control blood glucose and insulin metabolism, participate in cholesterol and triglyceride metabolism, and help with fermentation. The digestive tract breaks down carbohydrates upon consumption into monosaccharides including glucose. The polysaccharide glycogen represents the main storage form of glucose in the body. Glycogen is made and stored primarily in the cells of the liver and skeletal muscle, where it is stored until further energy is needed. (17)

In its 2002 report, the Institute of Medicine (IOM) established an RDA for carbohydrate of 130 g/d for adults and children aged ≥1 y. This value is based on the amount of sugars and starches required to provide the brain with an adequate supply of glucose. The IOM set an acceptable macronutrient distribution range (AMDR) for carbohydrates of 45–65% of total calories. (18)

The four classes of carbohydrates in food are:

- Monosaccharides: The most basic, fundamental unit of a carbohydrate. These are simple sugars, such as glucose, galactose, fructose, with the general chemical structure of $C_6H_{12}O_6$;
- Disaccharides: Compound sugars, such as sucrose and lactose, containing two monosaccharides with the elimination of a water molecule with the general chemical structure $C_{12}H_{22}O_{11}$;
- Oligosaccharides: Polymers, such as maltodextrins and raffinose, containing three to ten monosaccharides;
- Polysaccharides: Polymers, such as amylose and cellulose, containing long chains of monosaccharides connected through glycosidic bonds;

Different carbohydrates have different effects on raising blood glucose:

- Simple Carbohydrates: One or two sugars (monosaccharides or disaccharides) combined in a simple chemical structure. These are easily utilized for energy, and can cause a rapid rise in blood glucose and insulin secretion from the pancreas.
- Complex Carbohydrates: Three or more sugars (oligosaccharides or polysaccharides) bonded together in a more complex chemical structure. These take longer to digest and therefore have a more gradual effect on the increase in blood sugar.

3.1 Glycemic Index

The Glycemic Index (GI) is a kinetic parameter which reflects the ability of carbohydrate contained in consumed foods to raise blood glucose in vivo. Considerable epidemiologic evidence links consuming lower glycemic index (GI) diets with good health.

The glycemic index (GI) concept was introduced by Jenkins et al in the early 1980s as a ranking system for carbohydrates based on their immediate impact on blood glucose levels. (19) GI was originally designed for people with diabetes as a guide to food selection, advice being given to select foods with a low GI. (20) Lower GI foods were considered to confer benefit as a result of the relatively low glycemic response following ingestion compared with high GI foods.

The GI concept has been extended to also take into account the effect of the total amount of carbohydrate consumed. Thus glycemic load (GL), a product of GI and quantity of carbohydrate eaten, provides an indication of glucose available for energy or storage following a carbohydrate containing meal.

In addition to a role in the treatment of diabetes, low GI and GL diets have more recently been widely recommended for the prevention of chronic diseases including diabetes, obesity, cancer and heart disease and in the treatment of cardiovascular risk factors, especially dyslipidaemia. (21)

There are various research methods for assigning a GI value to food. In general, the number is based on how much a food item raises blood glucose levels compared with how much pure glucose (100) raises blood glucose. GI values are generally divided into three categories:

- Low GI: 1 to 55
- Medium GI: 56 to 69
- High GI: 70 and higher

Comparing these values, therefore, can help guide healthier food choices. For example, an English muffin made with white wheat flour has a GI value of 77. A whole-wheat English muffin has a GI value of 45.

Examples of foods with low, middle and high GI values include the following: (22)

- Low GI: Green vegetables, most fruits, raw carrots, kidney beans, chickpeas, lentils and bran breakfast cereals
- Medium GI: Sweet corn, bananas, raw pineapple, raisins, oat breakfast cereals, and multigrain, oat bran or rye bread
- High GI: White rice, white bread and potatoes

See appendix at the end of this chapter for a more complete table showing Glycemic Index (glucose = 100) for a range of foods (22)

4. Dietary fiber

Dietary fiber is a key component of a healthy diet as recommended by several nutritional guidelines. (23) Dietary fiber is defined as the edible parts of plants or analogous carbohydrates that are resistant to digestion and absorption in the human small intestine. (24)

Traditionally, dietary fiber was defined as the portions of plant foods that were resistant to digestion by human digestive enzymes; this included certain polysaccharides and lignin. More recently, the definition has been expanded to include oligosaccharides, such as inulin, and resistant starches. (25) Soluble and insoluble dietary fibers make up the two basic categories of dietary fibers. Cellulose, hemicellulose and lignin are not soluble in water whereas pectins, gums and mucilages become gummy in water. (26)

Dietary fiber intake provides many health benefits. Individuals with high intakes of dietary fiber appear to be at significantly lower risk for developing coronary heart disease, stroke, hypertension, type 2 diabetes, obesity, and certain gastrointestinal diseases. Increasing fiber intake can lower blood pressure and serum cholesterol levels. Increased intake of soluble fiber improves glycemia and insulin sensitivity in non-diabetic and diabetic individuals. Fiber supplementation in obese individuals significantly enhances weight loss. Increased fiber intake benefits a number of gastrointestinal disorders including the following: gastroesophageal reflux disease, duodenal ulcer, diverticulitis, constipation, and hemorrhoids. Dietary fiber intake provides similar benefits for children as for adults. The recommended dietary fiber intakes for children and adults are 14 g/1000 kcal. (25) However, average fiber intakes for US children and adults are less than half of the recommended levels.

Prebiotic fibers appear to enhance immune function. A prebiotic is a non-absorbable compound that, through its metabolization by microorganisms in the gut, modulates composition and the activity of the gut microbiota, thus conferring a beneficial physiologic effect on the host. (27) The consumption of prebiotics is difficult to measure since they are found in very diverse food groups, in wide ranges of supplements, and there isn't an analytic test or universally agreed-upon method. Estimated consumption in US and European diets is several grams a day for naturally occurring prebiotics: inulin and fructo-oligosaccharides. (28, 29)

Inulin is a prebiotic that occurs naturally in leeks, asparagus, onions, wheat, garlic, chicory, oats, soybeans, and Jerusalem artichokes. Fructo-oligosaccharides (FOS) are oligosaccharides that occur naturally in plants such as onion, chicory, garlic, asparagus, banana, artichoke, among many others. They are composed of linear chains of fructose units, linked by β (2-1) bonds. The number of fructose units ranges from 2 to 60 and often terminate in a glucose unit. Dietary FOS are not hydrolyzed by small intestinal glycosidases and reach the cecum structurally unchanged. There, they are metabolized by the intestinal microflora to form short-chain carboxylic acids, L -lactate, CO2, hydrogen and other metabolites. (30)

5. Lipids

Dietary lipids are found in foods from both plants and animals. There are two types of fatty acids of nutritional concern:

- Saturated fatty acids, found in higher proportions in animal products.
- Unsaturated fatty acids — Monounsaturated and polyunsaturated fatty acids are found in higher proportions in plants.

Saturated fatty acid (SAFA) intake occurs to some degree from all fat-containing foods, with especially high amounts in dairy products, butter, and meats. (31) Most dietary SAFA have 12-18 carbon atoms, with foods varying in the relative amounts of individual SAFA. Palmitic (C_{16}) and stearic acids (C_{18}) are predominant in butter, dairy and meat products; lauric (C_{12}) and myristic (C_{14}) acids in butter, dairy foods, coconut, and palm kernel oils. (32) In many Western countries, in particular, SAFA intakes exceed 10% of Calories. (31, 33)

Randomized controlled trials that lowered intake of dietary saturated fat and replaced it with polyunsaturated vegetable oil reduced CVD by approximately 30%, similar to the reduction achieved by statin treatment. (34) Similarly, consuming polyunsaturated and/or monounsaturated fats in preference to saturated fats and trans fatty acids has beneficial effects on insulin sensitivity and reduces the risk of Type 2 Diabetes Mellitus. (35) Many of the other pathologies addressed in this book also demonstrate an adverse reaction to saturated fat.

Coconut oil contains greater than 80% SAFA. A common misconception is that SAFAs in coconut oil are metabolized differently from long-chain SAFA ($\geq C_{12}$). However, coconut oil contains approximately 50% lauric acid and 15% myristic acid. (36) Studies have shown that coconut oil generally raised total and low-density lipoprotein cholesterol to a greater extent than cis unsaturated plant oils, but to a lesser extent than butter. (37) Observational evidence suggests that consumption of coconut flesh or squeezed coconut in the context of traditional dietary patterns does not lead to adverse cardiovascular outcomes. However, due to large differences in dietary and lifestyle patterns, these findings cannot be applied to a typical

Western diet. (37) Overall, the weight of the evidence from interventional studies to date suggests that replacing coconut oil with cis unsaturated fats would improve blood lipid profiles, leading to a reduction in risk factors for cardiovascular disease. (37)

Trans fat is an unsaturated fat found primarily in partially hydrogenated oils (and foods containing these oils) and in small amounts in some animal products. Trans unsaturated fatty acids are monounsaturated or polyunsaturated fatty acids containing at least one double bond in the trans configuration. (34) Clinical trials have consistently documented the adverse effects of trans fatty acids on the lipid risk factors for CVD. Replacement of calories from other types of fats with trans fatty acids raises LDL cholesterol, apolipoprotein B, triglycerides, and lipoprotein(a), as well as lowering HDL cholesterol and apolipoprotein A1. (38)

Essential fatty acids are addressed in a separate article in the Nutritional Considerations In-depth section.

6. Vitamins

The material in this section is adapted from the National Institutes of Health Fact Sheets. (39)

6.1 Vitamin A

Vitamin A is the name of a group of fat-soluble retinoids, including retinol, retinal, and retinyl esters. (40, 41, 42) Vitamin A is involved in immune function, vision, reproduction, and cellular communication. (40, 43, 44) Vitamin A is critical for vision as an essential component of rhodopsin, a protein that absorbs light in the retinal receptors, and because it supports the normal differentiation and functioning of the conjunctival membranes and cornea. (41, 43, 44) Vitamin A also supports cell growth and differentiation, playing a critical role in the normal formation and maintenance of the heart, lungs, kidneys, and other organs. (41)

Two forms of vitamin A are available in the human diet: preformed vitamin A (retinol and its esterified form, retinyl ester) and provitamin A carotenoids. (40, 41, 42, 43, 44) Preformed vitamin A is found in foods from animal sources, including dairy products, fish, and meat. The most important provitamin A carotenoid is beta-carotene. Other provitamin A carotenoids are alpha-carotene and beta-cryptoxanthin. The body converts these plant pigments into vitamin A. Both provitamin A and preformed vitamin A must be metabolized intracellularly to retinal and retinoic acid, the active forms of vitamin A, to support the vitamin's important biological functions. (41, 42) Other carotenoids found in food, such as lycopene, lutein, and zeaxanthin, are valuable phytochemicals but are not converted into vitamin A.

RDAs for vitamin A are given as retinol activity equivalents (RAE) to account for the different bioactivities of retinol and provitamin A carotenoids, all of which are converted by the body into retinol. 1 mcg RAE is equivalent to the following amounts: 1 mcg of retinol, 2 mcg of supplemental beta-carotene, 12 mcg of dietary beta-carotene, and 24 mcg of dietary alpha-carotene or beta-cryptoxanthin. (44)

Vitamin A is listed on many food and supplement labels in international units (IUs) even though nutrition scientists rarely use this measure. Conversions between IU and mcg RAE are as follows: (45)

- 1 IU retinol = 0.3 mcg RAE
- 1 IU supplemental beta-carotene = 0.3 mcg RAE

- 1 IU dietary beta-carotene = 0.05 mcg RAE
- 1 IU dietary alpha-carotene or beta-cryptoxanthin = 0.025 mcg RAE

Table 1: Recommended Dietary Allowances (RDAs) for Vitamin A (46)

Age	Male	Female	Pregnancy	Lactation
0–6 months*	400 mcg RAE	400 mcg RAE		
7–12 months*	500 mcg RAE	500 mcg RAE		
1–3 years	300 mcg RAE	300 mcg RAE		
4–8 years	400 mcg RAE	400 mcg RAE		
9–13 years	600 mcg RAE	600 mcg RAE		
14–18 years	900 mcg RAE	700 mcg RAE	750 mcg RAE	1,200 mcg RAE
19–50 years	900 mcg RAE	700 mcg RAE	770 mcg RAE	1,300 mcg RAE
51+ years	900 mcg RAE	700 mcg RAE		

Because vitamin A is fat soluble, the body stores excess amounts, primarily in the liver, and these levels can accumulate. Although excess preformed vitamin A can have significant toxicity (known as hypervitaminosis A), large amounts of beta-carotene and other provitamin A carotenoids are not associated with major adverse effects, thus offering a safer route to vitamin A. (47)

Excess beta-carotene is predominantly stored in the fat tissues of the body. The most common side effect of excessive beta-carotene consumption is carotenodermia, a physically harmless condition that presents as a conspicuous orange skin tint arising from deposition of the carotenoid in the outermost layer of the epidermis. (48) Carotenodermia is quickly reversible upon cessation of excessive intakes.

Retinol and carotenoid levels are typically measured in plasma, and plasma retinol levels are useful for assessing vitamin A inadequacy. However, their value for assessing marginal vitamin A status is limited because they do not decline until vitamin A levels in the liver are almost depleted. (42) Frank vitamin A deficiency is rare in the United States.

Table 2: Plant food sources of provitamin A

Food	mcg RAE per serving	IU per serving	Percent DV*
Sweet potato, baked in skin, 1 whole	1,403	28,058	561
Spinach, frozen, boiled, ½ cup	573	11,458	229
Carrots, raw, ½ cup	459	9,189	184
Pumpkin pie, commercially prepared, 1 piece	488	3,743	249
Cantaloupe, raw, ½ cup	135	2,706	54
Peppers, sweet, red, raw, ½ cup	117	2,332	47
Mangos, raw, 1 whole	112	2,240	45
Black-eyed peas (cowpeas), boiled, 1 cup	66	1,305	26
Apricots, dried, sulfured, 10 halves	63	1,261	25
Broccoli, boiled, ½ cup	60	1,208	24
Tomato juice, canned, ¾ cup	42	821	16
Ready-to-eat cereal, fortified with 10% of the DV for vitamin A, ¾–1 cup (more heavily fortified cereals might provide more of the DV)	127–149	500	10
Baked beans, canned, plain or vegetarian, 1 cup	13	274	5
Summer squash, all varieties, boiled, ½ cup	10	191	4
Pistachio nuts, dry roasted, 1 ounce	4	73	1

*DV = Daily Value.

Vitamin A can interact with certain medications, and some medications can have an adverse effect on vitamin A levels. A few examples are provided below. Individuals taking these and other medications on a regular basis should discuss their vitamin A status with their healthcare providers.

Orlistat (Alli®, Xenical®), a weight-loss treatment, can decrease the absorption of vitamin A, other fat-soluble vitamins, and beta-carotene, causing low plasma levels in some patients. (49) The manufacturers of Alli and Xenical recommend encouraging patients on orlistat to take a multivitamin supplement containing vitamin A and beta-carotene, as well as other fat-soluble vitamins. (50, 51)

Several synthetic retinoids derived from vitamin A are used orally as prescription medicines. Examples include the psoriasis treatment acitretin (Soriatane®) and bexarotene (Targretin®), used to treat the skin effects of T-cell lymphoma. Retinoids can increase the risk of hypervitaminosis A when taken in combination with vitamin A supplements. (49)

6.2 B Vitamins

The eight B vitamins: thiamine (B1), riboflavin (B2), niacin (B3), pantothenic acid (B5), vitamin B6, folate (B9) and vitamin B12, act as coenzymes in a substantial proportion of the enzymatic processes that underpin every aspect of cellular physiological functioning. As a coenzyme, the biologically active form of the vitamin binds within a protein "apoenzyme" creating a "holoenzyme", thereby increasing the resultant enzyme's competence in terms of the diversity of reactions that it can catalyze. (52)

The B vitamins themselves are not grouped on the basis of any chemical structural similarity, but rather with regards to their water solubility and the inter-related, cellular coenzyme functions that they play. (53) Overall, the plethora of functions undertaken by B vitamins can generally be subdivided into their roles in catabolic metabolism, leading to the generation of energy, and anabolic metabolism, resulting in the construction and transformation of bioactive molecules. (53)

Vitamin B_1 – Thiamin plays a central role in the generation of energy from carbohydrates. It is involved in RNA and DNA production, as well as nerve function. Its active form is a coenzyme called thiamin pyrophosphate(TPP), which takes part in the conversion of pyruvate to acetyl coenzyme A(CoA) in metabolism. (54)

Vitamin B_2 – Riboflavin is involved in the energy production for the electron transport chain, the citric acid cycle, as well as the catabolism of fatty acids (beta oxidation). (55)

Vitamin B_3 – Niacin is composed of two structures: nicotinic acid and nicotinamide. There are two co-enzyme forms of niacin: nicotinamide adenine dinucleotide(NAD) and nicotinamide adenine dinucleotide phosphate(NADP). Both play an important role in energy transfer reactions in the metabolism of glucose, fat and alcohol. (56) NAD carries hydrogens and their electrons during metabolic reactions, including the pathway from the citric acid cycle to the electron transport chain. NADP is a coenzyme in lipid and nucleic acid synthesis. (57)

Vitamin B_5 - Pantothenic acid is involved in the oxidation of fatty acids and carbohydrates. Coenzyme A, which can be synthesized from pantothenic acid, is involved in the synthesis of amino acids, fatty acids, ketones, cholesterol, (58) phospholipids, steroid hormones, neurotransmitters (such as acetylcholine), and antibodies. (59)

Vitamin B_6 – Pyridoxine is usually stored in the body as pyridoxal 5'-phosphate(PLP), which is the co-enzyme form of vitamin B_6. Pyridoxine is involved in the metabolism of amino acids and lipids; in the synthesis of neurotransmitters (60) and hemoglobin, as well as in the production of nicotinic acid. (61) Pyridoxine also plays an important role in gluconeogenesis.

Vitamin B_7 – Biotin plays a key role in the metabolism of lipids, proteins and carbohydrates. It is a critical co-enzyme of four carboxylases:

acetyl CoA carboxylase, which is involved in the synthesis of fatty acids from acetate; propionyl CoA carboxylase, involved in gluconeogenesis; β-methylcrotonyl CoA carboxylase, involved in the metabolism of leucin; and pyruvate CoA carboxylase, which is involved in the metabolism of energy, amino acids and cholesterol. (62)

Vitamin B_9 - Folic Acid acts as a co-enzyme in the form of tetrahydrofolate (THF), which is involved in the transfer of single-carbon units in the metabolism of nucleic acids and amino acids. THF is involved in pyrimidine nucleotide synthesis, so is needed for normal cell division, especially during pregnancy and infancy, which are times of rapid growth. Folate also aids in erythropoiesis. (57)

Vitamin B_{12} is addressed in a separate article in the Nutritional Considerations In-depth section.

In terms of their origins, the B vitamins are typically synthesized by plants, with their synthesis in plant chloroplasts, mitochondria and the cytosol carefully regulated to the plant's fluctuating requirements, with the exception of vitamin B_{12} which is synthesized by soil bacteria. (53) Therefore, a well-planned plant-based diet should allow the patient to get all the B vitamins they need. Supplements are readily available and may be indicated in patients following an overly restrictive plant-based diet.

Table 3: The B vitamins: nomenclature, dietary sources, coenzyme forms (roles) (53)

Vitamin	Generally Known as	Good Dietary Sources	RDA [1] (mg)	UL [2]	Principal Bioactive Coenzymes (and Principal Coenzyme Role (52))
B_1	Thiamin(e)	Cereals (esp. whole grain), brown rice, green vegetables, potatoes, pasta	1.2/1.1	–	Thiamine pyrophosphate (Generation of leaving group potential)
B_2	Riboflavin	Leafy vegetables, legumes, yeast, mushrooms	1.3/1.1	–	Flavoproteins: flavin adenine dinucleotide (FAD) or flavin mononucleotide (FMN) (redox reactions)
B_3	Niacin	Whole grain cereal, legumes, mushrooms, nuts	16/14	35 mg	Nicotinamide adenine dinucleotide (NAD) and its phosphate (NADP) (redox reactions)
B_5	Pantothenic acid	Whole grain cereals, broccoli	5	–	Co-enzyme A (CoA) (acyl activation and transfer)
B_6	Vitamin B_6 (referring to: pyridoxal, pyridoxamine, pyridoxine)	Legumes, nuts, bananas, potatoes	1.3/1.3 (1.7/1.5 >50 year)	100 mg	pyridoxal-5'-phosphate (PLP) and pyridoxamine-5'-phosphate (PMP) (Generation of leaving group potential)
B_7	Biotin	Leafy vegetables	30 (µg)	–	biotin (carboxylation reactions)
B_9	Folic acid/folate	Leafy vegetables, legumes, citrus fruits	400 (µg)	1000 µg	tetrahydrofolates inc. methyltetrahydrofolate *(One carbon transfer)*
B_{12}	Vitamin B_{12} (referring to: the cobalamins)	Supplemented plant-based foods, and supplements	2.4 (µg)	–	Methylcobalamin, adenosylcobalamin (vicinal rearrangements)

[1] Recommended Daily Allowance; [2] Upper limit — Food and Nutrition Board, Institute of Medicine, USA estimated "adequate intake" due to lack of data required to arrive at an RDA.

Table 4: The B Vitamins, symptoms of deficiency, and risk factors (over and above low consumption) (53)

Vitamin	Symptoms of Deficiency	Brain Specific Symptoms of Deficiency	Specific Risk Factors for Deficiency
B_1	Mild deficiency: general fatigue/weakness gastro-intestinal symptoms. (63) Deficiency: "Beri-beri"—Peripheral nerve damage and cardiovascular dysfunction leading to: pain, impaired sensory perception; swelling, weakness and pain in the limbs; shortness of breath, irregular heart rate, heart failure. (64)	Mild deficiency: irritability, emotional disturbances, confusion, disturbed sleep, memory loss. (63) Deficiency: Wernicke-Korsakoff syndrome (neurodegeneration, within the medial thalamus and cerebellum). Ataxia, abnormal motor function and eye movement, amnesia, apathy, confabulation. (64)	Alcohol abuse, obesity (63)
B_2	Weakness, oral pain/tenderness, burning/itching of the eyes, dermatitis, anemia. (65)	Fatigue, personality change, brain dysfunction. (65)	Inherited riboflavin malabsorption/utilization (10%–15% prevalence) (66)
B_3	Pellagra: dermatitis/photo dermatitis, alopecia, muscle weakness, twitching/burning in the extremities, altered gait, diarrhea. (67)	Depression, anxiety, progressing to vertigo, memory loss, paranoia, psychotic symptoms, aggression (Pellagrous insanity) (67)	Alcohol abuse
B_5	Numbness/burning sensations in extremities, dermatitis, diarrhea. (68)	Encephalopathy, behavior change, demyelination. (68)	
B_6	Anemia	Irritability, impaired alertness, depression, cognitive decline, dementia, autonomic dysfunction, convulsions. (69)	Alcohol abuse, age-related malabsorption, contraceptive medications. (70)

B_7	Seborrheic eczematous rash, tingling/burning of the extremities. (71)	Depression, lethargy, hallucinations, seizures. (71)	Type II diabetes, poor gluco-regulation (72)
B_9	Megaloblastic anaemia, peripheral neuropathy, spinal cord lesions, metabolic abnormalities. (73, 74)	Affective disorders , behavior changes, psychosis, cognitive impairment/ decline, dementia (inc Alzheimer's disease and vascular dementia). (73)	Common genetic polymorphisms (inc. MTHFR C667T) (75) Low Riboflavin and B_{12} (76)
B_{12}	See separate article on Vitamin B_{12}		

6.3 Vitamin C

The recognition of vitamin C is associated with the search for the cause of the hemorrhagic disease, scurvy. Isolated in 1928, vitamin C is essential for the development and maintenance of connective tissues. It plays an important role in bone formation, wound healing and the maintenance of healthy gums. Vitamin C plays an important role in a number of metabolic functions including the activation of the B vitamin, folic acid, the conversion of cholesterol to bile acids and the conversion of the amino acid, tryptophan, to the neurotransmitter, serotonin. It is an antioxidant that protects body from free radical damage. (77)

Deficiency of this vitamin is often associated with anemia, infections, bleeding gums, scurvy, poor wound healing, capillary hemorrhage, muscle degeneration, atherosclerotic plaques and neurotic disturbances. For the correction of deficiency, vitamin C is often supplemented in large doses and unlike fat soluble vitamins, toxicity is rare. (77) However, vitamin C deficiency and scurvy are rare in developed countries. (78)

A well-planned plant-based diet is unlikely to be deficient in in vitamin C as there are numerous plant sources. Vitamin C is found in citrus fruits, green peppers, red peppers, strawberries, tomatoes, broccoli, brussels sprouts, turnips and leafy vegetables. (77) Supplements typically contain vitamin C in the form of ascorbic acid, which has equivalent bioavailability to that of naturally occurring ascorbic acid in foods, such as orange juice and broccoli. (79, 80, 81) Other forms of vitamin C supplements include sodium ascorbate; calcium ascorbate; and other mineral ascorbates.

Table 5: Recommended Dietary Allowances for Vitamin C (78)

Age	Male	Female	Pregnancy	Lactation
0–6 months	40 mg*	40 mg*		
7–12 months	50 mg*	50 mg*		
1–3 years	15 mg	15 mg		
4–8 years	25 mg	25 mg		
9–13 years	45 mg	45 mg		
14–18 years	75 mg	65 mg	80 mg	115 mg
19+ years	90 mg	75 mg	85 mg	120 mg
Smokers	Individuals who smoke require 35 mg/day more vitamin C than nonsmokers.			

Table 6: Selected Food Sources of Vitamin C (32)

Food	Milligrams (mg) per serving	Percent (%) DV*
Red pepper, sweet, raw, ½ cup	95	158
Orange juice, ¾ cup	93	155
Orange, 1 medium	70	117
Grapefruit juice, ¾ cup	70	117
Kiwifruit, 1 medium	64	107
Green pepper, sweet, raw, ½ cup	60	100
Broccoli, cooked, ½ cup	51	85
Strawberries, fresh, sliced, ½ cup	49	82

Food	Milligrams (mg) per serving	Percent (%) DV*
Brussels sprouts, cooked, ½ cup	48	80
Grapefruit, ½ medium	39	65
Broccoli, raw, ½ cup	39	65
Tomato juice, ¾ cup	33	55
Cantaloupe, ½ cup	29	48
Cabbage, cooked, ½ cup	28	47
Cauliflower, raw, ½ cup	26	43
Potato, baked, 1 medium	17	28
Tomato, raw, 1 medium	17	28
Spinach, cooked, ½ cup	9	15
Green peas, frozen, cooked, ½ cup	8	13

Vitamin D is addressed in a separate article in the Nutritional Considerations In-depth section.

6. 4 Vitamin E

Vitamin E is found naturally in some foods, added to others, and available as a dietary supplement.

Vitamin E is the collective name for a group of fat-soluble compounds with distinctive antioxidant activities, specifically that stop the production of reactive oxygen species formed when fat undergoes oxidation. (82) Naturally occurring vitamin E exists in eight chemical forms (alpha-, beta-, gamma-, and delta-tocopherol and alpha-, beta-, gamma-, and delta-tocotrienol) that have varying levels of biological activity. (83) Alpha- (or α-) tocopherol is the only form that is recognized to meet human requirements.

In addition to its activities as an antioxidant, vitamin E is involved in immune function and, as shown primarily by in vitro studies of cells, cell signaling, regulation of gene expression, and other metabolic processes. (83) Alpha-tocopherol inhibits the activity of protein kinase C, an enzyme involved in cell proliferation and differentiation in smooth muscle cells, platelets, and monocytes. (78) Vitamin-E–replete endothelial cells lining the interior surface of blood vessels are better able to resist blood-cell components adhering to this surface. Vitamin E also increases the expression of two enzymes that suppress arachidonic acid metabolism, thereby increasing the release of prostacyclin from the endothelium, which, in turn, dilates blood vessels and inhibits platelet aggregation. (78)

Numerous foods provide vitamin E. Nuts, seeds, and vegetable oils are among the best sources of alpha-tocopherol, and significant amounts are available in green leafy vegetables and fortified cereals. Most vitamin E in American diets is in the form of gamma-tocopherol from soybean, canola, corn, and other vegetable oils and food products. (84) Frank vitamin E deficiency is rare and overt deficiency symptoms are unusual in otherwise healthy people. (78)

Table 7: Selected Food Sources of Vitamin E (Alpha-Tocopherol) (32)

Food	Milligrams (mg) per serving	Percent DV*
Wheat germ oil, 1 tablespoon	20.3	100
Sunflower seeds, dry roasted, 1 ounce	7.4	37
Almonds, dry roasted, 1 ounce	6.8	34
Sunflower oil, 1 tablespoon	5.6	28
Safflower oil, 1 tablespoon	4.6	25
Hazelnuts, dry roasted, 1 ounce	4.3	22
Peanut butter, 2 tablespoons	2.9	15
Peanuts, dry roasted, 1 ounce	2.2	11
Corn oil, 1 tablespoon	1.9	10
Spinach, boiled, ½ cup	1.9	10
Broccoli, chopped, boiled, ½ cup	1.2	6
Soybean oil, 1 tablespoon	1.1	6
Kiwifruit, 1 medium	1.1	6
Mango, sliced, ½ cup	0.7	4
Tomato, raw, 1 medium	0.7	4
Spinach, raw, 1 cup	0.6	3

DV = Daily Value

Table 8: Recommended Dietary Allowances for Vitamin E (Alpha-Tocopherol) (78)

Age	Males	Females	Pregnancy	Lactation
0–6 months*	4 mg (6 IU)	4 mg (6 IU)		
7–12 months*	5 mg (7.5 IU)	5 mg (7.5 IU)		
1–3 years	6 mg (9 IU)	6 mg (9 IU)		
4–8 years	7 mg (10.4 IU)	7 mg (10.4 IU)		
9–13 years	11 mg (16.4 IU)	11 mg (16.4 IU)		
14+ years	15 mg (22.4 IU)	15 mg (22.4 IU)	15 mg (22.4 IU)	19 mg (28.4 IU)

Because the digestive tract requires fat to absorb vitamin E, people with fat-malabsorption disorders are more likely to become deficient than people without such disorders. Deficiency symptoms include peripheral neuropathy, ataxia, skeletal myopathy, retinopathy, and impairment of the immune response. (78, 85) People with Crohn's disease, cystic fibrosis, or an inability to secrete bile from the liver into the digestive tract, for example, often pass greasy stools or have chronic diarrhea; as a result, they sometimes require water-soluble forms of vitamin E, such as tocopheryl polyethylene glycol-1000 succinate. (83)

In general, clinical trials have not provided evidence that routine use of vitamin E supplements prevents cardiovascular disease or reduces its morbidity and mortality. Most research results do not support the use of vitamin E supplements by healthy or mildly impaired individuals to maintain cognitive performance or slow its decline with normal aging. Evidence to date is insufficient to support taking vitamin E to prevent cancer. Patients should not exceed the upper limits listed in Table 9.

Table 9: Tolerable Upper Intake Levels for Vitamin E (78)

Age	Male	Female	Pregnancy	Lactation
1–3 years	200 mg (300 IU)	200 mg (300 IU)		
4–8 years	300 mg (450 IU)	300 mg (450 IU)		
9–13 years	600 mg (900 IU)	600 mg (900 IU)		
14–18 years	800 mg (1200 IU)	800 mg (1200 IU)	800 mg (1200 IU)	800 mg (1200 IU)
19+ years	1000 mg (1500 IU)	1000 mg (1500 IU)	1,000 mg (1500 IU)	1000 mg (1500 IU)

6.5 Vitamin K

"Vitamin K," the generic name for a family of compounds with a common chemical structure of 2-methyl-1,4-naphthoquinone, is a fat-soluble vitamin that is naturally present in some foods and is available as a dietary supplement. (86) These compounds include phylloquinone (vitamin K1) and a series of menaquinones (vitamin K2). (87) Menaquinones have unsaturated isoprenyl side chains and are designated as MK-4 through MK-13, based on the length of their side chain. (86, 87) MK-4, MK-7, and MK-9 are the most well-studied menaquinones.

Phylloquinone is present primarily in plant foods and is the main dietary form of vitamin K. (44) Menaquinones, which are predominantly of bacterial origin, are present in modest amounts in various animal-based and fermented foods. (86) Almost all menaquinones, in particular the long-chain menaquinones, are also produced by bacteria in the human gut. (88, 89) MK-4 is unique in that it is produced by the body from phylloquinone via a conversion process that does not involve bacterial action. (90)

Vitamin K interacts with a few medications. In addition, certain medications can have an adverse effect on vitamin K levels.

Vitamin K functions as a coenzyme for vitamin K-dependent carboxylase, an enzyme required for the synthesis of proteins involved in hemostasis (blood clotting) and bone metabolism, and other diverse physiological functions. (44, 88) Prothrombin (clotting factor II) is a vitamin K-dependent protein in plasma that is directly involved in blood clotting. Warfarin (Coumadin®) and some anticoagulants used primarily in Europe, antagonize the activity of vitamin K and, in turn, prothrombin. (91) For this reason, individuals who are taking these anticoagulants need to maintain consistent vitamin K intakes. However, many plant foods are very high in vitamin K. Patients being treated with Warfarin might require more careful monitoring.

Antibiotics can destroy vitamin K-producing bacteria in the gut, potentially decreasing vitamin K status. This effect might be more pronounced with cephalosporin antibiotics, such as cefoperazone (Cefobid®), because these antibiotics might also inhibit the action of vitamin K in the body. (89, 92) Vitamin K supplements are usually not needed unless antibiotic use is prolonged (beyond several weeks) and accompanied by poor vitamin K intake. (92)

Bile acid sequestrants, such as cholestyramine (Questran®) and colestipol (Colestid®), are used to reduce cholesterol levels by preventing reabsorption of bile acids. They can also reduce the absorption of vitamin K and other fat-soluble vitamins, although the clinical significance of this effect is not clear. (92, 93) Vitamin K status should be monitored in people taking these medications, especially when the drugs are used for many years. (93)

Orlistat is a weight-loss drug that is available as both an over-the-counter (Alli®) and prescription (Xenical®) medication. It reduces the body's absorption of dietary fat and in doing so, it can also reduce the absorption of fat-soluble vitamins, such as vitamin K. Combining orlistat with warfarin therapy might cause a significant increase in prothrombin time. (94) Otherwise, orlistat does not usually have a clinically significant effect on vitamin K status, although clinicians usually recommend that patients taking orlistat take a multivitamin supplement containing vitamin K. (95, 96, 97)

Osteocalcin is another vitamin K-dependent protein that is present in bone and may be involved in bone mineralization or turnover. (88)

People with malabsorption syndromes and other gastrointestinal disorders, such as cystic fibrosis, celiac disease, ulcerative colitis, and short bowel syndrome, might not absorb vitamin K properly. (44, 88, 98) Vitamin K status can also be low in patients who have undergone bariatric surgery, although clinical signs may not be present. (99) These individuals might need monitoring of vitamin K status and, in some cases, vitamin K supplementation.

In the circulation, vitamin K is carried mainly in lipoproteins. (100) Compared to the other fat-soluble vitamins, very small amounts of vitamin K circulate in the blood. Vitamin K is rapidly metabolized and excreted. Based on phylloquinone measurements, the body retains only about 30% to 40% of an oral physiological dose, while about 20% is excreted in the urine and 40% to 50% in the feces via bile. (87, 100) This rapid metabolism accounts for vitamin K's relatively low blood levels and tissue stores compared to those of the other fat-soluble vitamins. (100)

The Food and Nutrition Board did not establish upper limits for vitamin K because of its low potential for toxicity. (44) In its report, the FNB stated that "no adverse effects associated with vitamin K consumption from food or supplements have been reported in humans or animals."

Table 10: Adequate Intakes for Vitamin K (44)

Age	Male	Female	Pregnancy	Lactation
Birth to 6 months	2.0 mcg	2.0 mcg		
7–12 months	2.5 mcg	2.5 mcg		
1–3 years	30 mcg	30 mcg		
4–8 years	55 mcg	55 mcg		
9–13 years	60 mcg	60 mcg		
14–18 years	75 mcg	75 mcg	75 mcg	75 mcg
19+ years	120 mcg	90 mcg	90 mcg	90 mcg

Table 11: Selected Food Sources of Vitamin K (32, 101)

Food	Micrograms (mcg) per serving	Percent DV*
Collards, frozen, boiled, ½ cup	530	662
Turnip greens, frozen, boiled ½ cup	426	532
Spinach, raw, 1 cup	145	181
Kale, raw, 1 cup	113	141
Broccoli, chopped, boiled, ½ cup	110	138
Soybeans, roasted, ½ cup	43	54
Carrot juice, ¾ cup	28	34
Soybean oil, 1 tablespoon	25	31
Edamame, frozen, prepared, ½ cup	21	26
Pumpkin, canned, ½ cup	20	25
Pomegranate juice, ¾ cup	19	24

Okra, raw, ½ cup	16	20
Pine nuts, dried, 1 ounce	15	19
Blueberries, raw, ½ cup	14	18
Iceberg lettuce, raw, 1 cup	14	18
Grapes, ½ cup	11	14
Vegetable juice cocktail, ¾ cup	10	13
Canola oil, 1 tablespoon	10	13
Cashews, dry roasted, 1 ounce	10	13
Carrots, raw, 1 medium	8	10

7. Phytonutrients

Naturally occurring compounds found in foods of plant origin, known as phytonutrients or phytochemicals (phyto means plant in Greek), are thought to be partly responsible for the protective health benefits of plant-based foods and beverages, beyond those conferred by their vitamin and mineral contents. These phytonutrients, which are part of a large and varied group of chemical compounds, also are responsible for the color, flavor, and odor of plant foods, such as blueberries' dark hue, broccoli's bitter taste, and garlic's pungent odor.

Research strongly suggests that consuming foods rich in phytonutrients provides health benefits. (3, 102) Phytonutrients are reported to have antioxidant and anti-carcinogenic properties, as well as a spectrum of potential tumor-blocking activities. (103, 104) Studies show that there are as many as 100 different phytonutrients in just one serving of vegetables. (104) Each phytonutrient comes from a variety of plant sources, and has different effects and benefits on the body. Some researchers estimate that there are up to 4000 phytonutrients in existence. (104)

Phytonutrients are found in fruits, vegetables, whole grains, legumes, herbs, spices, nuts, and seeds and are classified according to their chemical structures and functional properties. They include flavonoids, flavonols, flavanols, proanthocyanidins, and procyanidins. Phytonutrients also include compounds such as salicylates, phytosterols, saponins, glucosinolates, polyphenols, protease inhibitors, monoterpenes, carotenoids, phytoestrogens, sulfides, terpenes, lectins, and many more.

Though the broadest groups of phytonutrients, such as flavonoids, isoflavones, or anthocyanidins, often are referred to as if they were a homogenous group, the individual compounds within each group have different chemical structures, are metabolized differently by the body, and may have different health effects. (105) In addition, part of the health benefits of a plant-based diet may result from additive and synergistic combinations of phytonutrients present in whole and minimally processed foods, which may be responsible for their potent antioxidant and anticancer activities. (106)

Studies have found that phytonutrients have the potential to stimulate the immune system, prevent toxic substances in the diet from becoming carcinogenic, reduce inflammation, prevent DNA damage and aid DNA repair, reduce oxidative damage to cells, slow the growth rate of cancer cells, trigger damaged cells to apoptosis before they can reproduce, help regulate intracellular signaling of hormones and gene expression, and activate insulin receptors. (107, 108) In addition, there likely are health effects of phytonutrients that researchers haven't yet recognized. (107)

Many other studies have focused on the antioxidant function of phytonutrients. For many of the phytonutrients in food, their antioxidant effects on cell signaling and gene expression may be more important for health benefits than direct antioxidant activity, effects that can be seen even with low concentrations of phytonutrients in plasma and tissues. (109)

There's little information on the average intake of phytonutrients among Americans. However, it shouldn't be surprising that the intake of phytonutrients is higher among people consuming a plant-based diet. (110)

References

1. Melina V, Craig W, Levin S. (2016) Position of the academy of nutrition and dietetics: vegetarian diets. *J Acad Nutr Diet.* 116(12):1970-80.
2. Martínez Steele E, Baraldi L, Louzada M, Moubarac J, Mozaffarian D, Monteiro C. (2016) Ultra-processed foods and added sugars in the US diet: evidence from a nationally representative cross-sectional study. *BMJ Open* 6(3):e009892.
3. Webb D. (2013) Phytochemicals' Role in Good Health. *Today's Dietitian* 15(9):70.
4. Karlsen M, Rogers G, Miki A, et al. (2019) Theoretical food and nutrient composition of whole-food plant-based and vegan diets compared to current dietary recommendations. *Nutrients 11*(3):625.
5. Mariotti F, Gardner C. (2019) Dietary protein and amino acids in vegetarian diets - a review. *Nutrients* 11(11):2661.
6. Mariotti F. (2017) Plant protein, animal protein, and protein quality. In: Mariotti F, ed. *Vegetarian and Plant-Based Diets in Health and Disease Prevention*. 1st ed. Cambridge, MA: Academic Press.
7. Sobiecki J, Appleby P, Bradbury K, Key T. (2016) High compliance with dietary recommendations in a cohort of meat eaters, fish eaters, vegetarians, and vegans: results from the European Prospective Investigation into Cancer and Nutrition-Oxford study. *Nutr Res* 36(5):464-477.
8. Schmidt J, Rinaldi S, Scalbert A, et al. (2016) Plasma concentrations and intakes of amino acids in male meat-eaters, fish-eaters, vegetarians and vegans: a cross-sectional analysis in the EPIC-Oxford cohort. *Eur J Clin Nutr* 70(3):306-312.
9. Allès B, Baudry J, Méjean C, et al. (2017) Comparison of Sociodemographic and Nutritional Characteristics between Self-Reported Vegetarians, Vegans, and Meat-Eaters from the NutriNet-Santé Study. *Nutrients* 9(9):E1023.
10. Rizzo N, Jaceldo-Siegl K, Sabate J, Fraser G. (2013) Nutrient profiles of vegetarian and nonvegetarian dietary patterns. *J Acad Nutr Diet* 113(12):1610-1619.
11. Clarys P, Deliens T, Huybrechts I, et al. (2014) Comparison of nutritional quality of the vegan, vegetarian, semi-vegetarian, pesco-vegetarian and omnivorous diet. *Nutrients* 6(3):1318-1332.

12. Nasset E. (1972) Amino acid homeostasis in the gut lumen and its nutritional significance. *World Rev Nutr Diet* 14:134-153.
13. Nasset E. (1957) Role of the digestive tract in the utilization of protein and amino acids. *JAMA* 164(2):172-177.
14. Fuller M, Reeds P. (1998) Nitrogen cycling in the gut. *Ann Rev Nutr* 18:385-411.
15. Badaloo A, Boyne M, Reid M, et al. (1999) Dietary protein, growth and urea kinetics in severely malnourished children and during recovery. *J Nutr* 129(5):969-979.
16. Millward D. (1999) The nutritional value of plant-based diets in relation to human amino acid and protein requirements. *Proc Nutr Soc* 58(2):249-260.
17. Holesh J, Martin A. (2019) Physiology, Carbohydrates. *StatPearls [Internet]*. Treasure Island (FL): StatPearls Publishing.
18. Institute of Medicine, Food and Nutrition Board. (2002) *Dietary Reference Intakes for energy, carbohydrate, fiber, fat, fatty acids, cholesterol, protein and amino acids*. Washington DC: National Academies Press.
19. Jenkins D, Wolever T, Taylor R, et al. (1981) Glycemic index of foods: a physiological basis for carbohydrate exchange. *Am J Clin Nutr* 34(3):362-366.
20. Jenkins D, Wolever T, Jenkins A, et al. (1983) The glycaemic index of foods tested in diabetic patients: a new basis for carbohydrate exchange favouring the use of legumes. *Diabetologia* 24(4):257-264.
21. Jenkins D, Kendall C, Augustin L, et al. (2002) Glycemic index: overview of implications in health and disease. *Am J Clin Nutr* 76(1):266S-273S.
22. Atkinson F, Foster-Powell K, Brand-Miller J. (2008) International tables of glycemic index and glycemic load values: 2008. *Diabetes Care* 31(12):2281-2283.
23. Lichtenstein A, Appel L, Brands M, et al. (2006) Diet and lifestyle recommendations revision 2006: a scientific statement from the American Heart Association Nutrition Committee. *Circulation* 114(1):82-96.
24. Park Y, Subar A, Hollenbeck A, Schatzkin A. (2011) Dietary fiber intake and mortality in the NIH-AARP diet and health study. *Arch Intern Med* 171(12):1061-1068.
25. Anderson J, Baird P, Davis RJ, et al. (2009) Health benefits of dietary fiber. *Nutr Rev* 67(4):188-205.
26. Dhingra D, M M, Rajput H, Patil R. (2012) Dietary fibre in foods: a review. *J Food Sci Technol* 49(3):255-266.
27. Bindels L, Delzenne N, Cani P, Walter J. (2015) Towards a more comprehensive concept for prebiotics. *Nat Rev Gastroenterol Hepatol* 12(5):303-310.
28. Moshfegh A, Friday J, Goldman J, Ahuja J. (1999) Presence of inulin and oligofructose in the diets of Americans. *J Nutr* 129(7 Suppl):1407S-1411S.
29. van Loo J, Coussement P, de Leenheer L, Hoebregs H, Smits G. (1995) On the presence of inulin and oligofructose as natural ingredients in the western diet. *Crit Rev Food Sci Nutr* 35(6):525-552.
30. Sabater-Molina M, Larqué E, Torrella F, Zamora S. (2009) Dietary fructooligosaccharides and potential benefits on health. *J Physiol Biochem* 65(3):315-328.
31. Eilander A, Harika R, Zock P. (2015) Intake and sources of dietary fatty acids in Europe: Are current population intakes of fats aligned with dietary recommendations? *Eur J Lipid Sci Technol* 117(9):1370-1377.
32. USDA. FoodData Central Search. *USDA Agricultural Research Service*.
33. Harika R, Eilander A, Alssema M, Osendarp S, Zock P. (2013) Intake of fatty acids in general populations worldwide does not meet dietary recommendations to prevent coronary heart disease: a systematic review of data from 40 countries. *Ann Nutr Metab* 63(3):229-238.

34. Sacks F, Lichtenstein A, Wu J, Appel L, Creager M, et al. (2017) Dietary Fats and Cardiovascular Disease: A Presidential Advisory From the American Heart Association. *Circulation* 136(3):e1-e23.

35. Risérus U, Willett W, Hu F. (2009) Dietary fats and the prevention of type 2 diabetes. *Prog Lipid Res* 48(1):44-51.

36. Nettleton J, Brouwer I, Geleijnse J, Hornstra G. (2017) Saturated Fat Consumption and Risk of Coronary Heart Disease and Ischemic Stroke: A Science Update. *Ann Nutr Metab* 70(1):26-33.

37. Eyres L, Eyres M, Chisholm A, Brown R. (2016) Coconut oil consumption and cardiovascular risk factors in humans. *Nutr Rev* 74(4):267-280.

38. Mozaffarian D, Clarke R. (2009) Quantitative effects on cardiovascular risk factors and coronary heart disease risk of replacing partially hydrogenated vegetable oils with other fats and oils. *Eur J Clin Nutr* 63(Suppl 2):S22-S33.

39. National Institutes of Health. Vitamin A Fact Sheet for Consumers. *National Institutes of Health Office of Dietary Supplements.*

40. Johnson E, Russell R. (2010) Beta-Carotene. In: Coates P, Betz J, Blackman M, et al, eds. *Encyclopedia of Dietary Supplements*. 2nd ed. London and New York: Informa Healthcare.

41. Ross C. (2010) Vitamin A. In: Coates P, Betz J, Blackman M, et al, eds. *Encyclopedia of Dietary Supplements*. 2nd ed. London and New York: Informa Healthcare.

42. Ross A. (2006) Vitamin A and Carotenoids. In: Shils M, Shike M, Ross A, Cabellero B, R C, eds. *Modern Nutrition in Health and Disease*. 10th ed. Baltimore, MD: Lippincott Williams & Wilkins.

43. Solomons N. (2006) Vitamin A. In: Bowman B, Russell R, eds. *Present Knowledge in Nutrition*. 9th ed. Washington DC: International Life Sciences Institute.

44. Institute of Medicine (US) Panel on Micronutrients. (2001) *Dietary Reference Intakes for Vitamin A, Vitamin K, Arsenic, Boron, Chromium, Copper, Iodine, Iron, Manganese, Molybdenum, Nickel, Silicon, Vanadium, and Zinc*. Washington DC: National Academies Press (US).

45. US FDA Center for Food Safety and Applied Nutrition. (2019) *Converting Units of Measure for Folate, Niacin, and Vitamins A, D, and E on the Nutrition and Supplement Facts Labels: Guidance for Industry*. Rockville, MD: US Department of Health and Human Services Food and Drug Administration.

46. Institute of Medicine, Food and Nutrition Board. (2001) *Dietary reference intakes for Vitamin A, Vitamin K, Arsenic, Boron, Chromium, Copper, Iodine, Iron, Manganese, Molybdenum, Nickel, Silicon, Vanadium, and Zinc*. Washington (DC): National Academies Press (US).

47. Grune T, Lietz G, Palou A, et al. (2010) Beta-carotene is an important vitamin A source for humans. *J Nutr* 140(12):2268S-2285S.

48. Stahl W, Heinrich U, Jungmann H, et al. (1998) Increased dermal carotenoid levels assessed by noninvasive reflection spectrophotometry correlate with serum levels in women ingesting Betatene. *J Nutr* 128(5):903-907.

49. Natural Medicines. (2011) Vitamin A. *Natural Medicines Therapeutic research*.

50. Genentech USA, Inc. (2015) Highlights of Prescribing Information - Xenical. *Food and Drug Administration*.

51. GlaxoSmithKline. (2018) Alli Drug Description. *Rx List*.

52. McCormick D. (2007) Bioorganic mechanisms important to coenzyme functions. In: Rucker R, Zempleni J, Suttie J, McCormick D, eds. *Handbook of Vitamins*. 4th ed. Boca Raton, FL: CRC Press.

53. Kennedy D. (2016) B Vitamins and the Brain: Mechanisms, Dose and Efficacy--A Review. *Nutrients* 8(2):68.

54. Fattal-Valevski A. (2011) Thiamine (Vitamin B1). *J Evid Based Complement Alternat Med* 16(1):12-20.

55. Alternative Medicine Review. (2008) Riboflavin. *Alternative Med Rev* 13(4):334-340.
56. Whitney E, Rolfes S, Crowe T, Cameron-Smith D, Walsh A. (2011) *Understanding Nutrition*. 12th ed ed. Melbourne, Aus: Cengage Learning.
57. Institute of Medicine (US). (1998) *Dietary Reference Intakes for Thiamin, Riboflavin, Niacin, Vitamin B6, Folate, Vitamin B12, Pantothenic Acid, Biotin, and Choline*. Washington, DC: National Academies Press.
58. University of Bristol. (2002) Pantothenic Acid. *University of Bristol School of Chemistry*.
59. Gropper S, Smith J, Groff J. (2009) *Advanced nutrition and human metabolism*. 5th ad ed. Belmont, CA: Cengage Learning.
60. Parra M, Stahl S, Hellmann H. (2018) Vitamin B6 and its role in cell metabolism and physiology. *Cells* 7(7):84.
61. University of Bristol. (2002) Vitamin B6 (Pyridoxine). *University of Bristol School of Chemistry*.
62. University of Bristol. (2002) Biotin. *University of Bristol School of Chemistry*.
63. Kerns J, Arundel C, Chawla L. (2015) Thiamin deficiency in people with obesity. *Adv Nutr* 6(2):147-153.
64. Bates C. Thiamine. (2007) In: Zempleni J, Rucker R, McCormick D, Suttie J, eds. *Handbook of Vitamins*. 4th ed. Boca Raton, FL: CRC Press.
65. Rivlin R. (2007) Riboflavin (vitamin B2). In: Zempleni J, Rucker R, McCormick D, Suttie J, eds. *Handbook of Vitamins*. 4th ed. Boca Raton, FL: CRC Press.
66. Sinigaglia-Coimbra R, Lopes A, Coimbra C. (2011) Riboflavin deficiency, brain function, and health. In: Preedy V, Watson R, Martin C, eds. *Handbook of Behavior, Food and Nutrition*. Berlin, Germany: Springer.
67. Kirkland J. (2007) Niacin. In: Zempleni J, Rucker R, McCormick D, Suttie J, eds. *Handbook of Vitamins*. 4th ed. Boca Raton, FL: CRC Press.
68. Rucker R, Bauerly K. (2013) Pantothenic acid. In: Zempleni J, Suttie J, Gregory J, Stover P, eds. *Handbook of Vitamins*. 5th ed. Boca Raton, FL: CRC Press.
69. Dakshinamurti S, Dakshinamurti K. (2013) Vitamin B6. In: Zempleni J, Suttie J, Gregory J, Stover P, eds. *Handbook of Vitamins*. 5th ed. Boca Raton, FL: CRC Press.
70. Morris M, Picciano M, Jacques P, Selhub J. (2008) Plasma pyridoxal 5'-phosphate in the US population: the National Health and Nutrition Examination Survey, 2003-2004. *Am J Clin Nutr* 87(5):1446-1454.
71. Mock D. Biotin. (2007) In: Zempleni J, Rucker R, McCormick D, Suttie J, eds. *Handbook of Vitamins*. 4th ed. Boca Raton, FL: CRC Press.
72. Via M. (2012) The malnutrition of obesity: micronutrient deficiencies that promote diabetes. *ISRN Endocrinol* 2012:103472.
73. Reynolds E. (2006) Vitamin B12, folic acid, and the nervous system. *Lancet Neurol* 5(11):949-960.
74. Green R, Miller J. (2007) Vitamin B12. In: Zempleni J, Rucker R, McCormick D, Suttie J, eds. *Handbook of Vitamins*. 4th ed. Boca Raton, FL: CRC Press.
75. Mitchell E, Conus N, Kaput J. (2014) B vitamin polymorphisms and behavior: evidence of associations with neurodevelopment, depression, schizophrenia, bipolar disorder and cognitive decline. *Neurosci Biobehav Rev* 47:307-320.
76. García-Minguillán C, Fernandez-Ballart J, Ceruelo S, et al. (2014) Riboflavin status modifies the effects of methylenetetrahydrofolate reductase (MTHFR) and methionine synthase reductase (MTRR) polymorphisms on homocysteine. *Genes Nutr* 9(6):435.
77. Chambial S, Dwivedi S, Shukla K, John P, Sharma P. (2013) Vitamin C in disease prevention and cure: an overview. *Indian J Clin Biochem* 28(4):314-328.
78. Institute of Medicine (US) Panel on Dietary Antioxidants and Related Compounds. (2000)

Dietary Reference Intakes for Vitamin C, Vitamin E, Selenium, and Carotenoids. Washington DC: National Academies Press.

79. Bates C. (1997) Bioavailability of vitamin C. *Eur J Clin Nutr* 51(Suppl 1):S28-S33.
80. Mangels A, Block G, Frey C, et al. (1993) The bioavailability to humans of ascorbic acid from oranges, orange juice and cooked broccoli is similar to that of synthetic ascorbic acid. *J Nutr* 123(6):1054-1061.
81. Gregory J. (1993) Ascorbic acid bioavailability in foods and supplements. *Nutr Rev* 51(10):301-303.
82. Verhagen H, Buijsse B, Jansen E, Bueno-de-Mesquita H. (2006) The state of antioxidant affairs. *Nutr Today* 41(6):244-250.
83. Traber M. (2006) Vitamin E. In: Shils M, Shike M, Ross A, Caballero B, Cousins R, eds. *Modern Nutrition in HEalth and Disease*. 10th ed. Baltimore, MD, USA: Lippincott Williams & Wilkins.
84. Dietrich M, Traber M, Jacques P, Cross C, Hu Y, Block G. (2006) Does gamma-tocopherol play a role in the primary prevention of heart disease and cancer? A review. *J Am Coll Nutr* 25(4):292-299.
85. Kowdley K, Mason J, Meydani S, Cornwall S, Grand R. (1992) Vitamin E deficiency and impaired cellular immunity related to intestinal fat malabsorption. *Gastroenterology* 102(6):2139-2142.
86. Booth S. (2012) Vitamin K: food composition and dietary intakes. *Food Nutr Res* 56:10.3402.
87. Ferland G. (2012) Vitamin K. In: Erdman J, Macdonald I, Zeisel S, eds. *Present knowledge in nutrition*. 10th ed. Washington DC: Wiley-Blackwell.
88. Suttie J. (2010) Vitamin K. In: Coates P, Betz J, Blackman M, GM C, Levine M, al e, eds. *Encyclopedia of Dietary Supplements*. 2nd ed. London and New York: Informa Healthcare.
89. Conly J, Stein K, Worobetz L, Rutledge-Harding S. (1994) The contribution of vitamin K2 (menaquinones) produced by the intestinal microflora to human nutritional requirements for vitamin K. *Am J Gastroenterol* 89(6):915-923.
90. Suttie J. (2014) Vitamin K. In: Ross A, Caballero B, Cousins R, Tucker K, Ziegler T, eds. *Modern Nutrition in Health and Disease*. 11th ed. Baltimore, MD: Lippincott Williams & Wilkins.
91. Ufer M. (2005) Comparative pharmacokinetics of vitamin K antagonists: warfarin, phenprocoumon and acenocoumarol. *Clin Pharmacokinet* 44(12):1227-1246.
92. Natural Medicines. (2014) Vitamin K. *Natural Medicines Comprehensive Database*.
93. Vroonhof K, van Rijn H, van Hattum J. (2003) Vitamin K deficiency and bleeding after long-term use of cholestyramine. *Neth J Med* 61(1):19-21.
94. MacWalter R, Fraser H, Armstrong K. (2003) Orlistat enhances warfarin effect. *Ann Pharmacother* 37(4):510-512.
95. McDuffie J, Calis K, Booth S, Uwaifo G, Yanovski J. (2002) Effects of orlistat on fat-soluble vitamins in obese adolescents. *Pharmacotherapy* 22(7):814-822.
96. Davidson M, Hauptman J DMFJHC, Heber D, et al. (1999) Weight control and risk factor reduction in obese subjects treated for 2 years with orlistat: a randomized controlled trial. *JAMA* 281(3):235-242.
97. US National Library of Medicine. (2014) Orlistat. *MedlinePlus*.
98. Jagannath V, Fedorowicz Z, Thaker V, Chang A. (2011) Vitamin K supplementation for cystic fibrosis. *Cochrane Database Syst Rev* 19(1):CD008482.
99. Heber D, Greenway F, Kaplan L, et al. (2010) Endocrine and nutritional management of the post-bariatric surgery patient: an Endocrine Society Clinical Practice Guideline. *J Clin Endocrinol Metab* 95(11):4823-4843.

100. Shearer M, Newman P. (2008) Metabolism and cell biology of vitamin K. *Thromb Haemost* 100(4):530-547.

101. Schurgers L, Vermeer C. (2000) Determination of phylloquinone and menaquinones in food. Effect of food matrix on circulating vitamin K concentrations. *Haemostasis* 30(6):298-307.

102. Arts I, Hollman P. (2005) Polyphenols and disease risk in epidemiologic studies. *Am J Clin Nutr* 81(1 Suppl):317S-325S.

103. Drewnowski A, Gomez-Carneros C. (2000) Bitter taste, phytonutrients, and the consumer: a review. *Am J Clin Nutr* 72(6):1424-1435.

104. Poe K. (2017) Plant-based diets and phytonutrients:potential health benefits and disease prevention. *iMedPub Journals* 9(6):7.

105. Erdman JJ, Balentine D, Arab L, et al. (2007) Flavonoids and heart health: proceedings of the ILSI North America Flavonoids Workshop, May 31-June 1, 2005, Washington, DC. *J Nutr* 137(3 Suppl 1):718S-737S.

106. Liu R. (2003) Health benefits of fruit and vegetables are from additive and synergistic combinations of phytochemicals. *Am J Clin Nutr* 78(3 Suppl):517S-520S.

107. World Cancer Research Fund/American Institute for Cancer Research. (2007) *Food, nutrition, physical activity, and the prevention of cancer: a global perspective*. Washington, DC: American Institute for Cancer Research.

108. Hanhineva K, Törrönen R, Bondia-Pons I, et al. (2010) Impact of dietary polyphenols on carbohydrate metabolism. *Int J Mol Sci* 11(4):1365-1402.

109. Gordon M. (2012) Significance of dietary antioxidants for health. *Int J Mol Sci* 13(1):173-179.

110. Murphy M, Barraj L, Herman D, Bi X, Cheatham R, Randolph R. (2012) Phytonutrient intake by adults in the United States in relation to fruit and vegetable consumption. *J Acad Nutr Diet* 112(2):222-229.

Appendix: Glycemic Index of Some Foods (22)

Food	Glycemic Index
High-Carbohydrate foods	
White wheat bread*	75 ± 2
Whole wheat/whole meal bread	74 ± 2
White rice, boiled*	73 ± 4
Unleavened wheat bread	70 ± 5
Brown rice, boiled	68 ± 4
Couscous†	65 ± 4
Wheat roti	62 ± 3
Rice noodles†	53 ± 7
Udon noodles	55 ± 7
Specialty grain bread	53 ± 2
Sweet corn	52 ± 5
Chapatti	52 ± 4
Spaghetti, white	49 ± 2
Spaghetti, whole meal	48 ± 5
Corn tortilla	46 ± 4
Barley	28 ± 2
Breakfast Cereals	
Cornflakes	81 ± 6
Instant oat porridge	79 ± 3
Rice porridge/congee	78 ± 9
Wheat flake biscuits	69 ± 2
Millet porridge	67 ± 5
Muesli	57 ± 2
Porridge, rolled oats	55 ± 2
Fruit and Fruit Products	
Watermelon, raw	76 ± 4
Pineapple, raw	59 ± 8
Mango, raw†	51 ± 5
Banana, raw†	51 ± 3
Orange juice	50 ± 2
Strawberry jam/jelly	49 ± 3
Peaches, canned†	43 ± 5
Orange, raw†	43 ± 3
Dates, raw	42 ± 4
Apple juice	41 ± 2
Apple, raw†	36 ± 2
Vegetables	
Potato, instant mash	87 ± 3
Potato, boiled	78 ± 4
Pumpkin, boiled	64 ± 7

Sweet potato, boiled	63 ± 6
Potato, french fries	63 ± 5
Plantain/green banana	55 ± 6
Taro, boiled	53 ± 2
Vegetable soup	48 ± 5
Carrots, boiled	39 ± 4
Dairy Alternatives	
Rice milk	86 ± 7
Soy milk	34 ± 4
Legumes	
Lentils	32 ± 5
Chickpeas	28 ± 9
Kidney beans	24 ± 4

Soya beans	16 ± 1
Snack Products	
Rice crackers/crisps	87 ± 2
Popcorn	65 ± 5
Soft drink/soda	59 ± 3
Potato crisps	56 ± 3
Chocolate	40 ± 3
Sugars	
Glucose	103 ± 3
Sucrose	65 ± 4
Honey	61 ± 3
Fructose	15 ± 4

Data are means ± SEM.

* Low-GI varieties were also identified.

† Average of all available data.

Advanced Research in Gastroenterology & Hepatology
ISSN: 2472-6400

Juniper Publishers
key to the Researchers

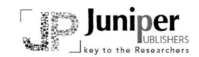

Mini Review
Volume 13 Issue 3 – July 2019
DOI: 10.19080/ARGH.2019.13.555862

Adv Res Gastroenterol Hepatol

Ensuring Adequate Vitamin B_{12} status on a Plant-Based Diet

Stewart D Rose* **and Amanda J Strombom**

Plant-Based Diets in Medicine, USA

Submission: June 18, 2019; **Published:** July 09, 2019

***Corresponding Author:** Stewart Rose, Plant-Based Diets in Medicine, 12819 SE 38th St, #427, Bellevue, WA 98006, USA

Abstract

Vitamin B_{12} is a water-soluble vitamin. All naturally occurring B_{12} is produced by bacteria in the soil. Animals ingest these bacteria along with their feed, resulting in their presence in animal-derived foods. It is also added to other foods as an enrichment, and is available as a dietary supplement.

Since patients on a plant-based diet eat no animal-derived foods, and only plant-foods cleaned of soil residue, they must rely on supplementation or fortified foods. Status is typically assessed via serum or plasma vitamin B_{12} levels. Injected Vitamin B_{12} appears to be equivalent to oral vitamin B_{12}, but there is no evidence that sublingual delivery offers any advantage over other oral preparations. Vitamin B_{12} has been demonstrated to be safe in doses up to 1,000 times the recommended dietary allowance and is safe in pregnancy.

It is vital that patients on a plant-based diet have adequate levels of Vitamin B_{12}. Vitamin B_{12} deficiency is characterized by megaloblastic anemia, fatigue, weakness, constipation, loss of appetite, and weight loss. Neurological changes, such as numbness and tingling in the hands and feet, can also occur. Due to conservation through enterohepatic recirculation, the body's stores of B_{12} may last the patient some time which can lead to complacency and give the patient a false sense of security. Therefore, the physician should emphasize the importance of vitamin B_{12} supplementation and the rationale for it.

Keywords:

B_{12} deficiency; Lactation; Megaloblastic anemia; Plant-based diet; Pregnancy; Supplementation; Vegan; Vegetarian; Vitamin B_{12}

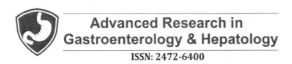

Abbreviations:

IF: Intrinsic Factor; Mcg: Micrograms; IOM: The Institute of Medicine; RDAs: Recommended Dietary Allowances; AI: Adequate Intake

1. Introduction

Vitamin B_{12} is a water-soluble vitamin that is naturally present in animal-derived foods. It is added to others and is available as a dietary supplement and a prescription medication. Vitamin B_{12} exists in several forms and contains the mineral cobalt, (1, 2, 3, 4) so compounds with vitamin B_{12} activity are collectively called "cobalamins". Methylcobalamin and 5-deoxyadenosylcobalamin are the forms of vitamin B_{12} that are active in human metabolism. (5)

Vitamin B_{12} is required for proper red blood cell formation, neurological function, and DNA synthesis. (1, 2, 3, 4, 5) Vitamin B_{12} functions as a cofactor for methionine synthase and L-methylmalonyl-CoA mutase. Methionine synthase catalyzes the conversion of homocysteine to methionine. (5, 6) Methionine is required for the formation of S-adenosylmethionine, a universal methyl donor for almost 100 different substrates, including DNA, RNA, hormones, proteins, and lipids. L-methylmalonyl-CoA mutase converts L-methylmalonyl-CoA to succinyl-CoA in the degradation of propionate, (3, 5, 6) an essential biochemical reaction in fat and protein metabolism. Succinyl-CoA is also required for hemoglobin synthesis. Thus maintaining adequate vitamin B_{12} status is vital for good health.

Vitamin B_{12}, bound to protein in animal-derived foods, is released by the activity of hydrochloric acid and gastric protease in the stomach. (5) When synthetic vitamin B_{12} is added to fortified foods and dietary supplements, it is already in free form and thus does not require this separation step. Free vitamin B_{12} then combines with intrinsic factor (IF), a glycoprotein secreted by the stomach's parietal cells, and the resulting complex undergoes absorption within the distal ileum by receptor-mediated endocytosis. (5, 7)

2. How much is needed?

Vitamin B_{12} status is typically assessed via serum or plasma vitamin B_{12} levels. Values below approximately 170–250 pg/mL (120–180 picomol/L) for adults (5) indicate a vitamin B_{12} deficiency. However, evidence suggests that serum vitamin B_{12} concentrations might not accurately reflect intracellular concentrations. (6) Elevated methylmalonic acid levels (values >0.4 micromol/L) might be a more reliable indicator of vitamin B_{12} status because they indicate a metabolic change that is highly specific to vitamin B_{12} deficiency. (5, 6, 7, 8, 9)

The following table lists the current RDAs for vitamin B_{12} in micrograms (mcg). (5) For infants aged 0 to 12 months, the Food and Nutrition Board established an adequate intake (AI) for vitamin B_{12} that is equivalent to the mean intake of vitamin B_{12} in healthy, breastfed infants.

How to cite this article: Rose S, Strombom A. Ensuring adequate vitamin B12 status on a plant-based diet. Adv Res Gastroentero Hepatol. 2019; 13(3): 555862.
DOI: 10.19080/ARGH.2019.13.555862

Recommended Dietary Allowances (RDAs) for Vitamin B_{12}

Life Stage	Age	Males (µg/day)	Females (µg/day)
Infants	0-6 months	0.4 (AI)	0.4 (AI)
Infants	7-12 months	0.5 (AI)	0.5 (AI)
Children	1-3 years	0.9	0.9
Children	4-8 years	1.2	1.2
Children	9-13 years	1.8	1.8
Adolescents	14-18 years	2.4	2.4
Adults	19-50 years	2.4	2.4
Adults	51 years and older	2.4*	2.4*
Pregnancy	all ages	–	2.6
Breast-feeding	all ages	–	2.8

*Vitamin B_{12} intake should be from supplements or fortified foods due to the age-related increase in food-bound malabsorption.

Approximately 56% of a 1mcg oral dose of vitamin B_{12} is absorbed, but absorption decreases drastically when the capacity of intrinsic factor is exceeded (at 1–2 mcg of vitamin B_{12}). (10) After the age of 50, the amount of intrinsic factor available is reduced, leading to malabsorption in many seniors. However, approximately 1% of oral vitamin B_{12} can be absorbed passively in the absence of intrinsic factor. (8, 9) For example, only about 5 mcg of a 500 mcg oral supplement is actually absorbed in healthy people. (10)

The bioavailability of sublingual vitamin B_{12} appears to be equivalent to oral vitamin B_{12}, but there is no evidence that sublingual delivery offers any advantage over oral preparations. (11) Given the lower cost and ease of administration of oral vitamin B_{12}, this might be a reasonable choice for replacement in many patients. (12)

Vitamin B_{12} has been demonstrated to be safe in doses up to 1,000 times the recommended dietary allowance and is safe in pregnancy. (5) The Institute of Medicine (IOM) did not establish an upper limit for vitamin B_{12} because of its low potential for toxicity. The IOM states that "no adverse effects have been associated with excess vitamin B_{12} intake from food and supplements in healthy individuals". (5) Findings from an intervention trial support these conclusions. In the HOPE 2 trial, vitamin B_{12} supplementation (in combination with folic acid and vitamin B_6) did not cause any serious adverse events when administered at doses of 1.0 mg for 5 years. (13)

3. Vitamin B_{12} for plant-based diet consumers

All naturally occurring B_{12} is produced by microorganisms. (14) The only organisms to produce vitamin B_{12} are certain species of bacteria. Some of these bacteria are found in the soil around the grasses that ruminants eat. They are taken into the animal, proliferate, form part of their gut flora, and continue to produce vitamin B_{12}. (14) Since patients on a plant-based diet eat no animal-derived foods, and only plant-foods cleaned of soil residue, they must rely on supplementation or fortified foods.

Fortified breakfast cereals are a readily available source of vitamin B_{12} with high bioavailability for vegetarians. (5, 8, 9, 15, 16) Some nutritional yeast products also contain vitamin B_{12}. Fortified foods vary in formulation between brands and over time, so it is important to read product labels regularly to determine which added nutrients they contain.

Several studies have shown varying prevalences of B_{12} deficiency with those on a plant-based diet. (17, 18, 19) For instance one study showed that (52%) of those following a plant-based diet were B_{12} deficient (<118 pmol/L). (20) However, other studies have found a lower incidence of B_{12} deficiency. (21) As expected, those taking B_{12} containing supplements have lower incidences of B_{12} deficiency. (20)

Vitamin B_{12} is secreted in bile and then most is reabsorbed via the enterohepatic circulation by ileal receptors which require IF. In healthy individuals most of this B_{12} is reabsorbed and available for metabolic functions. (5) This gives the body an effective mechanism to conserve its B_{12}, so deficiency can take as long as several years to present. This sometimes leads to complacency among patients following a plant-based diet. Development of vitamin B_{12} deficiency is likely to be more rapid in patients with pernicious anemia since IF is lacking. (5)

4. Vitamin B_{12} deficiency

Vitamin B_{12} deficiency is characterized by megaloblastic anemia, fatigue, weakness, constipation, loss of appetite, and weight loss. (2, 3, 22) Neurological changes, such as numbness and tingling in the hands and feet, can also occur. (5, 23) Additional symptoms of vitamin B_{12} deficiency include difficulty maintaining balance, depression, confusion, dementia, poor memory, and soreness of the mouth or tongue. (23) The neurological symptoms of vitamin B_{12} deficiency can occur without anemia, so early diagnosis and intervention is important to avoid irreversible damage. (6)

Large amounts of folic acid can mask the damaging effects of vitamin B_{12} deficiency by correcting the megaloblastic anemia caused by vitamin B_{12} deficiency (2, 24) without correcting the neurological damage that also occurs. (2, 24)

Vitamin B_{12} crosses the placenta during pregnancy and is present in breast milk. Exclusively breastfed infants of women who consume no animal products may have very limited reserves of vitamin B_{12} and they can develop vitamin B_{12} deficiency within months of birth. (5, 25) Undetected and untreated vitamin B_{12} deficiency in infants can result in severe and permanent neurological damage. During infancy, signs of a vitamin B_{12} deficiency include failure to thrive, movement disorders, developmental delays, and megaloblastic anemia. (26)

How to cite this article: Rose S, Strombom A. Ensuring adequate vitamin B12 status on a plant-based diet. Adv Res Gastroentero Hepatol. 2019; 13(3): 555862.
DOI: 10.19080/ARGH.2019.13.555862

5. Treating B_{12} deficiency

Vitamin B_{12} deficiency is sometimes treated with vitamin B_{12} injections, since this method bypasses potential barriers to absorption. However, high doses of oral vitamin B_{12} may also be effective. In a 2005 review of randomized controlled trials comparing oral with intramuscular vitamin B_{12}, patients who received high dosages of oral vitamin B_{12} (1 to 2 mg daily) for 90 to 120 days had an improvement in serum vitamin B_{12} similar to patients who received intramuscular injections. The authors concluded that 2,000 mcg of oral vitamin B_{12} daily, followed by a decreased daily dose of 1,000 mcg and then 1,000 mcg weekly, can be as effective as intramuscular administration. (8, 9) These results were consistent in patients regardless of the etiology of their vitamin B_{12} deficiency, including malabsorption states and pernicious anemia. Overall, an individual patient's ability to absorb vitamin B_{12} from the diet is the most important factor in determining whether vitamin B_{12} should be administered orally or via injection. (10)

The American Dietetic Association recommends supplemental vitamin B_{12} for vegans and lacto-ovo vegetarians during both pregnancy and lactation to ensure that enough vitamin B_{12} is transferred to the fetus and infant. (27) Pregnant and lactating women who follow strict vegetarian or vegan diets should consult with a pediatrician regarding vitamin B_{12} supplements for their infants and children. (5)

6. Discussion

In previous eras and under primitive conditions, man may have absorbed adequate vitamin B_{12} through the soil left on his food, when there was little to no washing and peeling. Now, however, patients following a plant-based, or vegan diet, must supplement with vitamin B_{12}. Due to conservation through enterohepatic recirculation, the body's stores of B_{12} may last the patient some time.

Some vegetarian and vegan patients are complacent when it comes to vitamin B_{12} supplementation. The long lag time until symptoms present can add to the complacency and some patients may become convinced they don't need supplemental B_{12}. Therefore, the physician should emphasize the importance of vitamin B_{12} supplementation and the rationale for it. The physicians should also make the patient aware of the consequences of deficiency.

Given the higher rate of B_{12} deficiency in vegans and vegetarians, they should have the lab work done initially. If a deficiency is found, or there is non-compliance with recommended supplementation, then more frequent lab work is called for.

Vitamin B_{12} deficiency is easy to prevent. Vitamin B_{12} is included in many multivitamins as well as being sold separately. While some foods are fortified with B_{12}, this cannot be relied upon due to dietary preference variations and commercial reformulation.

500mcg and 1,000mcg vitamin B_{12} supplements, as well as smaller doses, are widely available and affordable and can be used to prevent or treat deficiency, regardless of etiology, without the need for intramuscular injections. Considering the exceptionally low toxicity, vitamin B_{12} can be prescribed in generous doses if the clinician considers it best to err on the side of safety with a patient.

References

1. Herbert V, K D. (1994) *Vitamin B12 in Modern Nutrition in Health and Disease*. 8th ed ed. Baltimore, MD: Williams & Wilkins.

How to cite this article: Rose S, Strombom A. Ensuring adequate vitamin B12 status on a plant-based diet. Adv Res Gastroentero Hepatol. 2019; 13(3): 555862.
DOI: 10.19080/ARGH.2019.13.555862

2. Herbert V. (1996) *Vitamin B12 in Present Knowledge in Nutrition*. 17th Ed ed. Washington, DC: International Life Sciences Institute Press.
3. Combs G. (1992) Chapter 17 Vitamin B12. *The Vitamins: Fundamental aspects in nutrition and health*. Third Edition ed. Burlington, MA: Elsevier Academic Press.
4. Zittoun J, Zittoun R. (1999) Modern clinical testing strategies in cobalamin and folate deficiency. *Semin Hematol* 36(1):35-46.
5. Institute of Medicine (US). (1998) *Dietary Reference Intakes for Thiamin, Riboflavin, Niacin, Vitamin B6, Folate, Vitamin B12, Pantothenic Acid, Biotin, and Choline*. Washington, DC: National Academies Press.
6. Clarke R. (2008) B-vitamins and prevention of dementia. *PRoc Nutr Soc* 67(1):75-81.
7. Klee G. (2000) Cobalamin and folate evaluation: measurement of methylmalonic acid and homocysteine vs vitamin B(12) and folate. *Clin Chem* 46(8 Pt 2):1277-83.
8. Vidal-Alaball J, Butler C, Cannings-John R, et al. (2005) Oral vitamin B12 versus intramuscular vitamin B12 for vitamin B12 deficiency. *Cochrane Database Syst Rev* (3).
9. Butler C, Vidal-Alaball J, Cannings-John R, et al. (2006) Oral vitamin B12 versus intramuscular vitamin B12 for vitamin B12 deficiency: a systematic review of randomized controlled trials. *Fam Pract* 23(3):279-85.
10. Carmel R. (2008) How I treat cobalamin (vitamin B12) deficiency. *Blood* 112(6):2214-2221.
11. Sharabi A, Cohen E, Sulkes J, Garty M. (2003) Replacement therapy for vitamin B12 deficiency: comparison between the sublingual and oral route. *Br J Clin Pharmacol* 56(6):635-8.
12. Langan R, Zawistoski K. (2011) Update on Vitamin B12 Deficiency. *American Family Physician* 83(12):1425-1430.
13. Lonn E, Yusuf S, Arnold M, Sheridan P, Pogue J, et al. (2006) Homocysteine lowering with folic acid and B vitamins in vascular disease. *N Engl J Med* 354(15):1567-77.
14. Groff J, Gropper S, Hunt S. (1995) *Advanced nutrition and human metabolism*. 2nd ed ed. Minneapolis: West Publishing Comp.
15. Subar A, Krebs-Smith S, Cook A, Kahle L. (1998) Dietary sources of nutrients among US adults, 1989 to 1991. *J Am Diet Assoc* 98(5):537-47.
16. Tucker K, Rich S, Rosenberg I, et al. (2000) Plasma vitamin B-12 concentrations relate to intake source in the Framingham Offspring study. *Am J Clin Nutr* 71(2):514-22.
17. Wokes F, Badenoch J, Sinclair H. (1955) Human dietary deficiency of vitamin B12. *Am J Clin Nutr* 3(5):375-382.
18. Herrmann W, Schorr H, Purschwitz K, Rassoul F, Richter V. (2001) Total homocysteine, vitamin B(12), and total antioxidant status in vegetarians. *CLin Chem* 47(6):1094-101.
19. Herrmann W, Schorr H, Obeid R, Geisel J. (2003) Vitamin B-12 status, particularly holotranscobalamin II and methylmalonic acid concentrations, and hyperhomocysteinemia in vegetarians. *Am J Clin Nutr* 78(1):131-136.
20. Gilsing A, Crowe F, Lloyd-Wright, Z, et al. (2010) Serum concentrations of vitamin B12 and folate in British male omnivores, vegetarians and vegans: results from a cross-sectional analysis of the EPIC-Oxford cohort study. *Eur J Clin Nutr* 64(9):933-9.
21. Majchrzak D, Singer I, Männer M, et al. (2006) B-vitamin status and concentrations of homocysteine in Austrian omnivores, vegetarians and vegans. *Ann Nutr Metab* 50(6):485-91.
22. Bernard M, Nakonezny P, Kashner T. (1998) The effect of vitamin B12 deficiency on older veterans and its relationship to health. *J am Geriatr Soc* 46(10):1199-206.
23. Bottiglieri T. (1996) Folate, vitamin B12, and neuropsychiatric disorders. *Nutr Rev* 54(12):382-90.

How to cite this article: Rose S, Strombom A. Ensuring adequate vitamin B12 status on a plant-based diet. Adv Res Gastroentero Hepatol. 2019; 13(3): 555862.
DOI: 10.19080/ARGH.2019.13.555862

24. Chanarin I. (1994) Adverse effects of increased dietary folate. Relation to measures to reduce the incidence of neural tube defects. *Clin Invest Med* 17(3):244-252.
25. von Schenck U, Bender-Gotze C, Koletzko B. (1997) Persistence of neurological damage induced by dietary vitamin B12 deficiency in infancy. *Arch Dis Childhood* 77(2):137-9.
26. Bjørke Monsen A, Ueland P. (2003) Homocysteine and methylmalonic acid in diagnosis and risk assessment from infancy to adolescence. *Am J Clin Nutr* 78(1):7-21.
27. Kaiser L, Allen L, American Dietetic Association. (2008) Position of the American Dietetic Association: nutrition and lifestyle for a healthy pregnancy outcome. *J Am Diet Assoc* 108(3):553-61.

How to cite this article: Rose S, Strombom A. Ensuring adequate vitamin B12 status on a plant-based diet. Adv Res Gastroentero Hepatol. 2019; 13(3): 555862.
DOI: 10.19080/ARGH.2019.13.555862

Orthopedics and Rheumatology
Open Access Journal
ISSN: 2471-6804

Juniper Publishers
key to the Researchers

Review Article
Volume 15 Issue 3 - December 2019
DOI: 10.19080/OROAJ.2019.15.555913

Orth & Rheum Open Access J

Ensuring Adequate Vitamin D Status for Patients on a Plant-Based Diet

Stewart Rose* and Amanda Strombom

Plant-Based Diets in Medicine, USA

Submission: November 14, 2019; **Published:** December 03, 2019

***Corresponding author:** Stewart Rose, Plant-Based Diets in Medicine, 12819 SE 38th St, #427, Bellevue, WA 98006, USA

Abstract

Vitamin D is a fat-soluble vitamin that is naturally present in a few foods, added to others, and available as a dietary supplement. It is also produced endogenously when ultraviolet rays from sunlight strike the skin and trigger vitamin D synthesis.

The flesh of fatty fish (such as salmon, tuna, and mackerel) and fish liver oils are among the best sources of foods that contain vitamin D naturally. Small amounts of vitamin D are also found in beef liver, cheese and egg yolks. Almost all of the U.S. dairy milk supply is voluntarily fortified with 100 IU/cup.

Since patients following a plant-based diet don't consume any of these, there has been some concern that that they may run a higher risk of Vitamin D deficiency. However, studies show that on average their levels 25(OH) D are adequate. However, this shouldn't lead to complacency, since Vitamin D deficiency is widespread in the general population. Over 41% of people in a large study of all races, ethnicities and ages showed insufficient vitamin D levels. Those adults at greatest risk of vitamin D deficiency include patients with chronic illnesses, dark-pigmented skin, or poor nutrition.

Vegans obtain vitamin D from sunlight, from fortified foods and supplements. Patients should be informed that they must rely on these sources and so should make sure that their intake of these foods is adequate. While Vitamin D3 comes from animal sources, vitamin D2 comes from plant sources and is equivalent in daily dosing.

1. Physiology

Vitamin D is a fat-soluble vitamin that is naturally present in very few foods, added to others, and available as a dietary supplement. It is also produced endogenously when ultraviolet rays from sunlight strike the skin and trigger vitamin D synthesis. Vitamin D obtained from sun exposure, food, and supplements is biologically inert and must undergo two hydroxylations in the body for activation. The first occurs in the liver and converts vitamin D to 25-hydroxyvitamin D [25(OH)D], also known as calcidiol. The second occurs primarily in the kidney and forms the physiologically active 1,25-dihydroxyvitamin D [1,25(OH)2D], also known as calcitriol. (1)

Vitamin D promotes calcium absorption in the gut and maintains adequate serum calcium and phosphate concentrations to enable normal mineralization of bone and to prevent hypocalcemic tetany. It is also needed for bone growth and bone remodeling by osteoblasts and osteoclasts. (1, 2) Without sufficient vitamin D, bones can become thin, brittle, or misshapen. Vitamin D sufficiency prevents rickets in children and osteomalacia in adults. (1) Together with calcium, vitamin D also helps protect older adults from osteoporosis. (3)

Vitamin D also has other roles in the body, including modulation of cell growth, neuromuscular and immune function, and reduction of inflammation. (1, 4, 5) Many genes encoding proteins that regulate cell proliferation, differentiation, and apoptosis are modulated in part by vitamin D. (1) Many cells have vitamin D receptors, and some convert 25(OH)D to 1,25(OH)2D.

Given the high rate of bone development early in life, adequate serum concentrations of vitamin D are crucial for the developing child. There has also been a piquing interest in vitamin D in pediatric patients due to the recent epidemiologic reports suggesting that vitamin D may protect against autoimmune disease and play a role in innate immunity. (6)

2. UV Source

Most people meet at least some of their vitamin D needs through exposure to sunlight. (1, 2) Ultraviolet (UV) B radiation with a wavelength of 290–320 nanometers penetrates uncovered skin and converts cutaneous 7-dehydrocholesterol to previtamin D3, which in turn becomes vitamin D3. (1)

Season, time of day, length of day, cloud cover, smog, skin melanin content, and sunscreen are among the factors that affect UV radiation exposure and vitamin D synthesis. (1) Perhaps surprisingly, geographic latitude does not consistently predict average serum 25(OH)D levels in a population. Ample opportunities exist to form vitamin D (and store it in the liver and fat) from exposure to sunlight during the spring, summer, and fall months, even in the far north latitudes. (1) However, this requires spending adequate time outdoors in the sunshine, without blocking the UV radiation using clothing or sunscreen.

3. Food Sources

Very few foods in nature contain vitamin D. The flesh of fatty fish (such as salmon, tuna, and mackerel) and fish liver oils are among the best sources. (1, 7) Small amounts of vitamin D are found in beef liver, cheese, and egg yolks. Vitamin D in these foods is primarily in the form of vitamin D3 and its metabolite 25(OH)D3. (8) Some mushrooms provide vitamin D2 in variable amounts. (9, 10) Mushrooms with enhanced levels of vitamin D2 from being exposed to ultraviolet light under controlled conditions are also available.

Fortified foods provide most of the vitamin D in the American diet. (1, 9) Fortification of cow's milk with vitamin D began in the United States during

How to cite this article: Rose S, Strombom A. Ensuring adequate vitamin D status for patients on a plant-based diet. Ortho & Rheum Open Access J. 2019; 15(3): 555913.
DOI: 10.19080/OROAJ.2019.15.555913

the 1930s, largely as an effort to combat rickets, a major public health problem at the time. (9) Almost all milk available in the U.S. is now fortified with 100 IU/cup of vitamin D2. (11) In Canada, milk is fortified by law with 35–40 IU/100 mL, as is margarine at ≥530 IU/100 g. However, other dairy products made from milk, such as cheese and ice cream, are generally not fortified. Ready-to-eat breakfast cereals often contain added vitamin D, as do some brands of orange juice, yogurt, margarine and other food products. Dairy-free milks, and other dairy substitutes, often have vitamin D added to them.

Both the United States and Canada mandate the fortification of infant formula with vitamin D: 40–100 IU/100 kcal in the United States and 40–80 IU/100 kcal in Canada. (1)

4. Lactation

Vitamin D requirements cannot ordinarily be met by human milk alone, (1, 12) Breast milk contains very little vitamin D, an average of 22 units/L (range 15 to 50 units/L) in a vitamin D-sufficient mother. (13) The vitamin D content of human milk is related to the mother's vitamin D status, so mothers who supplement with high doses of vitamin D may have correspondingly high levels of this nutrient in their milk. (14) Recent studies suggest that maternal intake of higher than recommended doses of vitamin D (4000 to 6400 units daily) may achieve vitamin D concentrations in breast milk to provide sufficient vitamin D supplementation for breastfeeding infants. However, this approach is not recommended. (15, 14)

While the sun is a potential source of vitamin D, the AAP (American Academy of Pediatrics) advises keeping infants out of direct sunlight and having them wear protective clothing and sunscreen. (16)

5. Deficiency

The disease of rickets is fortunately rare today, but it does still occur. A review of reports of nutritional rickets found that a majority of cases occurred among young, breastfed African Americans. (17) A survey of Canadian pediatricians found the incidence of rickets in their patients to be 2.9 per 100,000; almost all those with rickets had been breastfed. (18) Due to the low vitamin D concentrations found in breast milk, and the advice to avoid the sun, the newest recommendation for exclusively and partially breastfed infants is to provide a supplement of 400 units per day to the infant (increased from 200 units per day). (3, 14)

While rickets is rare, unfortunately, Vitamin D deficiency remains a significant problem. Large percentages of people in all races, ethnicities, and ages show a high prevalence of Vitamin D deficiency. In one study, insufficient vitamin D levels were found in 41.6% of a large sample size. Race was identified as a significant risk factor, with African American adults having the highest prevalence rate of vitamin D deficiency at 82% followed by Hispanic adults at 63%. (19, 11, 20)

Those adults at greatest risk of vitamin D deficiency include patients with chronic illnesses (e.g., chronic kidney disease, cystic fibrosis, asthma, and sickle cell disease), dark-pigmented skin, poor nutrition. (6, 21) Chronic use of certain medications (e.g., glucocorticoids, cytochrome P450 3A4 inducers, anticonvulsants, and anti-retroviral agents) has also been associated with compromised vitamin D concentrations. (6)

6. Diagnosis

Serum concentration of 25(OH)D is the best indicator of vitamin D status. It reflects both

How to cite this article: Rose S, Strombom A. Ensuring adequate vitamin D status for patients on a plant-based diet. Ortho & Rheum Open Access J. 2019; 15(3): 555913.
DOI: 10.19080/OROAJ.2019.15.555913

vitamin D produced cutaneously and that obtained from food and supplements (1) and has a fairly long circulating half-life of 15 days [B]. 25(OH)D functions as a biomarker of exposure, but it is not clear to what extent 25(OH)D levels also serve as a biomarker of effect (i.e., relating to health status or outcomes). (1) Serum 25(OH)D levels do not indicate the amount of vitamin D stored in body tissues.

In contrast to 25(OH)D, circulating 1,25(OH)2D is generally not a good indicator of vitamin D status because it has a short half-life of 15 hours and serum concentrations are closely regulated by parathyroid hormone, calcium, and phosphate. (22) Levels of 1,25(OH)2D do not typically decrease until vitamin D deficiency is severe. (2, 6)

Desirable concentrations of Serum 25-Hydroxyvitamin D (25(OH)D)

Serum 25-Hydroxyvitamin D [25(OH)D] Concentrations and Health* (1)		
nmol/L**	**ng/mL***	**Health status**
<30	<12	Associated with vitamin D deficiency, leading to rickets in infants and children and osteomalacia in adults
30 to <50	12 to <20	Generally considered inadequate for bone and overall health in healthy individuals
≥50	≥20	Generally considered adequate for bone and overall health in healthy individuals
>125	>50	Emerging evidence links potential adverse effects to such high levels, particularly >150 nmol/L (>60 ng/mL)

* Serum concentrations of 25(OH)D are reported in both nanomoles per liter (nmol/L) and nanograms per milliliter (ng/mL).

** 1 nmol/L = 0.4 ng/mL

7. Vegans

While there has been some concern that vegans and vegetarians might have inadequate levels of 25(OH)D, studies have shown that vegans do have adequate levels. Therefore vegans do not run a risk of deficiency any higher than their meat-eating counterparts or require more monitoring or intervention.

A study of Danish vegans showed that they had an average 57nmol/l 25(OH)D. (23) This result is similar to a British study which showed that vegans had an average 25(OH)D of 56 nmol/l 25(OH)D. (24) An American study of a group containing both vegetarians and vegans showed an average level of 25(OH)D at 77nmol/l (25)

How to cite this article: Rose S, Strombom A. Ensuring adequate vitamin D status for patients on a plant-based diet. Ortho & Rheum Open Access J. 2019; 15(3): 555913.
DOI: 10.19080/OROAJ.2019.15.555913

8. Supplements D_2 vs D_3

In supplements and fortified foods, vitamin D is available in two forms, D_2 (ergocalciferol) and D_3 (cholecalciferol) that differ chemically only in their side-chain structure. Vitamin D_2 is manufactured by the UV irradiation of ergosterol in yeast, and vitamin D_3 is manufactured by the irradiation of 7-dehydrocholesterol from lanolin and the chemical conversion of cholesterol. (6)

Vitamin D_2 has been the mainstay for the prevention and treatment of vitamin D deficiency in children and adults for more than 90 years. (6, 26) As little as 100 IU vitamin D_2 was found to be effective in the prevention of rickets. (26, 27, 28) It is commonly used for supplementation and food fortification. Vitamin D_2 is more acceptable to those on a plant-based diet because it is not derived from animals.

Vitamin D_3 is the endogenous form of vitamin D produced by keratinocytes in the skin in response to ultraviolet B radiation from sunlight. Both forms of vitamin D are hydroxylated in the liver to 25(OH)D.

It has been suggested that vitamin D_3 may be superior to vitamin D_2 in sustaining adequate 25(OH)D values in adults (29, 30) because 25(OH) D_2 may bind less avidly to vitamin D binding protein and be cleared more rapidly than 25(OH)D_3. However, others have found that regular supplementation with both forms of vitamin D, at common doses of say 1000 IU daily, were equally effective in maintaining 25(OH)D levels. (31, 32)

In children, both vitamins D_2 and D_3 similarly increase serum 25(OH)D concentrations in rachitic and healthy children. (33) Even if vitamin D_3 was more efficacious than vitamin D_2 under special circumstances, it can still be used with equal efficacy by simply raising the dose of D_2.

Both vitamin D_2 and vitamin D_3 are available as supplements, but only vitamin D_2 is available as a pharmaceutical preparation because its use predated the Food and Drug Administration and was thus grandfathered as a pharmaceutical drug. Vitamin D_3 was commercially developed in the 1950s and has not been approved as a pharmaceutical agent in the United States, but it is used in food supplementation and vitamin supplements.

9. Toxicity

Vitamin D toxicity can cause non-specific symptoms such as anorexia, weight loss, polyuria, and heart arrhythmias. More seriously, it can also raise blood levels of calcium which leads to vascular and tissue calcification, with subsequent damage to the heart, blood vessels, and kidneys. (1) A serum 25(OH)D concentration consistently >500 nmol/L (>200 ng/mL) is considered to be potentially toxic. (22)

Excessive sun exposure does not result in vitamin D toxicity because the sustained heat on the skin is thought to photodegrade previtamin D_3 and vitamin D_3 as it is formed. (6) In addition, thermal activation of previtamin D_3 in the skin gives rise to various non-vitamin D forms that limit formation of vitamin D_3 itself. Some vitamin D_3 is also converted to nonactive forms. (1) Intakes of vitamin D from food that are high enough to cause toxicity are very unlikely. Toxicity is much more likely to occur from high intakes of dietary supplements containing vitamin D.

Most reports suggest a toxicity threshold for vitamin D of 10,000 to 40,000 IU/day and serum 25(OH)D levels of 500–600 nmol/L (200–240 ng/

How to cite this article: Rose S, Strombom A. Ensuring adequate vitamin D status for patients on a plant-based diet. Ortho & Rheum Open Access J. 2019; 15(3): 555913.
DOI: 10.19080/OROAJ.2019.15.555913

mL). While symptoms of toxicity are unlikely at daily intakes below 10,000 IU/day, the FNB pointed to emerging science from national survey data, observational studies, and clinical trials suggesting that even lower vitamin D intakes and serum 25(OH)D levels might have adverse health effects over time. The FNB concluded that serum 25(OH) D levels above approximately 125–150 nmol/L (50–60 ng/mL) should be avoided, as even lower serum levels (approximately 75–120 nmol/L or 30–48 ng/mL) are associated with increases in all-cause mortality, greater risk of cancer at some sites like the pancreas, greater risk of cardiovascular events, and more falls and fractures among the elderly. The FNB committee cited research which found that vitamin D intakes of 5,000 IU/day achieved serum 25(OH)D concentrations between 100–150 nmol/L (40–60 ng/mL), but no greater. Applying an uncertainty factor of 20% to this intake value gave an upper limit of 4,000 IU which the FNB applied to children aged 9 and older and adults, with corresponding lower amounts for younger children. (34)

10. Discussion

Vitamin D deficiency is widespread. With declining milk consumption levels, and more care being taken to limit sun exposure, this problem is likely to get worse across the US population.

Concern by some physicians that those patients who follow a vegan diet need different measures for the prevention and treatment of vitamin D deficiency seems unwarranted. Studies of vegans have shown that, on average, their 25(OH)D levels are within the recommended range. They are, therefore, not any more likely to be vitamin D deficient than any other patient. The vegan patients should maintain their 25(OH)D in the recommended range the same as any other patient.

Vitamin D_2 is as effective as Vitamin D_3 for the prevention and treatment of vitamin D deficiency, as well as for preventing related disease such as rickets, so vegan patients can safely be treated with Vitamin D_2.

Research on vitamin D and other pathologies such as cancer and diabetes are ongoing. We await their results. In the meantime, maintaining adequate levels of 25(OH)D in patients may be preventing pathologies other than osteomalacia and rickets.

References

1. Institute of Medicine Food and Nutrition Board. (2010) *Dietary Reference Intakes for Calcium and Vitamin D*. Washington DC.
2. Cranney C, Horsley T, O'Donnell S, et al. (2007) *Effectiveness and safety of vitamin D in relation to bone health*. Rockville, MD: Evid Rep Technol Assess (Full Rep). (158):1-235.
3. Misra M, Pacaud D, Petryk A, Collett-Solberg P, Kappy M, et al. (2008) Vitamin D deficiency in children and its management: review of current knowledge and recommendations. *Pediatrics* 122(2):398-417.
4. Holick M. Vitamin D. In: Shils M, Shike M, Ross A, Caballero B, Cousins R, eds. (2005) *Modern Nutrition in Health and Disease*. Tenth Edition ed. Philadelphia, PA: Lippincott Williams & Wilkins.
5. Norman A, Henry H. (2006) Vitamin D. In: Bowman B, Russell R, eds. *Present Knowledge in Nutrition*. 9th ed. Washington DC: ILSI Press.
6. Holick M. (2007) Vitamin D Deficiency. *New Eng J Med* 357:266-281.
7. US Department of Agriculture, Agricultural Research Service. (2011) *USDA National Nutrient Database for Standard Reference*: Nutrient Data Laboratory. Release 24.

How to cite this article: Rose S, Strombom A. Ensuring adequate vitamin D status for patients on a plant-based diet. Ortho & Rheum Open Access J. 2019; 15(3): 555913.
DOI: 10.19080/OROAJ.2019.15.555913

8. Ovesen L, Brot C, Jakobsen J. (2003) Food contents and biological activity of 25-hydroxyvitamin D: a vitamin D metabolite to be reckoned with? *Ann Nutr Metab* 47(3-4):107-113.
9. Calvo M, Whiting S, Barton C. (2004) Vitamin D fortification in the United States and Canada: current status and data needs. *Am J Clin Nutr* 80(6 Suppl):1710S-1716S.
10. Mattila P, Piironen V, Uusi-Rauva E, Koivistoinen P. (1994) Vitamin D Contents in Edible Mushrooms. *Agric Food Chem* 42(11):2449-2453.
11. Parva N, Tadepalli S, Singh P, et al. (2018) Prevalence of Vitamin D Deficiency and Associated Risk Factors in the US Population (2011-2012). *Cureus* 10(6):e2741.
12. Picciano M. (2001) Nutrient composition of human milk. *Pediatr Clin North Am* 48(1):53-67.
13. Leerbeck E, Søndergaard H. (1980) The total content of vitamin D in human milk and cow's milk. *Br J Nutr* 44(1):7-12.
14. Wagner C, FR G, (2008) American Academy of Pediatrics Section on Breastfeeding. Prevention of rickets and vitamin D deficiency in infants, children, and adolescents. *Pediatrics* 122(5):1142-1152.
15. Basile L, Taylor S, Wagner C, Horst R, Hollis B. (2006) The effect of high-dose vitamin D supplementation on serum vitamin D levels and milk calcium concentration in lactating women and their infants. *Breastfeed Med* 1(1):27-35.
16. American Academy of Pediatrics Committee on Environmental Health. (1999) Ultraviolet light: a hazard to children. *Pediatrics* 104(2 Pt 1):326-333.
17. Weisberg P, Scanlon K, Li R, Cogswell M. (2004) Nutritional rickets among children in the United States: review of cases reported between 1986 and 2003. *Am J Clin Nutr* 80(6 Suppl):1697S-1705S.
18. Ward L, Gaboury I, Ladhani M, Zlotkin S. (2007) Vitamin D–deficiency rickets among children in Canada. *Can Med Assoc J* 177(2):161-166.
19. Forrest K, Stuhldreher W. (2011) Prevalence and correlates of vitamin D deficiency in US adults. *Nutr Res* 31(1):48-54.
20. Lebrun J, Moffatt M, Mundy R, et al. (1993) Vitamin D deficiency in a Manitoba community. *Can J Pub Health* 84(6):394-396.
21. Zhou C, Assem M, Tay J, Watkins P, Blumberg B et al. (2006) Steroid and xenobiotic receptor and vitamin D receptor crosstalk mediates CYP24 expression and drug-induced osteomalacia. *J Clin Invest* 116(6):1703-12.
22. Jones G. (2008) Pharmacokinetics of vitamin D toxicity. *Am J Clin Nutr* 88(2):582S-586S.
23. Hansen T, Madsen M, Jørgensen N, et al. (2018) Bone turnover, calcium homeostasis, and vitamin D status in Danish vegans. *Eur J Clin Nutr* 72(7):1046-1054.
24. Crowe F, Steur M, Allen N, Appleby P, Travis R, Key T. (2011) Plasma concentrations of 25-hydroxyvitamin D in meat eaters, fish eaters, vegetarians and vegans: results from the EPIC-Oxford study. *Public Health Nutr* 14(2):340-346.
25. Chan J, Jaceldo-Siegl K, Fraser G. (2009) Serum 25-hydroxyvitamin D status of vegetarians, partial vegetarians, and nonvegetarians: the Adventist Health Study-2. *Am J Clin Nutr* 89(5):1686S-1692S.
26. Eliot M, Park E. (1938) Rickets. *Brennerman's Practice of Pediatrics*. Vol 1. Hagerstown, MD: WF Prior.
27. Holick M. (2006) Resurrection of Vitamin D deficiency and rickets. *J Clin Invest* 116(8):2062-2072.
28. Jeans P. (1950) Vitamin D. *JAMA* 143:177-181.
29. Armas L, Hollis B, Heaney R. (2004) Vitamin D2 is much less effective than vitamin D3 in humans. *J Clin Endocrinol Metab* 89(11):5387-5391.

How to cite this article: Rose S, Strombom A. Ensuring adequate vitamin D status for patients on a plant-based diet. Ortho & Rheum Open Access J. 2019; 15(3): 555913.
DOI: 10.19080/OROAJ.2019.15.555913

30. Trang H, Cole D, Rubin L, Pierratos A, Siu S, Vieth R. (1998) Evidence that vitamin D3 increases serum 25-hydroxyvitamin D more efficiently than does vitamin D2. *Am J Clin Nutr* 68(4):854-858.

31. Holick M, Biancuzzo R, Chen T, et al. (2008) Vitamin D2 is as effective as vitamin D3 in maintaining circulating concentrations of 25-hydroxyvitamin D. *J Clin Endocrinol Metab* 93(3):677-681.

32. Gordon C, Williams A, Feldman H, et al. (2008) Treatment of Hypovitaminosis D in Infants and Toddlers. *J Clin Endocrinol Metab* 93(7):2716-2721.

33. Thacher T, Fischer P, Obadofin M, Levine M, Singh R, Pettifor J. (2010) Comparison of metabolism of vitamins D2 and D3 in children with nutritional rickets. *J Bone Miner Res* 25(9):1988-1995.

34. National Institutes of Health Office of Dietary Supplements. (2018) Vitamin D Fact Sheet for Health Professionals. *Factsheets*.

How to cite this article: Rose S, Strombom A. Ensuring adequate vitamin D status for patients on a plant-based diet. Ortho & Rheum Open Access J. 2019; 15(3): 555913.
DOI: 10.19080/OROAJ.2019.15.555913

Advanced Research in Gastroenterology & Hepatology
ISSN: 2472-6400

Juniper Publishers
key to the Researchers

Mini Review
Volume 13 Issue 4 - July 2019
DOI: 10.19080/ARGH.2019.13.555867

Adv Res Gastroenterol Hepatol

Ensuring Adequate Iron Status in Vegetarians and Vegans

Stewart D Rose* **and Amanda J Strombom**

Plant-Based Diets in Medicine, USA

Submission: June 18, 2019; **Published:** July 26, 2019

***Corresponding Author:** Stewart Rose, Plant-Based Diets in Medicine, 12819 SE 38th St, #427, Bellevue, WA 98006, USA

Abstract

Many people, including some physicians, are concerned about iron deficiency anemia in patients consuming a plant-based diet. However, studies show that the risk of anemia in vegetarian and vegan patients is no greater than in omnivorous patients.

Plant foods contain only non-heme iron, whereas meat contains both the heme and non-heme iron. There used to be a concern that non-heme iron would be poorly absorbed resulting in iron deficiency anemia. However, non-heme is well absorbed in most vegetarian patients and vegan because other plant foods, containing substances such as vitamin C and citric acid, can greatly enhance its absorption. Furthermore, non-heme iron absorption increases whenever iron stores are low.

Adequate iron levels can easily be maintained in the vegan patient with a little planning. Consuming foods high in iron along with foods that enhance non-heme iron absorption, will prevent iron deficiency anemia in vegan and vegetarian patients. Because both groups of foods are widely available, this should not be difficult to accomplish.

Patients that are already anemic can be treated by increasing their consumption of iron rich and iron enhancing foods. Supplements are sometimes required. In these cases, iron supplements can be prescribed in the same manner as with omnivorous patients.

Keywords:

Anemia; Deficiency; Heme iron; Hepcidin; Iron; Non-heme iron; Plant-based diet; Supplements; Vegetarian; Vegan; Plant foods; Enterocytes; Macrophages; Synaptogenesis; Myelinization; Oxidative phosphorylation; Cytochromes, Sulfuric Proteins

1. Iron Sources

There are two types of iron in food: heme and non-heme iron. In animal products, 40% of the total iron content is heme iron and 60% non-heme iron. (1) Plant foods contain only non-heme iron. Many breakfast cereals and some breads are also fortified with iron. (2)

Plant foods that naturally contain iron, are wholegrain cereals and breads; dried beans and legumes; dark green leafy vegetables; dried fruits; and nuts and seeds. (3)

Table 1: Sources of Iron in plant foods

Food	Serving Size	Iron (mg)
Vegetables and Fruit:		
Spinach, cooked	125mL (1/2 cup)	2.0-3.4
Tomato puree	125mL (1/2 cup)	2.4
Edamame, baby soybeans, cooked	125mL (1/2 cup)	2.2
Asparagus, raw	6 spears	2.1
Hearts of palm, canned	125mL (1/2 cup)	2.0
Potato with skin, cooked	1 medium	1.3-1.9
Snow peas, cooked	125mL (1/2 cup)	1.7
Turnip or beet greens, cooked	125mL (1/2 cup)	1.5-1.7
Prune juice	125mL (1/2 cup)	1.6
Apricots, dried	60mL (1/4 cup)	1.6
Beets, canned	125mL (1/2 cup)	1.6
Kale, cooked	125mL (1/2 cup)	1.3
Green peas, cooked	125mL (1/2 cup)	1.3
Tomato sauce	125mL (1/2 cup)	1.3
Grain Products:		
Oatmeal, instant cooked	175mL (3/4 cup)	4.5-6.6
Cream of wheat, all types, cooked	175mL (3/4 cup)	5.7-5.8

How to cite this article: Rose S, Strombom A. Ensuring adequate iron status in vegetarians and vegans. Adv Res Gastroentero Hepatol. 2019; 13(4): 555867.
DOI: 10.19080/ARGH.2019.13.555867

Cereal, dry all types	30g (check product label for serving size)	4.0-4.3
Granola bar, oats, fruit and nut	32g (1 bar)	1.2-2.7
Legumes, nuts and seeds:		
Tofu, cooked	150g (3/4 cup)	2.4-8.0
Soybeans, mature, cooked	175mL (3/4 cup)	6.5
Lentils, cooked	175mL (3/4 cup)	4.1-4.9
Beans (white, kidney, navy, pinto, black, adzuki), cooked	175mL (3/4 cup)	2.6-4.9
Pumpkin or squash seeds, roasted	60mL (1/4 cup)	1.4-4.7
Peas (chickpeas, black-eyed, split), cooked	175mL (3/4 cup)	1.9-3.5
Tempeh/fermented soy product, cooked	150g (3/4 cup)	3.2
Meatless sausage, chicken, meatballs, fish sticks, cooked	75g (2.5 oz)	1.5-2.8
Baked beans, canned	175mL (3/4 cup)	2.2
Nuts (cashews, almonds, hazelnuts, macadamia, pistachio), without shell, raw	60mL (1/4 cup)	1.3-2.2
Sesame seeds, roasted	15mL (1 Tbsp)	1.4
Meatless luncheon slices	75g (2.5oz)	1.4
Hummus	60mL (1/4 cup)	1.5
Almond butter	30mL (2 Tbsp)	1.1

Source: Canadian Nutrient File 2015

2. Physiology and Pathology

Iron is a transition metal and has multiple functions in more than 180 biochemical reactions in the human body, including electron transport in redox reactions (cytochromes, sulfuric proteins), redox catalytic functions (cytochrome p450, catalase, peroxidase) and reversible storage and transport of O_2 (hemoglobin, myoglobin). It also plays an important role in the production of neurotransmitters, and is essential in synaptogenesis and myelinization. Oxidative phosphorylation is the most critical biochemical pathway in which iron is involved. (4, 5, 6)

Iron deficiency anemia usually develops slowly. As iron levels decline in the stores (iron deficiency) and in the circulation (iron restricted erythropoiesis), becoming insufficient for the full hemoglobinization of mature erythroblasts (iron deficiency anemia), the liver peptide hormone hepcidin is transcriptionally suppressed. (7) Indeed serum hepcidin levels are significantly lower in young women with a negative iron balance compared with males and postmenopausal women, and are even undetectable in serum of individuals with iron deficiency anemia. (8, 9, 10) The decrease of hepcidin enhances iron release into plasma through ferroportin from both enterocytes and macrophages in the attempt to maintain normal transferrin. (7)

2.1 Absorption

The amount of non-heme iron absorbed is primarily determined by the body's need for iron — people with the lowest iron stores will absorb more and excrete less. (2, 11) Humans can adapt successfully to a wide range of iron requirements and intakes. (12) If iron intake is low, vegetarians adapt by excreting less fecal ferritin. (11) In pregnant women who need the most iron, absorption can increase by 60% relative to normal. (12, 13) Non-heme iron is nearly as well absorbed as heme iron in people with very low iron stores. (12) There is apparently no advantage in storing more than a minimal amount of iron. (14)

Absorption is increased as much as three to six-fold with the addition of 50 mg of vitamin C per meal. (3) Vitamin C facilitates the conversion of Fe^{3+} (ferric) to Fe^{2+} (ferrous) iron, the form in which iron is best absorbed. This process is carefully regulated by the gut. Vegetarians typically have high intakes of vitamin C from a wide variety of fruits and vegetables.

Other common organic acids such as citric and malic, (15) as well as vitamin A and β-carotene, also enhance non-heme iron absorption. (15, 16)

This Vitamin C table shows that even modest servings of fruits and vegetables supply adequate vitamin C to enhance iron absorption:

Table 2: Selected Food Sources of Vitamin C

Food	Milligrams (mg) per serving	Percent (%) DV*
Red pepper, sweet, raw, ½ cup	95	158
Orange juice, ¾ cup	93	155
Orange, 1 medium	70	117
Grapefruit juice, ¾ cup	70	117
Kiwifruit, 1 medium	64	107
Green pepper, sweet, raw, ½ cup	60	100
Broccoli, cooked, ½ cup	51	85

How to cite this article: Rose S, Strombom A. Ensuring adequate iron status in vegetarians and vegans. Adv Res Gastroentero Hepatol. 2019; 13(4): 555867.
DOI: 10.19080/ARGH.2019.13.555867

Table 2: Selected Food Sources of Vitamin C

Food	Milligrams (mg) per serving	Percent (%) DV*
Strawberries, fresh, sliced, ½ cup	49	82
Brussels sprouts, cooked, ½ cup	48	80
Grapefruit, ½ medium	39	65
Broccoli, raw, ½ cup	39	65
Tomato juice, ¾ cup	33	55
Cantaloupe, ½ cup	29	48
Cabbage, cooked, ½ cup	28	47
Cauliflower, raw, ½ cup	26	43

U.S. Department of Agriculture, Agricultural Research Service. 2011. USDA National Nutrient Database for Standard Reference, Release 24. Nutrient Data Laboratory.

2.2 Inhibitors of absorption

There used to be some concern about tea consumption and iron absorption. However, tea consumption does not influence iron status in Western populations in which most people have adequate iron stores as determined by serum ferritin concentrations. Only in individuals with marginal iron status, may there be a negative association between tea consumption and iron status. (17)

There has also been a theoretical concern about the larger intake of phytates that comes from following a plant-based diet inhibiting absorption of some minerals, such as iron. However, it turns out that the intestinal flora of vegetarians act to degrade phytate, thus allowing for good absorption of minerals. One recent study concludes that, "it was the vegetarians' microbiota that particularly degraded up to 100% phytate to myo-inositol phosphate products." (18)

While some studies have found that oxalic acid (present in spinach, silverbeet and beetroot leaves) may inhibit iron absorption, recent studies suggest that its effects are relatively insignificant. (19) Calcium has also been considered an inhibitor of both heme and non-heme iron absorption, but recent research suggests that, over a long period of time, calcium has a limited effect on iron absorption (possibly due to an adaptive physiological response) (20) Nevertheless, it may be best to avoid consuming large calcium supplements with meals.

3. Clinical Considerations

Vegetarians and vegans who eat a varied and well-balanced diet are not at any greater risk of iron deficiency anemia than non-vegetarians, even though iron stores of vegetarians may be lower than in non vegetarians. (3, 21, 22, 23)

Iron deficiency anemia occurs in 5–12% of otherwise healthy premenopausal women (24, 25) and is usually due to menstrual loss, increased demands in pregnancy and breast feeding, or dietary deficiency. (26) Blood loss from the GI tract is the most common cause in adult men and postmenopausal women. (27, 28, 29, 30, 31, 32)

Gastrointestinal conditions, such as celiac disease and inflammatory bowel disease, as well as chronic kidney disease, cancer, and chronic heart failure increase the risk for anemia and iron deficiency. (33, 34, 35, 36, 37, 38, 39, 40, 41) Underlying conditions should be treated concurrently.

The diagnostic criteria for anemia in iron deficiency anemia vary between studies: Hgb less than 10–11.5 g/dl for women and less than 12.5–13.8 g/dl for men. The lower limit of the normal range of hemoglobin concentration, for the laboratory performing the test, should therefore be used to define anemia. (42)

For anemic patients, both the mean corpuscular volume (MCV) and the mean corpuscular hemoglobin concentration (MCHC) will also have values below the normal range for the laboratory performing the test. Reference range values for MCV and MCHC are 83-97 fL and 32-36 g/dL, respectively.

Serum ferritin concentration is a valuable test for iron deficiency anemia. (43) A serum ferritin concentration of less than 12 μg/dl is diagnostic of iron deficiency anemia. (44) However, elevated ferritin levels are usually due to causes such as acute or chronic inflammation, chronic alcohol consumption, liver disease, renal failure, metabolic syndrome, or malignancy rather than iron overload, (45) so serum ferritin may be above 12–15 μg/dl in patients with iron deficiency anemia and concurrent chronic inflammation, malignancy, or hepatic disease. If the concentration is greater than 100 μg/dl, iron deficiency anemia is almost certainly not present. (44)

To avoid false negative results (high ferritin levels in spite of iron deficiency), an acute phase reaction should be excluded by taking a history and measuring the C-reactive protein or erythrocyte sedimentation rate. (45)

The cornerstone of preventing iron deficiency in patients following a plant-based diet is to instruct patients to include plant foods high in iron in their diet. These foods can also be used to treat mild deficiencies while they can serve as an adjunct to iron supplementation. Patients should also be counseled to include iron absorption enhancers in the prevention and treatment of iron deficiency anemia.

Treatment of an underlying cause should prevent further iron loss, but all anemic patients should have iron supplementation both to correct anemia and replenish body stores. (46) This is achieved affordably with ferrous sulfate 200 mg twice daily. Lower doses may be as effective and better tolerated (47, 48) and should be considered in patients not tolerating traditional doses. Other iron compounds (eg, ferrous fumarate, ferrous gluconate) or formulations (iron suspensions) may also be tolerated better than ferrous sulfate. Oral iron should be continued for 3 months after the iron deficiency has been corrected so that stores are replenished. (49)

Intestinal iron absorption is limited. The maximum rate of absorption of 100 mg of oral iron supplement is 20% to 25% and is reached only in the

How to cite this article: Rose S, Strombom A. Ensuring adequate iron status in vegetarians and vegans. Adv Res Gastroentero Hepatol. 2019; 13(4): 555867.
DOI: 10.19080/ARGH.2019.13.555867

late stage of iron deficiency. Latent iron deficiency and iron deficiency anemia correspond to mean absorption rates of 10% and 13%, respectively, whereas healthy males absorb 5% and healthy females 5.6%. (50, 49)

Dose-dependent gastrointestinal side effects of iron supplementation hinder compliance and result in nonadherence in up to 50% of patients. (51) For those intolerant or not responding to oral iron, three parenteral preparations are available (49)

4. Discussion

Patients following a plant-based diet, and their physicians, need not be concerned that a plant-based diet will lead to iron deficiency anemia any more than an omnivorous diet will. However, that doesn't mean that iron deficiency anemia shouldn't be tested for when indicated. Iron deficiency is prevalent in the general population; an average of 5.6% of the U.S. population met the criteria for anemia and 1.5% for moderate-severe anemia. (52) Menstruating and pregnant women are at particular risk. (52)

The vegetarian and vegan patient should be instructed as to which plant foods are high in iron and how to enhance absorption. Plenty of foods that are high in iron can be chosen. If this is not enough and anemia results, then supplements are available and can be employed the same way as with omnivorous patients.

There are now several million Americans who follow either a vegan or vegetarian diet. Many physicians have started to prescribe a plant-based diet for the prevention and treatment of several diseases such as coronary artery disease and type 2 diabetes. By prescribing a diet that has ample iron-containing foods, along with the foods that enhance absorption, the physician can help ensure an adequate iron status in their patients following a plant-based diet.

References

1. Beard J, Dawson H, Piñero D. (1996) Iron metabolism: a comprehensive review. *Nutr Rev* 54(10):295-317.
2. Hurrell R, Egli I. (2010) Iron bioavailability and dietary reference values. *Am J Clin Nutr* 91(5):1461S-1467S.
3. Saunders A, Craig W, Baines S, Posen J. (2013) Iron and vegetarian diets. *Med J Aust* 199(4 Suppl):S11-S16.
4. Clénin G. (2017) The treatment of iron deficiency without anaemia (in otherwise healthy persons). *Swiss Med Wkly* 147:w14434.
5. Ganz T. (2007) Molecular control of iron transport. *J Am Soc Nephrol*. 18(2):394-400.
6. Löffler G, Petrides P. (1998) *Biochemie und Pathobiochemie*. 6th Edition ed. Berlin Heidelberg: Springer-Lehrbuch.
7. Camaschella C, Hoffbrand A, Hershko C. (2016) Iron metabolism iron deficiency and disorders of haem synthesis. In: Hoffbrand V, Higgs D, Keeling D, Mehta A, eds. *Postgraduate Haematology*. 7th ed. Oxford: Wiley-Blackwell.
8. Traglia M, Girelli D, Biino G, et al. (2011) Association of HFE and TMPRSS6 genetic variants with iron and erythrocyte parameters is only in part dependent on serum hepcidin concentrations. *J Med Genet* 48(9):629-634.
9. Galesloot T, Vermeulen S, Geurts-Moespot A, et al. (2011) Serum hepcidin: reference ranges and biochemical correlates in the general population. *Blood* 117(25):e218-225.
10. Camaschella C. (2015) Iron deficiency: new insights into diagnosis and treatment. *Hematology, Am Soc Hematol Educ Program* 2015:8-13.
11. Hunt J. (2003) Bioavailability of iron, zinc, and other trace minerals from vegetarian diets. *Am J Clin Nutr* 78(3 Suppl):633S-639S.

How to cite this article: Rose S, Strombom A. Ensuring adequate iron status in vegetarians and vegans. Adv Res Gastroentero Hepatol. 2019; 13(4): 555867.
DOI: 10.19080/ARGH.2019.13.555867

12. Hunt J, Roughead Z. (1999) Nonheme-iron absorption, fecal ferritin excretion, and blood indexes of iron status in women consuming controlled lactoovovegetarian diets for 8 wk. *Am J Clin Nutr* 69(5):944-952.
13. Whittaker P, Barrett J, Lind T. (2001) The erythrocyte incorporation of absorbed non-haem iron in pregnant women. *Br J Nutr* 86(3):323-329.
14. Siimes M, Refino C, Dallman P. (1980) Manifestation of iron deficiency at various levels of dietary iron intake. *Am J Clin Nutr* 33(3):570-574.
15. Gillooly M, Bothwell T, Torrance J, et al. (1983) The effects of organic acids, phytates and polyphenols on the absorption of iron from vegetables. *Br J Nutr* 49(3):331-342.
16. García-Casal M, Layrisse M, Solano L, et al. (1998) Vitamin A and beta-carotene can improve nonheme iron absorption from rice, wheat and corn by. *J Nutr* 128(3):646-650.
17. Temme E, Van Hoydonck P. (2002) Tea consumption and iron status. *Eur J Clin Nutr* 56(5):379-386.
18. Markiewicz L, Honke J, Haros M, Świątecka D, Wróblewska B. (2013) Diet shapes the ability of human intestinal microbiota to degrade phytate- in vitro studies. *J Appl Microbiol* 115(1):247-259.
19. Storcksdieck S, Walczyk T, Renggli S, Hurrell R. (2008) Oxalic acid does not influence nonhaem iron absorption in humans: a comparison of kale and spinach meals. *Eur J Clin Nutr* 62:336-341.
20. Mølgaard C, Kaestel P, Michaelsen K. (2005) Long-term calcium supplementation does not affect the iron status of 12–14-y-old girls. *Am J Clin Nutr* 82(1):98-102.
21. Craig W. (1994) Iron status of vegetarians. *Am J Clin Nutr* 59(5 Suppl):1233S-1237S.
22. Haddad E, Berk LKJ, Hubbard R, Peters W. (1999) Dietary intake and biochemical, hematologic, and immune status of vegans compared with nonvegetarians. *Am J Clin Nutr* 70(3 Suppl):586S-593S.
23. Elorinne A, Alfthan G, Erlund I, et al. (2016) Food and Nutrient Intake and Nutritional Status of Finnish Vegans and Non-Vegetarians. *PLoS One* 11(2):e0148235.
24. World Health Organization. (1992) Maternal Health and Safe Motherhood Programme & World Health Organization. Nutrition Programme. *The Prevalence of Anaemia in Women: A Tabulation of Available Information, 2nd ed.* Geneva: World Health Organization.
25. Looker A, Dallman P, Carroll M, Gunter E, Johnson C. (1997) Prevalence of iron deficiency in the United States. *JAMA* 277(12):973-976.
26. Allen L. (1997) Pregnancy and iron deficiency: unresolved issues. *Nutr Rev* 55(4):91-101.
27. Kepczyk T, Kadakia S. (1995) Prospective evaluation of gastrointestinal tract in patients with iron-deficiency anemia. *Dig Dis Sci* 40(6):1283-1289.
28. Rockey D, Cello JP. (1993) Evaluation of the gastro-intestinal tract in patients with iron-deficiency anemia. *New Eng J Med* 329:1691-1695.
29. Cook I, Pavli P, Riley JW, Goulston K, Dent O. (1986) Gastrointestinal investigation of iron deficiency anaemia. *Br Med J (Clin Res Ed)* 292(6532):1380-1382.
30. Zuckerman G, Benitez J. (1992) A prospective study of bidirectional endoscopy (colonoscopy and upper endoscopy) in the evaluation of patients with occult gastrointestinal bleeding. *Am J Gastroenterol* 87(1):62-66.
31. Hardwick R, Armstrong C. (1997) Synchronous upper and lower gastrointestinal endoscopy is an effective method of investigating iron-deficiency anaemia. *Br J Surg* 84(12):1725-1728.
32. James M, Chen C, Goddard W, Scott B, Goddard A. (2005) Risk factors for gastrointestinal malignancy in patients with iron-deficiency anaemia. *Eur J Gastroenterol Hepatol* 17(11):1197-1203.

How to cite this article: Rose S, Strombom A. Ensuring adequate iron status in vegetarians and vegans. Adv Res Gastroentero Hepatol. 2019; 13(4): 555867.
DOI: 10.19080/ARGH.2019.13.555867

33. Hershko C, Hoffbrand A, Keret D, et al. (2005) Role of autoimmune gastritis, Helicobacter pylori and celiac disease in refractory or unexplained iron deficiency anemia. *Haematologica* 90(5):585-595.

34. Corazza G, Valentini R, Andreani M, et al. (1995) Subclinical coeliac disease is a frequent cause of iron-deficiency anaemia. *Scand J Gastroenterol* 30(2):153-156.

35. Kulnigg S, Gasche C. (2006) Systematic review: managing anaemia in Crohn's disease. *Aliment Pharmacol Ther* 24(11-12):1507-1523.

36. Gasche C. (2000) Anemia in IBD: the overlooked villain. *Inflamm Bowel Dis* 6(2):142-150.

37. De Nicola L, Minutolo R, Chiodini P, et al. (2010) Prevalence and prognosis of mild anemia in non-dialysis chronic kidney disease: a prospective cohort study in outpatient renal clinics. *Am J Nephrol* 32(6):533-540.

38. Minutolo R, Locatelli F, Gallieni M, et al. (2013) Anaemia management in non-dialysis chronic kidney disease (CKD) patients: a multicentre prospective study in renal clinics. *Nephrol Dial Transplant* 28(12):3035-45.

39. Baribeault D, Auerbach M. (2011) Iron replacement therapy in cancer-related anemia. *Am J Health Syst Pharm* 68(10 Suppl 1):S4-S14.

40. Jankowska E, Rozentryt P, Witkowska A, et al. (2010) Iron deficiency: an ominous sign in patients with systolic chronic heart failure. *Eur Heart J* 31(15):1872-1880.

41. Klip I, Comin-Colet J, Voors A, et al. (2013) Iron deficiency in chronic heart failure: an international pooled analysis. *Am Heart J* 165(4):575-582.

42. Goddard A, James M, McIntyre A, Scott B. (2011) Guidelines for the management of iron deficiency anaemia. *Gut* 60(10):1309-1316.

43. Guyatt G, Oxman A, Ali M, Willan A, McIlroy W, Patterson C. (1992) Laboratory diagnosis of iron-deficiency anemia: an overview. *J Gen Intern Med* 7(2):145-153.

44. Cook J, Baynes R, Skikne B. (1992) Iron deficiency and the measurement of iron status. *Nutr Res Rev* 5(1):198-202.

45. Koperdanova M, Cullis J. (2015) Interpreting raised serum ferritin levels. *BMJ* 351:h3692.

46. Smith A. (1997) Prescribing iron. *Prescribers' J* 37:82-87.

47. Crosby W, O'Neil-Cutting M. (1984) A small dose iron tolerance test as an indicator of mild iron deficiency. *JAMA* 251(15):1986-1987.

48. Joosten E, Vander Elst B, Billen J. (1997) Small-dose iron absorption testing in anemic and non-anemic elderly hospitalised patients. *Eur J Haematol* 58(2):99-103.

49. Jimenez K, Kulnigg-Dabsch S, Gasche C. (2015) Management of Iron Deficiency Anemia. *Gastroenterol Hapatol (NY)* 11(4):241-250.

50. Werner E, Kaltwasser J, Ihm P. (1976) [Intestinal absorption from therapeutic iron doses (author's transl)]. *Arzneimittelforschung* 26(11):2093-2100.

51. Tolkien Z, Stecher L, Mander A, Pereira D, Powell J. (2015) Ferrous sulfate supplementation causes significant gastrointestinal side-effects in adults: a systematic review and meta-analysis. *PLoS One* 10(2):e0117383.

52. Le C. (2016) The Prevalence of Anemia and Moderate-Severe Anemia in the US Population (NHANES 2003-2012). *PLoS One* 11(11):e0166635.

How to cite this article: Rose S, Strombom A. Ensuring adequate iron status in vegetarians and vegans. Adv Res Gastroentero Hepatol. 2019; 13(4): 555867.
DOI: 10.19080/ARGH.2019.13.555867

Orthopedics and Rheumatology
Open Access Journal
ISSN: 2471-6804

Juniper PUBLISHERS key to the Researchers

Review Article
Volume 15 Issue 1 - October 2019
DOI: 10.19080/OROAJ.2019.15.555903

Orth & Rheum Open Access J

Ensuring Adequate Calcium intake on a Plant-Based Diet

Stewart Rose* and Amanda Strombom

Plant-Based Diets in Medicine, USA

Submission: October 04, 2019; **Published:** October 16, 2019

***Corresponding author:** Stewart Rose, Plant-Based Diets in Medicine, 12819 SE 38th St, #427, Bellevue, WA 98006, USA

Abstract

Patients on a plant-based diet consume no dairy products and so must get their calcium from plant foods. Fortunately, a number of plant foods can supply the calcium needed. However, care needs to be taken to obtain calcium from foods that have a low oxalate content and therefore are more bioavailable. Concern about reduced bioavailability due to phytate is less of an issue for those on a plant-based diet because they develop bacterial flora that effectively degrades it.

Epidemiologic studies show that people on a plant-based diet achieve a bone mineral density equal to their omnivore counterparts if their calcium intake is adequate. However, plant-based diets vary in their content. While some patients on a plant-based diet achieve adequate calcium intake, many don't.

In order to ensure adequate calcium intake, patients need to be counseled to emphasize foods with a high calcium content. Patients should also be counseled on dietary factors that decrease calcium retention, particularly sodium. Almost half the American public take calcium supplements. This can be helpful for patients on a plant-based diet.

Obtaining calcium from plant foods has the advantage of avoiding the saturated fat and cholesterol in dairy products, and providing other nutrients, including fiber and phytonutrients, absent in dairy.

1. Physiology

Calcium (Ca) is the most abundant mineral in the body. The only source of calcium is from the diet. It is found in some foods, added to others, available as a dietary supplement, and present in some medicines (such as antacids). Calcium is required for vascular contraction and vasodilation, muscle function, nerve transmission, intracellular signaling and hormonal secretion, although less than 1% of total body calcium is needed to support these critical metabolic functions. The remaining 99% of the body's calcium supply is stored in the bones and teeth where it supports their structure and function. (1)

Serum calcium is very tightly regulated and does not fluctuate with changes in dietary intakes. The body uses bone tissue as a reservoir for, and source of calcium, to maintain constant concentrations of calcium in blood, muscle, and intercellular fluids. (1)

Calcium insufficiency manifests as decreased bone mass and osteoporotic fracture. In the rapidly growing child, calcium deficiency causes rickets. Low levels of intestinal calcium resulting from low dietary intakes have also been associated with increased risk of kidney stones and colon cancer. (2) This is probably due to the decreased binding and increased absorption of oxalic acid, the main constituent of kidney stones, and of carcinogens such as bile acids. (3)

Calcium's metabolism is regulated by 3 major transport systems: intestinal absorption, renal reabsorption, and bone metabolism. Calcium transport in these tissues is regulated by a homeostatic hormonal system that involves parathyroid hormone, 1,25 dihydroxyvitamin D, ionized calcium, and the calcium sensing receptor. (1, 3)

1.1 Intestinal absorption

The transfer of calcium across the intestinal barrier occurs through both saturable (transcellular) and non-saturable (paracellular diffusion) pathways. (4, 5, 6, 7, 8) The saturable component of Ca absorption is prevalent in the proximal small intestine (i.e. duodenum and jejunum) and is under nutritional and physiological regulation. This is an energy dependent pathway whereby Ca movement from the mucosal-to-serosal side of the intestinal barrier can occur against a concentration gradient. (9, 8)

In contrast, passive transport occurs throughout the length of the intestine and is a non-saturable, linear function of luminal Ca concentration (e.g. 13% of luminal load per hour in humans.) (7, 8) The non-saturable portion of Ca absorption in the human ileum is vitamin D sensitive, (7, 8) as is the saturable pathway to a lesser degree.

In the case of low intake of calcium, the saturable transport pathway is up-regulated, a process mediated by increased renal production of 1,25 dihydroxyvitamin D (1,25(OH)2 D). **(10)** Dawson-Hughes et al. found that in women, the efficiency of Ca absorption increased by 32% within one week of reducing dietary Ca intake from 2000 mg/d to 300 mg/d. (11) Consistent with this, low vitamin D status, as well as deletion/mutation of the vitamin D receptor (VDR) or 25 hydroxyvitamin D-1α hydroxylase (CYP27B1) genes, limit Ca absorption by reducing the saturable pathway.

1.2 Bone metabolism

Calcium metabolism is regulated in large part by the parathyroid hormone (PTH)–vitamin D endocrine system, which is characterized by a series of homeostatic feedback loops. The rapid release of mineral from the bone is essential to maintain adequate levels of ionized calcium in serum. During vitamin D deficiency states, bone metabolism is significantly affected as a result of reduced active calcium absorption. This leads to increased PTH secretion as the calcium sensing receptor in the parathyroid gland senses changes in circulating ionic calcium. Increased PTH levels

How to cite this article: Rose S, Strombom A. Ensuring adequate calcium intake on a plant-based diet. Ortho & Rheum Open Access J. 2019; 15(1): 555903.
DOI: 10.19080/OROAJ.2019.15.555903

induce enzyme activity (1α-hydroxylase) in the kidney, which converts vitamin D to its active hormonal form, calcitriol. In turn, calcitriol stimulates enhanced calcium absorption from the gut. Not surprisingly, the interplay between the dynamics of calcium and vitamin D often complicates the interpretation of data relative to calcium requirements, deficiency states, and excess intake. (1)

In addition to the well-established effects that estrogen has on bone and bone cells, (12, 13, 14) estrogen can influence Ca metabolism in several ways. (15) In a comparison of pre and post-menopausal women, Heaney et al. found that calcium balance fell significantly in post-menopausal women and that this was due to both a reduction in calcium absorption and an increase in urinary calcium loss. (12) Estrogen loss can reduce the serum level of 1,25(OH)2 D, but this can be reversed by estrogen repletion and is accompanied by an increase in fractional calcium absorption. (16)

1.3 Renal reabsorption

Calcium leaves the body mainly in urine and feces, but also in other body tissues and fluids, such as sweat. Calcium excretion in the urine is a function of the balance between the calcium load filtered by the kidneys and the efficiency of reabsorption from the renal tubules. (17) Nearly 98 percent of filtered calcium (i.e., glomerular filtrate) is reabsorbed by either passive or active processes occurring at four sites in the kidney, each contributing to maintaining neutral calcium balance. Seventy percent of the filtered calcium is reabsorbed passively in the proximal tubule.

Active calcium transport is regulated by the calcium sensing receptor located in the ascending loop of Henle, where, in response to high calcium levels in the extracellular fluid, active reabsorption in the loop is blocked through actions of the calcium sensing receptor. In contrast, when the filtered calcium load is low, the calcium sensing receptor is activated, and a greater fraction of the filtered calcium is reabsorbed. In the distal tubule, the ion channels known as transient receptor potential cation channel vanilloid family member 5 (TRPV5) control active calcium transport and this process is regulated by calcitriol and estradiol. Finally, the collecting duct also can participate in passive calcium transport, although the relative percentage of total calcium reabsorption in the collecting duct is low. Overall, a typical daily calcium loss for a healthy adult man or woman via renal excretion is 5 mmol/day. (18)

Disruption of any of these mechanisms leads to abnormal calcium homeostasis. In chronic kidney disease, disturbances in calcium homeostasis are common and, as GFR decreases, disturbances in calcium homeostasis increase. (19)

Healthy vegans who have a lower than desirable Ca intake can still maintain sufficient Ca status through the activation of the saturable pathway and through increased renal absorption.

2. Epidemiology

2.1 Bone density

Several studies have shown that vegans have the same bone density (BMD) and fracture rates as omnivores. (20, 21, 22, 23) However some studies did not. (24) The differences may be a result of different diets within the spectrum of plant based diets. Some vegan diets have higher intakes of calcium than others. This may be particularly true of east Asian plant-based diets.

In one study of those who follow a plant-based diet, subjects who had at least 525 mg calcium per

How to cite this article: Rose S, Strombom A. Ensuring adequate calcium intake on a plant-based diet. Ortho & Rheum Open Access J. 2019; 15(1): 555903.
DOI: 10.19080/OROAJ.2019.15.555903

day had the same fracture risk as omnivores, but, those whose intake was less than 525 mg per day had a higher risk of fracture. (25) So it appears that at a Ca intake level of 525 mg and above, the fracture rates of vegans are equivalent to the fracture rate of omnivores.

With aging and after menopause, fractional calcium absorption has been reported to decline on average by 0.21 percent per year after 40 years of age. (1)

2.2 Nutrition

Many plant foods are a good source of calcium and the absorption of calcium from them is often better than from dairy products. However, oxalic acid, found naturally in some plants, binds to calcium and can inhibit its absorption. (1) The high bioavailability of calcium from low oxalate vegetables, relative to milk, suggests two things. First, the fibers in the vegetables do not inhibit calcium absorption. This has been confirmed with purified fibers. (26, 27) Second, low oxalate vegetables may contain calcium absorption enhancers that have not yet been identified. (26)

In general, calcium absorption is inversely proportional to the oxalic acid content of the food. Thus, calcium bioavailability is low from both American and Chinese varieties of spinach (5%) and rhubarb, intermediate from sweet potatoes (25%), and high from low oxalate vegetables such as kale (50%), broccoli (62%), and bok choy (54%). A notable exception to this generalization is soybeans. Soybeans are rich in both oxalate and phytate, yet soy products have relatively high calcium bioavailability. (26)

High intake of fruits and vegetables have been associated with a benefit to bone health. (28, 29, 30) Potassium levels in fruits and vegetables have been a leading candidate for this benefit. However, in a large Scottish study, flavonoid intake was more strongly related to bone health than fruit and vegetable intake in general. (31) Flavonoids are polyphenolic compounds, some of which have specific effects on osteoblasts or osteoclasts that reduce age-related bone loss. (32) Observational studies have limited ability to distinguish the effect of potassium on bone in the context of many other constituents that may influence bone such as flavonoids.

It must also be remembered that some fruits and vegetables have specific positive effects on bone metabolism, which are independent of the alkalizing action of vegetarian diets. For example, the consumption of onions, (33) and of tomatoes, berries, salad greens and green vegetables may be significantly correlated with lower bone resorption and higher BMD of the lumbar spine in humans. (34) Blue fruits, such as plums and blueberries were also shown to inhibit bone resorption and to increase BMD in humans. (35, 36)

2.3 Antinutrients

Urinary calcium losses account for 50% of the variability in calcium retention. (37) Of the nutritional factors thought to influence urinary calcium losses (protein, caffeine and sodium intake), sodium appears to be the most important factor. Because sodium and calcium share some of the same transport systems in the proximal tubule, each 2300mg sodium excreted by the kidney pulls 40–60mg calcium out with it. (38)

How to cite this article: Rose S, Strombom A. Ensuring adequate calcium intake on a plant-based diet. Ortho & Rheum Open Access J. 2019; 15(1): 555903.
DOI: 10.19080/OROAJ.2019.15.555903

High protein intake also increases calcium excretion and was therefore thought to negatively affect calcium status. (26, 39) However, more recent research suggests that high protein intake also increases intestinal calcium absorption, effectively offsetting its effect on calcium excretion, so whole body calcium retention remains substantially unchanged. (40)

In a double-blind, placebo-controlled trial, Berger-Lux et al. showed that a coffee intake in excess of 1000 mL could induce an extra calcium loss of 1.6 mmol calcium/day, whereas intakes of 1-2 cups of coffee per day would have little impact on calcium balance. (41) Other studies reported differing results, but relied on estimating caffeine consumption from food-composition tables. (42) Although caffeine consumed in high amounts acutely increases urinary calcium, the effect on 24-hr urinary calcium was negligible. (41) On average, a cup (240 mL) of coffee decreases calcium retention by only 2–3mg. (26) Thus, even heavy consumption of caffeine has a modest effect on calcium loss for most people.

The effect of phosphate on calcium excretion is minimal. Several observational studies suggest that consumption of carbonated soft drinks with high levels of phosphate is associated with reduced bone mass and increased fracture risk. However, the effect is probably due to replacing milk with soda rather than the phosphorus itself. (43, 44)

There has long been a theoretical concern about the larger intake of phytates in plant foods inhibiting mineral absorption of some minerals, such as calcium in those following a vegetarian diet. However, there was little evidence of deficiency commonly occurring in practice. Part of the answer lies in the microbiota of the vegetarian. It turns out that their flora act to degrade phytate, thus allowing for good absorption of minerals. One recent study concludes that, "it was the vegetarians' microbiota that particularly degraded up to 100% phytate to myo-inositol phosphate products." A diet rich in phytate increases the potential of intestinal microbiota to degrade phytate. The co-operation of both aerobic and anaerobic bacteria is essential for the complete phytate degradation. (45)

3. Clinical considerations.

Here are the current U.S. recommended dietary allowances (RDAs):

Table 1: Recommended Dietary Allowances for Calcium (1)

Age	Male	Female	Pregnant	Lactating
0-6 months	200 mg	200 mg		
7-12 months	260 mg	260 mg		
1-3 years	700 mg	700 mg		
4-8 years	1,000 mg	1,000 mg		
9-13 years	1,300 mg	1,300 mg		
14-18 years	1,300 mg	1,300 mg	1,300 mg	1,300 mg
19-50 years	1,000 mg	1,000 mg	1,000 mg	1,000 mg
51-70 years	1,000 mg	1,000 mg		
71+ years	1,200 mg	1,200 mg		

These RDAs are not universally recommended and vary from country to country. For instance, in the United Kingdom the RDAs are around half the U.S. levels. Given the data on fracture rates (25) the United Kingdom RDAs appear to be adequate.

Table 2: Calcium content of various foods

Food	Calcium (mg/100 cal serving)	Absorption Rate
Bok Choy	870 mg	High
Collard Greens	609 mg	Medium
Orange Juice (calc fortified)	320 mg	High
Tofu (set with calcium)	287 mg	Medium
Kale	270 mg	High
Broccoli	215 mg	High
Cow's milk (for comparison)	188 mg	Medium
Sesame seeds	170 mg	Medium
Cabbage	160 mg	High
White Beans	72 mg	Medium
Tempeh	55 mg	Medium

How to cite this article: Rose S, Strombom A. Ensuring adequate calcium intake on a plant-based diet. Ortho & Rheum Open Access J. 2019; 15(1): 555903.
DOI: 10.19080/OROAJ.2019.15.555903

To meet the recommendations generous portions of plant foods should be eaten. Even so, some people will still need help in reaching recommended intakes of calcium. In these cases, supplements will prove very helpful.

3.1 Calcium Supplements

About 43% of the U.S. population (including almost 70% of older women) uses dietary supplements containing calcium, increasing calcium intakes on average by about 330 mg/day among supplement users. (1, 46)

The two main forms of calcium in supplements are carbonate and citrate. Calcium carbonate is more commonly available and is both inexpensive and convenient. Due to its dependence on stomach acid for absorption, calcium carbonate is absorbed most efficiently when taken with food, whereas calcium citrate is absorbed equally well when taken with or without food. (47) Calcium citrate is also useful for people with achlorhydria, inflammatory bowel disease, or absorption disorders. (1) Calcium citrate or malate is a well-absorbed form of calcium found in some fortified juices. (48) Other calcium forms in supplements or fortified foods include gluconate, lactate, and phosphate.

The percentage of calcium absorbed depends on the total amount of elemental calcium consumed at one time; as the amount increases, the percentage absorption decreases. Absorption is highest in doses less than 500mg. (1) So, for example, one who takes 1,000mg/day of calcium from supplements might split the dose and take 500mg at two separate times during the day.

Some individuals who take calcium supplements might experience gastrointestinal side effects including gas, bloating, constipation, or a combination of these symptoms. Calcium carbonate appears to cause more of these side effects than calcium citrate, (1) so consideration of the form of calcium supplement is warranted if these side effects are reported. Other strategies to alleviate symptoms include spreading out the calcium dose throughout the day and/or taking the supplement with meals.

3.2 Medication Interactions

Calcium supplements have the potential to interact with several types of medications. Individuals taking these medications on a regular basis should discuss their calcium intake with their healthcare providers.

Calcium can decrease absorption of the following drugs when taken together: bisphosphonates, benzodiazephines, the fluoroquinolone and tetracycline classes of antibiotics, levothyroxine, phenytoin, and tiludronate disodium. (49, 50, 51)

Thiazide-type diuretics can interact with calcium carbonate and vitamin D supplements, increasing the risks of hypercalcemia and hypercalciuria. (50)

Both aluminum- and magnesium-containing antacids increase urinary calcium excretion. Mineral oil and stimulant laxatives decrease calcium absorption. Glucocorticoids, such as prednisone, can cause calcium depletion and eventually osteoporosis when they are used for months. (50)

Studies on human subjects have shown that calcium (Ca) can inhibit iron (Fe) absorption, regardless of whether it is given as Ca salts or in food products. This has caused concern as increased Ca intake commonly is recommended for children and women, the same populations that are at risk of Fe deficiency. However, a thorough review of studies on humans in which Ca intake was substantially increased for long periods shows no changes in hematological measures or indicators of iron status. (52)

4. Discussion

The patient on a plant-based diet needs calcium the same as their omnivore counterparts. Calcium needs can be met with plant foods, so dairy consumption is not necessary.

In fact, obtaining calcium from plant food sources is preferable, in that they provide fiber, vitamins, minerals and phytonutrients, without the price tag of saturated fat and risk for the lactose intolerant. Vegetables also have the advantage of providing phytonutrients which have been associated with greater bone mineral density.

Patients should be counseled on which foods are high in bioavailable calcium. Apart from this, patient advice is the same as for omnivores. Special note should be made to avoid excessive sodium.

References

1. Institute of Medicine Food and Nutrition Board. (2010) *Dietary Reference Intakes for Calcium and Vitamin D*. Washington DC.
2. Shils M, Shike M. (2006) *Modern nutrition in health and disease*. 10th ed ed. Philadelphia: Lippincott Williams & Wilkins.
3. Weaver C, Peacock M. (2011) Calcium. *Advances in Nutrition*. 2(3):290–292.
4. Wasserman R, Taylor A. (1969) Some aspects of the intestinal absorption of calcium, with special reference to vitamin D. In: Comar C, Bronner F, eds. *Mineral Metabolism, An advanced treatise*. New York: Academic Press.
5. Pansu D, Bellaton C, Bronner F. (1981) Effect of Ca intake on saturable and nonsaturable components of duodenal Ca transport. *Am J Physiol*. 240(1):G32-37.
6. Heaney R, Saville P, Recker R. (1975) Calcium absorption as a function of calcium intake. *J Lab Clin Med*. 85(6):881-890.
7. Sheikh M, Schiller L, Fordtran J. (1990) In vivo intestinal absorption of calcium in humans. *Miner Electrolyte Metab*. 16(2-3):130-146.
8. Fleet J, Schoch R. (2010) Molecular mechanisms for regulation of intestinal calcium absorption by vitamin D and other factors. *Crit Rev Clin Lab Sci*. 47(4):181-195.
9. Favus M, Angeid-Backman E, Breyer M, Coe F. (1983) Effects of trifluoperazine, ouabain, and ethacrynic acid on intestinal calcium transport. *Am J Physiol*. 244(2):G111-G115.
10. Favus M, Walling M, Kimberg D. (1974) Effects of dietary calcium restriction and chronic thyroparathyroidectomy on the metabolism of (3H)25-hydroxyvitamin D3 and the active transport of calcium by rat intestine. *J Clin Invest*. 53:1139-1148.
11. Dawson-Hughes B, Harris S, Kramich C, Dallal G, Rasmussen H. (1993) Calcium retention and hormone levels in black and white women on high- and low-calcium diets. *J Bone Min Res*. 8(7):779-787.
12. Heaney R, Recker R, Saville P. (1978) Menopausal changes in bone remodeling. *J Lab Clin Med*. 92(6):964-970.
13. Hofbauer L, Khosla S, Dunstan C, Lacey D, Spelsberg T, et al. (1999) Estrogen stimulates gene expression and protein production of osteoprotegerin in human osteoblastic cells. *Endocrinology*. 140(9):4367-4370.
14. Sarma U, Edwards M, Motoyoshi K, Flanagan A. (1998) Inhibition of bone resorption by 17β-estradiol in human bone marrow cultures. *J Cell Physiol*. 175(1):99-108.
15. Riggs B, Khosla S, Melton L. (2002) Sex steroids and the construction and conservation of the adult skeleton. *Endocr Rev*. 23(3):279-302.
16. Gallagher J, Riggs B, DeLuca H. (1980) Effect of estrogen on calcium absorption and serum vitamin D metabolites in postmenopausal

How to cite this article: Rose S, Strombom A. Ensuring adequate calcium intake on a plant-based diet. Ortho & Rheum Open Access J. 2019; 15(1): 555903.
DOI: 10.19080/OROAJ.2019.15.555903

osteoporosis. *J Clin Endocrinol Metab*. 51(6):1359-1364.

17. Peacock M. (1988) Renal excretion of calcium. In: Nordin BEC, ed. *Calcium in Human Biology*. 1st ed. London: Springer-Verlag.
18. McCormick C. (2002) Passive diffusion does not play a major role in the absorption of dietary calcium in normal adults. *J Nutr*. 132(11):3428-3430.
19. Goodman W. (2005) Calcium and phosphorus metabolism in patients who have chronic kidney disease. *Med Clin North Am*. 89(3):631-647.
20. Ho-Pham L, Nguyen N, Nguyen T. (2009) Effect of vegetarian diets on bone mineral density: a Bayesian meta-analysis. *Am J Clin Nutr*. 90(4):943-950.
21. Knurick J, Johnston C, Wherry S, Aguayo I. (2015) Comparison of correlates of bone mineral density in individuals adhering to lacto-ovo, vegan, or omnivore diets: a cross-sectional investigation. *Nutrients*. 7(5):3416-3426.
22. Ho-Pham L, Vu B, Lai T, Nguyen N, Nguyen T. (2012) Vegetarianism, bone loss, fracture and vitamin D: a longitudinal study in Asian vegans and non-vegans. *Eur J Clin Nutr*. 66(1):75-82.
23. Ho-Pham L, Nguyen P, Le T, Doan T, Tran N, et al. (2009) Veganism, bone mineral density, and body composition: a study in Buddhist nuns. *Osteoporos Int*. 20(12):2087-2093.
24. Iguacel I, Miguel-Berges M, Gómez-Bruton A, Moreno L, Julián C. (2019) Veganism, vegetarianism, bone mineral density, and fracture risk: a systematic review and meta-analysis. *Nutr Rev*. 77(1):1-18.
25. Appleby P, Roddam A, Allen N, Key T. (2007) Comparative fracture risk in vegetarians and nonvegetarians in EPIC-Oxford. *Eur J Clin Nutr*. 61(12):1400-1406.
26. Weaver C, Proulx W, Heaney R. (1999) Choices for achieving adequate dietary calcium with a vegetarian diet. *Am J Clin Nutr*. 70(3 Suppl):543S-548S.
27. Heaney R, Weaver C. (1995) Effect of psyllium on absorption of co-ingested calcium. *J Am Geriatr Soc*. 43(3):261-263.
28. Tucker K, Hannan M, Chen H, Cupples L, Wilson P, et al. (1999) Potassium, magnesium, and fruit and vegetable intakes are associated with greater bone mineral density in elderly men and women. *Am J Clin Nutr*. 69(4):727-736.
29. Prynne C, Mishra G, O'Connell M, Muniz G, Laskey M, et al. (2006) Fruit and vegetable intakes and bone mineral status: a cross sectional study in 5 age and sex cohorts. *Am J Clin Nutr*. 83(6):1420-1428.
30. Chen Y, Ho S, Woo J. (2006) Greater fruit and vegetable intake is associated with increased bone mass among postmenopausal Chinese women. *Br J Nutr*. 96(4):745-751.
31. Hardcastle A, Aucott L, Reid D, Macdonald H. (2011) Associations between dietary flavonoid intakes and bone health in a Scottish population. *J Bone Miner Res*. 26(5):941-947.
32. Weaver C, Alekel D, Ward W, Ronis M. (2012) Flavonoid intake and bone health. *J Nutr Gerontol Geriatr*. 31(3):239-253.
33. Matheson E, Mainous A, Carnemolla M. (2009) The association between onion consumption and bone density in perimenopausal and postmenopausal non-Hispanic white women 50 years and older. *Menopause*. 16(4):756-759.
34. Macdonald H, Hardcastle A.(2010) Dietary patterns and bone health. In: Burckhardt P, Dawson-Hughes B, Weaver C, eds. *Nutritional Influences on Bone Health*. 1st ed. London: Spinger.
35. Hooshmand S, Chai S, Saadat R, Payton M, Brummel-Smith K, et al. (2011) Comparative effects of dried plum and dried apple on bone in postmenopausal women. *Br J Nutr*. 106(6):923-930.
36. Davicco M, Puel C, Lebecque P, Coxam V. (2013) Blueberry in Calcium- and Vitamin D-Enriched Fermented Milk Is Able to Modulate Bone Metabolism in

Postmenopausal Women. In: Burckhardt P, Dawson-Hughes B, Weaver C, eds. *Nutritional Influences on Bone Health*. 8th ed. London: Springer.

37. NIH Consensus Development Panel on optimal calcium intake. (1994) Optimal calcium intake. *JAMA*. 272(24):1942-1948.
38. Nordin B, Need A, Morris H, Horowitz M. (1993) The nature and significance of the relationship between urinary sodium and urinary calcium in women. *J Nutr*. 123(9):1615-1622.
39. Heaney R. (1996) Bone mass, nutrition, and other lifestyle factors. *Nutr Rev*. 54(4 Pt 2):S3-10.
40. Kerstetter J, O'Brien K, Caseria D, Wall D, Insogna K. (2005) The impact of dietary protein on calcium absorption and kinetic measures of bone turnover in women. *J Clin Endocrinol Metab*. 90(1):26-31.
41. Hasling C, Søndergaard K, Charles P, Mosekilde L. (1992) Calcium metabolism in postmenopausal osteoporotic women is determined by dietary calcium and coffee intake. *J Nutr*. 122(5):1119-1126.
42. Barger-Lux M, Heaney R, Stegman M. (1990) Effects of moderate caffeine intake on the calcium economy of premenopausal women. *Am J Clin Nutr*. 52(4):722-725.
43. Calvo M. (1993) Dietary phosphorus, calcium metabolism and bone. *J Nutr*. 123(9):1627-1633.
44. Heaney R, Rafferty K. (2001) Carbonated beverages and urinary calcium excretion. *Am J Clin Nutr*. 74(3):343-347.
45. Markiewicz L, Honke J, Haros M, Świątecka D, Wróblewska B. (2013) Diet shapes the ability of human intestinal microbiota to degrade phytate–in vitro studies. *J Appl Microbiol*. 115(1):247-259.
46. Bailey R, Dodd K, Goldman J, Gahche J, Dwyer J, et al. (2010) Estimation of total usual calcium and vitamin D intakes in the United States. *J Nutr*. 140(4):817-822.
47. Straub D. (2007) Calcium supplementation in clinical practice: a review of forms, doses, and indications. *Nutr Clin Pract*. 22(3):288-296.
48. Andon M, Peacock M, Kanerva R, De Castro J. (1996) Calcium absorption from apple and orange juice fortified with calcium citrate malate (CCM). *J Am Coll Nutr*. 15(3):313-316.
49. Shannon M, Wilson B, Stang C. (2000) *Health Professionals Drug Guide*. Stamford, CT: Appleton and Lange.
50. Jellin J, Gregory P, Batz F, Hitchens K. (2000) *Pharmacist's letter/Prescriber's letter Natural medicines comprehensive database*. 3rd ed ed. Stockton, CA: Therapeutic Research Facility.
51. Peters M, Leonard M, Licata A. (2001) Role of alendronate and risedronate in preventing and treating osteoporosis. *Cleve Clin J Med*. 68(11):945-51.
52. Lönnerdal B. (2010) Calcium and iron absorption–mechanisms and public health relevance. *Int J Vitam Nutr Res*. 80(4-5):293-299.

How to cite this article: Rose S, Strombom A. Ensuring adequate calcium intake on a plant-based diet. Ortho & Rheum Open Access J. 2019; 15(1): 555903.
DOI: 10.19080/OROAJ.2019.15.555903

Advanced Research in Gastroenterology & Hepatology
ISSN: 2472-6400

Juniper Publishers
key to the Researchers

Review Article
Volume 14 Issue 3 - December 2019
DOI: 10.19080/ARGH.2019.14.555887

Adv Res Gastroenterol Hepatol

Ensuring Adequate Zinc status in Vegans and Vegetarians

Stewart D Rose and Amanda J Strombom*

Plant-Based Diets in Medicine, USA

Submission: November 22, 2019; **Published:** December 18, 2019

***Corresponding Author:** Amanda Strombom, Plant-Based Diets in Medicine, 12819 SE 38th St, #427, Bellevue, WA 98006, USA

Abstract

Zinc is an essential mineral that is naturally present in some foods, added to others, and available as a dietary supplement. It is involved in numerous aspects of cellular metabolism, and also supports normal growth and development. Frequent intake of zinc is required to maintain a steady state because the body has no specialized zinc storage system.

Zinc is available from many plant foods. Protein increases zinc absorption. Because of this, foods high in protein and zinc, such as legumes and nuts, are good choices. Zinc deficiency is characterized by growth retardation, loss of appetite, and impaired immune function.

Zinc nutritional status is difficult to measure adequately using laboratory tests. Clinical effects of zinc deficiency can be present in the absence of abnormal laboratory indices. Adverse health effects have not been commonly demonstrated with varied, plant-based diets consumed in developed countries.

Supplements are an option for those with potential deficiencies. Both zinc gluconate and zinc citrate are well-absorbed. However, zinc supplements have the potential to interact with several types of medications.

Keywords:

Nutritional status; Zinc; Zinc gluconate; Zinc citrate; Medications; Plant foods; Cellular metabolism; Immune function; Protein synthesis; Lactic dehydrogenase; Protein; Growth retardation; Loss of appetite; Impaired immune function

1. Introduction

Zinc is an essential mineral that is naturally present in some foods, added to others, and available as a dietary supplement. Zinc is involved in numerous aspects of cellular metabolism. It is required for the catalytic activity of approximately 100 enzymes, (1, 2) and it plays a role in immune function, (3, 4) protein synthesis, (4) wound healing, (5) DNA synthesis, (2, 4) and cell division. (4)

Zinc also supports normal growth and development during pregnancy, childhood, and adolescence (6, 7, 8) and is required for proper sense of taste and smell. (9) Importantly, Zinc is an integral part of carbonic anhydrase and lactic dehydrogenase. (10)

A frequent intake of zinc is required to maintain a steady state because the body has no specialized zinc storage system. (11)

Table 1: Recommended Dietary Allowances (RDAs) for Zinc (2)

Age	Male	Female	Pregnancy	Lactation
0–6 months	2 mg*	2 mg*		
7–12 months	3 mg	3 mg		
1–3 years	3 mg	3 mg		
4–8 years	5 mg	5 mg		
9–13 years	8 mg	8 mg		
14–18 years	11 mg	9 mg	12 mg	13 mg
19+ years	11 mg	8 mg	11 mg	12 mg

* Adequate Intake (AI)

2. Zinc food sources

Table 2: A list of representative plant-based foods

Food	Serving Size	Amount of Zinc
Wheat Germ	**1 ounce**	**3.4 mg**
Baked beans, canned, plain or vegetarian	**½ cup**	**2.9 mg**
Pumpkin seeds, dried	**1 ounce**	**2.2 mg**
Tofu	**½ cup**	**2.0 mg**
Cashews, dry roasted	**1 ounce**	**1.6 mg**
Chickpeas, cooked	**½ cup**	**1.3 mg**
Oatmeal, instant, plain, prepared with water	**1 packet**	**1.1 mg**

How to cite this article: Rose S, Strombom A. Ensuring adequate zinc status in vegans and vegetarians. Adv Res Gastroentero Hepatol. 2019; 14(3): 555887.
DOI: 10.19080/ARGH.2019.14.555887

Protein increases zinc absorption. Because of this, foods high in protein and zinc, such as legumes and nuts, are good choices. (12) If a food doesn't have much protein, it can still be accompanied by one that does in order to enhance absorption.

3. Zinc deficiency

Zinc deficiency is characterized by growth retardation, loss of appetite, and impaired immune function. In more severe cases, zinc deficiency causes hair loss, diarrhea, delayed sexual maturation, impotence, hypogonadism in males, and eye and skin lesions. (2, 8, 13, 14) Weight loss, delayed healing of wounds, taste abnormalities, and mental lethargy can also occur. (8, 5, 15, 16, 17, 18, 19) Many of these symptoms are non-specific and often associated with other health conditions; therefore, a medical examination is necessary to ascertain whether a zinc deficiency is present.

4. Diagnosis

Zinc nutritional status is difficult to measure adequately using laboratory tests (2, 20, 21) due to its distribution throughout the body as a component of various proteins and nucleic acids. (22) Plasma or serum zinc levels are the most commonly used indices for evaluating zinc deficiency, but these levels do not necessarily reflect cellular zinc status due to tight homeostatic control mechanisms. (8) Clinical effects of zinc deficiency can be present in the absence of abnormal laboratory indices. (8)

5. Zinc deficiency risk in vegetarians and vegans

The zinc deficiencies commonly associated with plant-based diets in impoverished nations are not associated with vegetarian diets in wealthier countries. (20) Adverse health effects have not been demonstrated with varied, plant-based diets consumed in developed countries. (23)

Well-planned vegetarian diets can provide adequate amounts of zinc from plant sources. Vegetarians appear to adapt to lower zinc intakes by increased absorption and retention of zinc. Studies show vegetarians have similar serum zinc concentrations to, and no greater risk of zinc deficiency than, non-vegetarians despite differences in zinc intake. (24)

A meta study showed that zinc intake by vegetarians was only slightly lower than their omnivorous counterparts. It showed vegans to have only a slightly lower serum zinc level than non-vegetarians, a difference of 1.17 ± 0.45 μmol/l. (25) Average serum zinc levels are from 10 to 15 μmol/l. (26) Therefore the clinical relevance may be minimal. Existing data indicate no differences in serum zinc or growth between young vegetarian and omnivorous children. (27)

Pregnant women are vulnerable to a low zinc status due to the additional zinc demands associated with pregnancy and fetal development. A meta study found the pregnant vegetarian women consume on average, about 1.4mg per day less than their omnivorous pregnant women. (28) Supplements may be necessary for pregnant women.

Although vegans have lower zinc intake than omnivores, they do not differ from the nonvegetarians in functional immunocompetence as assessed by natural killer cell cytotoxic activity. (29) It appears that there may be facilitators of zinc absorption and compensatory mechanisms to help vegetarians adapt to a lower intake of zinc. (30)

How to cite this article: Rose S, Strombom A. Ensuring adequate zinc status in vegans and vegetarians. Adv Res Gastroentero Hepatol. 2019; 14(3): 555887.
DOI: 10.19080/ARGH.2019.14.555887

There has long been a theoretical concern about the larger intake of phytates in plant foods inhibiting mineral absorption of some minerals, such as zinc, in those following a vegetarian diet. However, there was little evidence of deficiency commonly occurring in practice. Part of the answer lies in the microbiota of the vegetarian. It turns out that their flora act to degrade phytate, thus allowing for good absorption of minerals. One recent study concludes that, "it was the vegetarians' microbiota that particularly degraded up to 100% phytate to myo-inositol phosphate products." A diet rich in phytate increases the potential of intestinal microbiota to degrade phytate. The co-operation of both aerobic and anaerobic bacteria is essential for the complete phytate degradation. (31)

The vegetarian diet compared with a meat-based diets resulted in lower amounts of absorbed Zn due to a higher content of Zn in the meat diets, but no difference was observed in the fractional absorption of zinc despite a high intake of phytates. (32) The presence of garlic and onion very significantly increased the bioavailability of zinc from grains. (33)

6. Zinc Supplements

Both zinc gluconate and zinc citrate are well-absorbed. (34) Zinc picolinate is also thought to well absorbed. (35) However, zinc oxide, which is used in many supplements because it's cheaper, may not be well absorbed by some people. (34) Note that in the case of zinc, the Supplement Facts panel on the supplement container is required to list the elemental zinc content, as opposed to the compound.

7. Interactions with Medications

Zinc supplements have the potential to interact with several types of medications:

Antibiotics: Both quinolone antibiotics (such as Cipro®) and tetracycline antibiotics (such as Achromycin® and Sumycin®) interact with zinc in the gastrointestinal tract, inhibiting the absorption of both zinc and the antibiotic. (36, 37) Taking the antibiotic at least 2 hours before or 4–6 hours after taking a zinc supplement minimizes this interaction. (38)

Penicillamine: Zinc can reduce the absorption and action of penicillamine, a drug used to treat rheumatoid arthritis. (39) To minimize this interaction, individuals should take zinc supplements at least 2 hours before or after taking penicillamine. (37)

Diuretics: Thiazide diuretics such as chlorthalidone (Hygroton®) and hydrochlorothiazide (Esidrix® and HydroDIURIL®) increase urinary zinc excretion by as much as 60%. (40) Prolonged use of thiazide diuretics could deplete zinc tissue levels, so clinicians should monitor zinc status in patients taking these medications.

References

1. Sandstead H. (1994) Understanding zinc: recent observations and interpretations. *J Lab Clin Med.* 124(3):322-327.
2. Institute of Medicine (US) Panel on Micronutrients. (2001) *Dietary Reference Intakes for Vitamin A, Vitamin K, Arsenic, Boron, Chromium, Copper, Iodine, Iron, Manganese, Molybdenum, Nickel, Silicon, Vanadium, and Zinc.* Washington DC: National Academies Press (US)
3. Solomons N. (1998) Mild human zinc deficiency produces an imbalance between cell-mediated and humoral immunity. *Nutr Rev.* 56(1 Pt 1):27-28.
4. Prasad A. (1995) Zinc: an overview. *Nutrition.* 11(1 Suppl):93-99.

How to cite this article: Rose S, Strombom A. Ensuring adequate zinc status in vegans and vegetarians. Adv Res Gastroentero Hepatol. 2019; 14(3): 555887.
DOI: 10.19080/ARGH.2019.14.555887

5. Heyneman C. (1996) Zinc deficiency and taste disorders. *Ann Pharmacother*. 30(2):186-187.
6. Simmer K, Thompson R. (1985) Zinc in the fetus and newborn. *Acta Paediatr Scand Suppl*. 319:158-163.
7. Fabris N, Mocchegiani E. (1995) Zinc, human diseases and aging. *Aging (Milano)*. 7(2):77-93.
8. Maret W, Sandstead H. (2006) Zinc requirements and the risks and benefits of zinc supplementation. *J Trace Elem Med Biol*. 20(1):3-18.
9. Prasad A, Beck F, Grabowski S, Kaplan J, Mathog R. (1997) Zinc deficiency: changes in cytokine production and T-cell subpopulations in patients with head and neck cancer and in noncancer subjects. *Proc Assoc Am Physicians*. 109(1):68-77.
10. Hall J. (2015) *Guyton and Hall Textbook of Medical Physiology*. 13th Edition ed: Saunders
11. Rink L, Gabriel P. (2000) Zinc and the immune system. *Proc Nutr Soc*. 59(4):541-552.
12. Messina V, Mangels A. (2001) Considerations in planning vegan diets: children. *J Am Diet Assoc*. 101(6):661-669.
13. Prasad A. (2004) Zinc deficiency: its characterization and treatment. *Met Ions Biol Syst*. 41:103-37.
14. Wang L, Busbey S. (2005) Images in clinical medicine. Acquired acrodermatitis enteropathica. *N Engl J Med*. 352(11):1121.
15. Hambidge K. (1989) Mild Zinc Deficiency in Human Subjects. In: Mills C, ed. *Zinc in Human Biology*. New York, NY: Springer-Verlag
16. King J, Cousins R. (2005) Zinc. In: Shils M, Shike M, Ross A, Caballero B, Cousins R, eds. *Modern Nutrition in Health and Disease*. 10th ed. Baltimore, MD: Lippincott Williams & Wilkins
17. Krasovec M, Frenk E. (1996) Acrodermatitis enteropathica secondary to Crohn's disease. *Dermatology*. 193(4):361-363.
18. Ploysangam A, Falciglia G, Brehm B. (1997) Effect of marginal zinc deficiency on human growth and development. *J Trop Pediatr*. 43(4):192-198.
19. Nishi Y. (1996) Zinc and growth. *J Am Coll Nutr*. 15(4):340-344.
20. Hunt J. (2003) Bioavailability of iron, zinc, and other trace minerals from vegetarian diets. *Am J Clin Nutr*. 78(3 Suppl):633S-639S.
21. Van Wouwe J. (1995) Clinical and laboratory assessment of zinc deficiency in Dutch children. A review. *Biol Trace Elem Res*. 49:211-225.
22. Hambidge K, Krebs N. (2007) Zinc deficiency: a special challenge. *J Nutr*. 137(4):1101-1105.
23. Hunt J. (2002) Moving toward a plant-based diet: are iron and zinc at risk? *Nutr Rev*. 60(5 Pt 1):127-134.
24. Saunders A, Craig W, Baines S. (2013) Zinc and vegetarian diets. *Med J Aust*. 199(4 Suppl):S17-S21.
25. Foster M, Chu A, Petocz P, Samman S. (2013) Effect of vegetarian diets on zinc status: a systematic review and meta-analysis of studies in humans. *J Sci Food Agri*. 93(10):2362-2371.
26. Institute of Medicine of National Academies of Science. (2006) *Dietary Reference Intakes: the essentail guide to nutrient requirements*. Washington DC: National Academies Press
27. Gibson R, Heath A, Szymlek-Gay E. (2014) Is iron and zinc nutrition a concern for vegetarian infants and young children in industrialized countries? *Am J Clin Nutr*. 100(Suppl 1):459S-468S.
28. Foster M, Herulah U, Prasad A, Petocz P, Samman S. (2015) Zinc Status of Vegetarians during Pregnancy: A Systematic Review of Observational Studies and Meta-Analysis of Zinc Intake. *Nutrients*. 7(6):4512-4525.
29. Haddad E, Berk LKJ, Hubbard R, Peters W. (1999) Dietary intake and biochemical, hematologic, and immune status of vegans compared with nonvegetarians. *Am J Clin Nutr*. 70(3 Suppl):586S-593S.

How to cite this article: Rose S, Strombom A. Ensuring adequate zinc status in vegans and vegetarians. Adv Res Gastroentero Hepatol. 2019; 14(3): 555887.
DOI: 10.19080/ARGH.2019.14.555887

30. Gibson R. (1994) Content and bioavailability of trace elements in vegetarian diets. *Am J Clin Nutr*. 59(5 Suppl):1223S-1232S.

31. Markiewicz L, Honke J, Haros M, Świątecka D, Wróblewska B. (2013) Diet shapes the ability of human intestinal microbiota to degrade phytate–in vitro studies. *J Appl Microbiol*. 115(1):247-259.

32. Kristensen M, Hels O, Morberg C, Marving J, Bügel S, et al. (2006) Total zinc absorption in young women, but not fractional zinc absorption, differs between vegetarian and meat-based diets with equal phytic acid content. *Br J Nutr*. 95(5):963-967.

33. Gautam S, Platel K, Srinivasan K. (2010) Higher bioaccessibility of iron and zinc from food grains in the presence of garlic and onion. *J Agric Food Chem*. 58(14):8426-8429.

34. Wegmüller R, Tay F, Zeder C, Brnic M, Hurrell R. (2014) Zinc absorption by young adults from supplemental zinc citrate is comparable with that from zinc gluconate and higher than from zinc oxide. *J Nutr*. 144(2):132-136.

35. Barrie S, Wright J, Pizzorno J, Kutter E, Barron P. (1987) Comparative absorption of zinc picolinate, zinc citrate and zinc gluconate in humans. *Agents Actions*. 21(1-2):223-228.

36. Lomaestro B, Bailie G. (1995) Absorption interactions with fluoroquinolones. 1995 update. *Drug Saf*. 12(5):314-333.

37. Penttilä O, Hurme H, Neuvonen P. (1975) Effect of zinc sulphate on the absorption of tetracycline and doxycycline in man. *Eur J Clin Pharmacol*. 9(2-3):131-134.

38. Therapeutic research center. (2019) Zinc. *Natural Medicines Comprehensive Database*.

39. Brewer G, Yuzbasiyan-Gurkan V, Johnson V, Dick R, Wang Y. (1993) Treatment of Wilson's disease with zinc: XI. Interaction with other anticopper agents. *J Am Coll Nutr*. 12(1):26-30.

40. Wester P. (1980) Urinary zinc excretion during treatment with different diuretics. *Acta Med Scand*. 208(3):209-12.

How to cite this article: Rose S, Strombom A. Ensuring adequate zinc status in vegans and vegetarians. Adv Res Gastroentero Hepatol. 2019; 14(3): 555887.
DOI: 10.19080/ARGH.2019.14.555887

Advanced Research in Gastroenterology & Hepatology
ISSN: 2472-6400

Juniper Publishers
key to the Researchers

Review Article
Adv Res Gastroenterol Hepatol
Volume 15 Issue 1 - March 2020

DOI: 10.19080/ARGH.2020.15.555897

Ensuring Adequate Essential Fatty Acid status in Vegetarians

Stewart D Rose and Amanda J Strombom*

Plant-Based Diets in Medicine, USA

Submission: February 03, 2020; **Published:** March 06, 2020

***Corresponding Author:** Amanda Strombom, Plant-Based Diets in Medicine, 12819 SE 38th St, #427, Bellevue, WA 98006, USA

Abstract

Omega-3 and omega-6 fatty acids are essential in the human diet, in that they cannot be synthesized physiologically. The Omega-3 fatty acid, DHA, is highly concentrated in the brain and is important for brain function. Omega-6 fatty acids are also important. They lower harmful LDL cholesterol, boost HDL, and help keep blood sugar in check by improving the body's sensitivity to insulin. The latest evidence shows that both omega 3 and omega 6 fatty acids are healthy. Therefore omega 6 fatty acids intake does not need to be reduced. However, an increase in Omega 3 fatty acids (ALA) consumption may be necessary in some patients.

Omega-3 fatty acids are present in some plant foods as alpha-linolenic acid (ALA), which can be converted by the body into DHA. Omega-6 fatty acids are found in many plant foods in the form of linolenic acid (LA). Evidence suggests that ALA-derived DHA is sufficient to maintain brain DHA levels and preserve function. There is no evidence of adverse effects on health or cognitive function with lower DHA ingestion levels in vegans. While fish oils provide a source of EPA and DHA which don't require conversion, the most recent science doesn't confirm the benefits of fish oil supplements for the prevention and treatment of coronary artery disease.

A good supply of ALA is essential for a healthy plant-based diet. This can easily be obtained from plant foods. Patients should warned about the unsubstantiated cardiovascular health claims of fish oil products.

Keywords:

ALA; DHA; Essential fatty acids; Fish oil; LA; Omega-3; Omega-6; Plant-based; Vegan; Vegetarian

Nutritional Considerations In-depth – Essential Fatty Acids

Abbreviations:

PUFAs: Polyunsaturated Essential Fatty Acids; Omega-3s: Omega-3 Fatty Acids; ALA: Alpha-Linolenic Acid; EPA: Eicosapentaenoic Acid; DHA: Docosahexaenoic Acid; AHA: American Heart Association; CHD: Coronary Heart Disease; EAR: Estimated Average Requirements; AI: Adequate Intake; RDA: Recommended Dietary Allowance

1. Introduction

The two major classes of polyunsaturated essential fatty acids (PUFAs) are the omega-3 and omega-6 fatty acids. Like all fatty acids, PUFAs consist of long chains of carbon atoms with a carboxyl group at one end of the chain and a methyl group at the other. PUFAs are distinguished from saturated and monounsaturated fatty acids by the presence of two or more double bonds between carbons within the fatty acid chain. (1, 2, 3)

Both omega-3 and omega-6 fatty acids are essential in that they cannot be synthesized physiologically. Omega-3 fatty acids (omega-3s) have a carbon–carbon double bond located three carbons from the methyl end of the chain. Omega-3s, sometimes referred to as "n-3s," are present in some plant foods such as soy, flaxseed oil, canola oil, and walnuts, in the form of alpha-linolenic acid (ALA). In animal foods such as oily fish, they are found in the form of eicosapentaenoic acid (EPA) and docosahexaenoic acid (DHA). These are not considered to be essential since they can be converted from ALA. (4) Humans can synthesize DHA from ingested ALA, although this is not an efficient process. The human conversion rate of ALA to EPA and DHA is about 5%–8% (1, 2, 3), which seems to be sufficient provided and adequate amount of ALA is ingested.

Omega-6 fatty acids have a carbon-carbon double bond located six carbons from the methyl end of the chain. Omega-6s, "n-6s," are found in plant foods such as soy, corn, safflower and sunflower oils, nuts and seeds, in the form of linolenic acid (LA). Most humans (except those with inborn errors of metabolism) can convert LA to arachidonic acid (ARA or AA).

2. Benefits of Omega-3 and Omega-6 fatty acids

The omega-3 fatty acid, Docosahexaenoic acid (DHA), is highly concentrated in the brain and is important for brain function, in part by regulation of cell survival and neuroinflammation. (5, 6, 7, 8, 9) DHA is the main n-3 PUFA in the brain as it is concentrated at levels of about 10,000 nmol/g brain (10–15% of brain fatty acids or about 5g in an adult brain), (10) at least 50-fold more than EPA and 200-fold more than ALA (11, 12, 13).

Omega-6 fatty acids are also important. They lower harmful LDL cholesterol and boost protective HDL. They help keep hyperglycemia in check by improving the body's sensitivity to insulin. (14)

Some linolenic acid is converted to arachidonic acid, a building block for molecules that can promote inflammation, blood clotting, and the constriction of blood vessels. This fact led to concern that the consumption of omega-6 fatty acids should be limited. However, it turns out that very little LA is converted into ARA, even when LA is abundant in the diet, and ARA is also converted into molecules that calm inflammation and fight blood clots. (15)

In a science advisory by the American Heart Association (AHA), nine independent researchers

How to cite this article: Rose SD. Strombom AJ. Ensuring adequate essential fatty acid status in vegetarians and vegans. Adv Res Gastroentero Hepatol, 2020;15(1): 555897.
DOI: 10.19080/ARGH.2020.15.555897

from around the country found that data from dozens of studies support the cardiovascular benefits of consuming omega-6 fatty acids. (15) This advisory was undertaken to summarize the current evidence on the consumption of omega-6 PUFAs, particularly LA, with respect to coronary heart disease (CHD) risk. Aggregate data from randomized trials, case-control and cohort studies, and long-term animal feeding experiments indicate that the consumption of at least 5% to 10% of energy from omega-6 PUFAs reduces the risk of CHD relative to lower intakes. The data also suggest that higher intakes appear to be safe and may be even more beneficial (as part of a low–saturated-fat, low-cholesterol diet). In summary, the AHA supports an omega-6 PUFA intake of at least 5% to 10% of energy in the context of other AHA lifestyle and dietary recommendations. To reduce omega-6 PUFA intakes from their current levels would be more likely to increase than to decrease risk for CHD.

The AHA reviewers found that eating more omega-6 fatty acids didn't promote inflammation. Instead, eating more omega-6 fatty acids either reduced markers of inflammation or left them unchanged. Omega-6 fatty acids also lower LDL cholesterol, and are protective against heart disease. So, both omega-6 and omega-3 fatty acids are healthful. (15)

Many other studies have showed that rates of heart disease went down as consumption of omega-6 fatty acids went up. A meta-analysis of six randomized trials found that replacing saturated fat with omega-6 fatty acids reduced the risk of heart attacks and other coronary events by 24%. A separate report published in the American Journal of Clinical Nutrition, that pooled the results of 11 large cohorts, showed that replacing saturated fatty acids with polyunsaturated fatty acids (including omega-6 and omega-3 fatty acids) reduced heart disease rates more than did replacing them with monounsaturated fatty acids or carbohydrates. (16)

While there is a theory that omega-3 fatty acids are better for our health than omega-6 fatty acids, this is not supported by the latest evidence. Some people have incorrectly thought that the ratio of n-3 to n-6 fatty acids is important. However the omega-3 to omega-6 ratio is basically the "good divided by the good," so it is of no value in evaluating diet quality or predicting disease. (17) In the Health Professionals Follow-up Study, for example, the ratio of omega-6 to omega-3 fatty acids wasn't linked with risk of heart disease because both of these were beneficial. (18) Rather than cutting down on beneficial omega 6, the patient would be better served by simply increasing their intake of ALA (omega 3).

3. Nutritional Requirements

Since the National Academy of Sciences concluded that there is inadequate information to set Estimated Average Requirements (EAR) or the Recommended Dietary Allowance (RDA) for either LA or ALA for healthy individuals, the Adequate Intake (AI) is used. The present essential fatty acid AI is based on "the highest median intake of LA and ALA in United States adults, where a deficiency is basically nonexistent in non-institutionalized populations" (19).

How to cite this article: Rose SD. Strombom AJ. Ensuring adequate essential fatty acid status in vegetarians and vegans. Adv Res Gastroentero Hepatol, 2020;15(1): 555897.
DOI: 10.19080/ARGH.2020.15.555897

Table 1: Adequate Intake of Omega-3 fatty acids (20)

Age	Male	Female	Pregnancy	Lactation
Birth to 6 months*	0.5 g	0.5 g		
7–12 months*	0.5 g	0.5 g		
1–3 years**	0.7 g	0.7 g		
4–8 years**	0.9 g	0.9 g		
9–13 years**	1.2 g	1.0 g		
14–18 years**	1.6 g	1.1 g	1.4 g	1.3 g
19-50 years**	1.6 g	1.1 g	1.4 g	1.3 g
51+ years**	1.6 g	1.1 g		

* All omega-3 polyunsaturated fatty acids present in human milk can contribute to the AI for infants.

**As ALA

Table 2: Adequate Intake of Omega-6 fatty acids (20)

Age	Male	Female	Pregnancy	Lactation
Birth to 6 months*	4.4 g	4.4 g		
7–12 months*	4.6 g	4.6 g		
1–3 years**	7 g	7 g		
4–8 years**	10 g	10 g		
9–13 years**	12 g	10 g		
14–18 years**	16 g	11 g	13 g	13 g
19-50 years**	17 g	12 g	13 g	13 g
51+ years**	14 g	11g		

* The various omega-6 polyunsaturated fatty acids (PUFA) present in human milk can contribute to the AI for infants.

** As LA

How to cite this article: Rose SD. Strombom AJ. Ensuring adequate essential fatty acid status in vegetarians and vegans. Adv Res Gastroentero Hepatol, 2020;15(1): 555897.
DOI: 10.19080/ARGH.2020.15.555897

However, it is unknown if the AIs are beneficial or physiologically adequate because dose-response data studies are lacking, Essential fatty acid status is not usually clinically tested, and absence of deficiency symptoms is not necessarily evidence of adequacy.

The rate of DHA uptake into the brain is assumed to be replacing DHA that is metabolized in the brain, and therefore, can be used as an estimate for the brain DHA requirement. It has been reported that the brain DHA uptake rate in humans is between 2.4 and 3.8 mg/day (4, 21, 22).

Based on current estimates of ALA consumption in adult males of 1700 mg/day, the percent conversion of ALA to DHA would need to be 0.14–0.22% to match the brain DHA requirement (22). Therefore, it is possible that even a small amount of DHA synthesis may be sufficient to meet adult brain DHA uptake demands.

In pre-menopausal women, there is evidence that significant changes in DHA status can occur independent of changes in n-3 PUFA intake, likely through increased synthesis of DHA from ALA. For example, women have higher DHA in plasma phospholipids and erythrocytes compared with men (23), which is associated with much higher rates of DHA synthesis in women (1, 2, 24)

Studies of premenopausal women reported a higher capacity of ALA conversion, and a more efficient conversion of ALA to EPA and DHA compared to men (1). In 21 days, women incorporated 700 mg of radioactive labeled [U-13C]-ALA, and resulted in a net fractional ALA interconversion of 21% of EPA, 6% of docosapentaenoic acid (can be converted to DHA), and 9% of DHA in plasma which led the researchers to postulate that increased conversion was due to either an estrogen catalyzed conversion or an increased need for EPA and DHA during pregnancy and fetal development (1).

One study did not find any associations between dietary EPA, DHA, or the n–6 PUFA and birth weight. In contrast, the results indicate a growth-promoting effect of ALA intake, with the increase in birth weight being independent of gestational age at birth. It is noteworthy that no specific function has been assigned to ALA itself other than serving as a source of energy or conversion to EPA and DHA. Therefore, any mechanisms of improvement in birth weight are most likely via desaturation and elongation to its longer-chain derivatives.

Although conversion rates of ALA into the longer-chain EPA and DHA are modest with the estimated fractional conversion reported to be less than 5% (3), increased ALA intake has demonstrated to increase proportions of long-chain n–3 fatty acids in plasma and cell lipids to reproduce beneficial effects. (25) Specifically, in pregnancy, the levels of DHA and ARA increase in cord blood in relation to circulating levels of ALA and LA in maternal blood (26)

4. Fish Oil Supplements

Sales of fish oil supplements reached $1.84 billion in 2018 indicating widespread use. However, the most recent science doesn't confirm the benefits of fish oil supplements for the prevention and treatment of coronary artery disease.

The initial reasoning for recommending fish oil supplements was based on studies of the Eskimo. It was mistakenly thought that the Eskimo suffered less from atherosclerosis and from coronary artery disease in particular. However, it is now known that the Eskimo do not have lower rates of coronary artery disease. One study concluded that the "Greenland Eskimos and the Canadian and Alaskan Inuit have CAD as often as the non-Eskimo populations." (27) Another study showed "Eskimos have CHD despite high consumption of omega-3 fatty acids." (28)

A meta study of the efficacy of fish oil summarizes their results as follows:

"All of the studies included were the gold-standard kind of clinical trial — with people assigned at random to either take fish oil or a placebo. The studies ranged in length from one to nearly five years. The authors detected no reduction in any cardiovascular events, such as heart attacks, sudden death, angina, heart failures, strokes, or death, no matter what dose of fish oil used." Sang Mi Kwak, MD et al, (29)

5. EFA status in vegans

The most plentiful dietary n-6 polyunsaturated essential fatty acid is LA. Omega-6 fatty acid food sources commonly consumed by vegans include nuts, seeds, certain vegetables, and vegetables oils such as soybean oil, safflower oil, and corn oil among others. Therefore, any diet that is plant-based leads to a high dietary intake of LA. (19)

Ensuring adequate essential fatty acids in vegans therefore focuses on obtaining an adequate intake of the omega 3 fatty acid, ALA.

There is evidence that DHA synthesis from ALA can be sufficient to maintain brain function. For example, vegetarians and vegans, in which DHA derived from ALA is the sole source of DHA, have DHA levels comparable to omnivores. (30) Some studies show that their DHA levels are lower than omnivores, (31, 32, 33) but have neurological disease rates comparable to omnivores (34, 35, 36, 37), suggesting that ALA-derived DHA is sufficient to maintain brain function in these individuals. In addition, dietary ALA, with no DHA, is sufficient to completely restore brain DHA in rats (38) and non-human primates (39) Taken together, evidence suggests that ALA-derived DHA is sufficient to maintain brain DHA levels and preserve function. (40) There is no evidence of adverse effects on health or cognitive function with lower DHA ingestion levels in vegans. (31)

One study showed that vegetarians give birth to infants with less DHA in their plasma and cord artery phospholipids but this did not appear to be independently related to the outcome of pregnancy. (41)

6. Clinical considerations

How to cite this article: Rose SD. Strombom AJ. Ensuring adequate essential fatty acid status in vegetarians and vegans. Adv Res Gastroentero Hepatol, 2020;15(1): 555897.
DOI: 10.19080/ARGH.2020.15.555897

Table 3: Sources of n-6 and n-3 in plant-foods. (19)

Nutrient		Energy	Protein	Total Lipid	n-6	n-3	CHO	Total Fiber
	Unit	Kcal	g	g	g	g	g	g
Oil, Canola	100g	884	0	100	18.64	9.137	0	0
Oil, Flaxseed/Linseed (Panos)	100g	884	0.110	99.98	14.25	53.37	0	0
Oil, Soybean	100g	763	0	100	50.42	6.789	0	0
Oil, Walnut	100g	884	0	100	52.90	10.40	0	0
Almonds Raw	100g	579	21.15	49.93	12.30	0.003	21.55	12.50
Amaranth	100g	371	13.65	7.020	2.736	0.042	65.25	6.70
Avocados, Raw, California	100g	167	1.960	15.41	1.674	0.111	8.640	6.80
Black Walnuts Dried	100g	619	24.06	59.33	33.80	2.680	9.580	6.80
Brazil Nuts, Dried	100g	659	14.32	67.10	23.859	0.018	11.74	7.50
Brown Rice Cooked	100g	123	2.740	0.970	0.355	0.011	25.58	1.60
Bulgur Cooked	100g	83	3.08	0.240	0.094	0.004	18.58	4.50
Cashews Raw	100g	553	18.22	43.85	7.782	0.062	30.19	3.30
Chia Seeds Dried	100g	486	16.54	30.74	5.840	17.80	42.12	34.4
English Walnuts Dried	100g	654	15.23	65.21	38.09	9.08	13.71	6.70
Flaxseed Raw	100g	534	18.29	42.16	5.903	22.81	28.88	27.3
Hempseed Hulled	100g	553	31.56	48.75	1.340	8.864	8.670	4.00
Millet Cooked	100g	119	3.510	1.000	0.480	0.028	23.67	1.300
Oat Bran Cooked	100g	40	3.210	0.860	0.324	0.015	11.44	2.60
Pistachio Raw	100g	560	20.16	45.32	13.10	0.210	27.17	10.60
Poppy Seeds	100g	525	17.99	41.56	28.30	0.273	28.13	19.50
Quinoa	100g	368	14.12	6.070	2.977	0.260	64.16	7.00
Rye	100g	338	10.34	1.630	0.659	0.108	75.86	15.1
Sesame Seeds dried	100g	573	17.73	49.67	21.375	0.376	23.45	11.8
Soybeans Raw	100g	446	36.49	19.94	9.925	1.330	30.16	9.30
Soybeans, Boiled	100g	141	12.35	6.400	2.657	0.354	11.05	4.20
Sunflower Seeds	100g	584	20.78	51.50	23.05 *	0.06 **	20.00	8.60

Generally, if a patient's food history doesn't include good sources of ALA then foods that are good sources of ALA should be prescribed. If the patient isn't compliant, then supplements can be prescribed. While the conversion of ALA to DHA rates in women are higher, if the intake of rich sources of ALA are not being consumed then supplements should be prescribed. Infant formula is available enriched with DHA.

Plant-based sources of omega-3s from algal oil usually provide around 100–300 mg DHA and some contain EPA as well. These supplements typically contain omega-3s in the triglyceride form (42). According to a small study, the bioavailability of DHA from algal oil is equivalent to that from cooked salmon (43) In one study vegans responded robustly to a relatively low dose of a vegan DHA and EPA supplement. (30)

7. Discussion

A good supply of ALA is essential for a healthy plant-based diet. This can easily be obtained from plant foods. Patients should warned about the unsubstantiated cardiovascular health claims of fish oil products.

References

1. Burdge GC, Wootton SA. (2002) Conversion of alpha-linolenic acid to eicosapentaenoic, docosapentaenoic and docosahexaenoic acids in young women. *Br J Nutr*. 88(4):411-420.
2. Burdge GC, Jones AE, Wootton SA. (2002) Eicosapentaenoic and docosapentaenoic acids are the principal products of alpha-linolenic acid metabolism in young men. *Br J Nutr*. 88(4):355-363.
3. Brenna JT. (2002) Efficiency of conversion of alpha-linolenic acid to long chain n-3 fatty acids in man. *Curr Opin Clin Nutr Metab Care*. 5(2):127-132.
4. Umhau JC, Zhou W, Carson RE, Rapoport SI, Polozova A, et al. (2009) Imaging incorporation of circulating docosahexaenoic acid into the human brain using positron emission tomography. *J Lipid Res*. 50(7):1259-1268.
5. Orr SK, Palumbo S, Bosetti F, Mount HT, Kan JX, et al. (2013) Unesterified docosahexaenoic acid is protective in neuroinflammation. *J Neurochem*. 127(3):378-393.
6. Bazan NG, Molina MF, Gordon WC. (2011) Docosahexaenoic acid signalolipidomics in nutrition: significance in aging, neuroinflammation, macular degeneration, Alzheimer's, and other neurodegenerative diseases. *Annu Rev Nutr*. 31:321-351.
7. Desai A, Kevala K, Kim HY. (2014) Depletion of brain docosahexaenoic acid impairs recovery from traumatic brain injury. *PLoS One*. 9(1):e86472.
8. Lukiw WJ, Cui JG, Marcheselli VL, Bodker M, Botkjaer A, et al. (2005) A role for docosahexaenoic acid-derived neuroprotectin D1 in neural cell survival and Alzheimer disease. *J Clin Invest*. 115(10):2774-2783.
9. Akbar M, Calderon F, Wen Z, Kim HY. (2005) Docosahexaenoic acid: a positive modulator of Akt signaling in neuronal survival. *Proc Natl Acad Sci U S A*. 102(31):10858-10863.
10. Martinez M. (1992) Abnormal profiles of polyunsaturated fatty acids in the brain, liver, kidney and retina of patients with peroxisomal disorders. *Brain Res*. 583(1-2):171-182.
11. Igarashi M, Ma K, Gao F, Kim H, Greenstein D, et al. (2009) Brain lipid concentrations in bipolar disorder. *J Psychiatr Res*. 44(3):177-182.
12. Chen CT, Domenichiello AF, Trépanier MO, Liu Z, Masoodi M, et al. (2013) The low levels of eicosapentaenoic acid in rat brain phospholipids are maintained via multiple redundant mechanisms. *J Lipid Res*. 54(9):2410-2422.
13. Brenna JT, Salem NJ, Sinclair AJ, Cunnane SC, the International Society for the Study of Fatty Acids and Lipids I. (2009) Alpha-Linolenic acid

How to cite this article: Rose SD. Strombom AJ. Ensuring adequate essential fatty acid status in vegetarians and vegans. Adv Res Gastroentero Hepatol, 2020;15(1): 555897.
DOI: 10.19080/ARGH.2020.15.555897

supplementation and conversion to n-3 long-chain polyunsaturated fatty acids in humans. *Prostaglandins Leukot Essent Fatty Acids*. 80(2-3):85-91.

14. Strombom A, Rose S. (2017) The prevention and treatment of Type II Diabetes Mellitus with a plant-based diet. *Endocrin Metab Int J*. 5(5):00138.
15. Harris WS, Mozaffarian D, Rimm E, Kris-Etherton P, Rudel L, et al. (2009) Omega-6 fatty acids and risk for cardiovascular disease: a science advisory from the American Heart Association Nutrition Subcommittee of the Council on Nutrition, Physical Activity, and Metabolism; Council on Cardiovascular Nursing; and Council on Epidem. *Circulation*. 119(6):902-907.
16. Harvard Heart Letter. (2019) No need to avoid healthy omega-6 fats. *Harvard Health Publishing*.
17. Ask the expert: Omega-3 fatty acids. *Harward T. H. Chan: School of public health*.
18. Mozaffarian D, Ascherio A, Hu FB, Stampfer M, Willett W, et al. (2005) Interplay between different polyunsaturated fatty acids and risk of coronary heart disease in men. *Circulation*. 111(2):157-164.
19. Burns-Whitmore B, Froyen E, Heskey C, Parker T, Pablo GS. (2019) Alpha-Linolenic and Linoleic Fatty Acids in the Vegan Diet: Do They Require Dietary Reference Intake/Adequate Intake Special Consideration? *Nutrients*. 11(10):2365.
20. Institute of Medicine (IOM). (2005) Dietary fats: Total fat and fatty acids. *Dietary Reference Intakes for Energy, Carbohydrate, Fiber, Fat, Fatty Acids, Cholesterol, Protein, and Amino Acids*. Washington, DC: National Academics Press.
21. Umhau JC, Zhou W, Thada S, Demar J, Hussein N, et al. (2013) Brain Docosahexaenoic Acid [DHA] Incorporation and Blood Flow Are Increased in Chronic Alcoholics: A Positron Emission Tomography Study Corrected for Cerebral Atrophy. *PLoS ONE* 8(2013):e75333.
22. Barceló-Coblijna G, Murphy EJ. (2009) Alpha-linolenic acid and its conversion to longer chain n-3 fatty acids: benefits for human health and a role in maintaining tissue n-3 fatty acid levels. *Prog Lipid Res*. 48(6):355-374.
23. Lohner S, Fekete K, Marosvölgyi T, Decsi T. (2013) Gender differences in the long-chain polyunsaturated fatty acid status: systematic review of 51 publications. *Ann Nutr Metab*. 62(2):98-112.
24. Pawlosky R, Hibbeln J, Lin Y, Salem N. (2003) n-3 fatty acid metabolism in women. *Br J Nutr*. 90(5):993-994.
25. Finnegan Y, Minihane A, Leigh-Firbank E, Kew S, Meijer G, et al. (2003) Plant- and marine-derived n-3 polyunsaturated fatty acids have differential effects on fasting and postprandial blood lipid concentrations and on the susceptibility of LDL to oxidative modification in moderately hyperlipidemic subjects. *Am J Clin Nutr*. 77(4):783-795.
26. Bobiński R, Mikulska M. (2015) The ins and outs of maternal-fetal fatty acid metabolism. *Acta Biochim Pol*. 62(3):499-507.
27. Fodor JG, Helis E, Yazdekhasti N, Vohnout B. (2014) "Fishing" for the origins of the "Eskimos and heart disease" story: facts or wishful thinking? *Can J Cardiol*. 30(8):864-868.
28. Ebbesson SOE, Risica PM, Ebbesson LOE, Kennish JM. (2005) Eskimos have CHD despite high consumption of omega-3 fatty acids: the Alaska Siberia project. *Int J Circumpolar Health*. 64(4):387-395.
29. Kwak S, Myung S, Lee Y, Seo H, Group KMaS. (2012) Efficacy of omega-3 fatty acid supplements (eicosapentaenoic acid and docosahexaenoic acid) in the secondary prevention of cardiovascular disease: a meta-analysis of randomized, double-blind, placebo-controlled trials. *Arch Intern Med*. 172(9):686-694.
30. Sarter B, Kelsey KS, Schwartz TA, Harris WS. (2015) Blood docosahexaenoic acid and eicosapentaenoic acid in vegans: Associations with age and gender and effects of an

algal-derived omega-3 fatty acid supplement. *Clin Nutr*. 34(2):212-218.

31. Welch AA, Shakya-Shrestha S, Lentjes MA, Wareham NJ, Khaw KT. (2010) Dietary intake and status of n-3 polyunsaturated fatty acids in a population of fish-eating and non-fish-eating meat-eaters, vegetarians, and vegans and the product-precursor ratio [corrected] of α-linolenic acid to long-chain n-3 polyunsaturated fatty ac. *Am J Clin Nutr*. 92(5):1040-1051.
32. Rosell MS, Lloyd-Wright Z, Appleby PN, Sanders TA, Allen NE, et al. (2005) Long-chain n-3 polyunsaturated fatty acids in plasma in British meat-eating, vegetarian, and vegan men. *Am J Clin Nutr*. 82(2):327-334.
33. Mann N, Pirotta Y, O'Connell S, Li D, Kelly F, et al. (2006) Fatty acid composition of habitual omnivore and vegetarian diets. *Lipids*. 41(7):637-646.
34. Giem P, Beeson W, Fraser G. (1993) The incidence of dementia and intake of animal products: preliminary findings from the Adventist Health Study. *Neuroepidemiology*. 12(1):28-36.
35. McCarty MF. (2001) Does a vegan diet reduce risk for Parkinson's disease? *Med Hypothese*. 57(3):318-323.
36. Orlich MJ, Singh PN, Sabaté J, Jaceldo-Siegl K, Fan J, et al. (2013) Vegetarian dietary patterns and mortality in Adventist Health Study 2. *JAMA Intern Med*. 173(13):1230-1238.
37. Beezhold BL, Johnston CS, Daigle DR. (2010) Vegetarian diets are associated with healthy mood states: a cross-sectional study in seventh day adventist adults. *Nutr J*. 9:26.
38. André A, Juanéda P, Sébédio JL, Chardigny JM. (2005) Effects of aging and dietary n-3 fatty acids on rat brain phospholipids: focus on plasmalogens. *Lipids*. 40(8): 799-806.
39. Anderson GJ, Neuringer M, Lin DS, Connor WE. (2005) Can prenatal N-3 fatty acid deficiency be completely reversed after birth? Effects on retinal and brain biochemistry and visual function in rhesus monkeys. *Pediatr Res*. 58(5):865-872.
40. Domenichiello AF, Kitson AP, Bazinet RP. (2015) Is docosahexaenoic acid synthesis from α-linolenic acid sufficient to supply the adult brain? *Progress in Lipid Research*. 59:54-66.
41. Reddy S, Sanders T, Obeid O. (1994) The influence of maternal vegetarian diet on essential fatty acid status of the newborn. *Eur J Clin Nutr*. 48(5):358-368.
42. ConsumerLab.com. *Product review: fish oil and omega-3 fatty acid supplements review (including krill, algae, calamari, green-lipped mussel oil).*
43. Arterburn LM, Oken HA, Hall EB, Hamersley J, Kuratko CN, et al. (2008) Algal-oil capsules and cooked salmon: nutritionally equivalent sources of docosahexaenoic acid. *J Am Diet Assoc*. 108(7):1204-1209.

How to cite this article: Rose SD. Strombom AJ. Ensuring adequate essential fatty acid status in vegetarians and vegans. Adv Res Gastroentero Hepatol, 2020;15(1): 555897.
DOI: 10.19080/ARGH.2020.15.555897